MW00844841

Advance Praise for *Hostility to Hospitality*

"With courage and compassion, *Hostility to Hospitality* explores the broad dimensions of science, history, culture, philosophy, and religion to rediscover the true essence of health care. This astonishing and provocative analysis serves to reunite the secular and sacred for the benefit of all in a time of need."

—**Howard K. Koh, MD, MPH,**
Harvey V. Fineberg Professor of the Practice of Public Health Leadership,
Harvard T.H. Chan School of Public Health, Harvard Kennedy School,
Cambridge, MA

"In a series of thoughtful and evidence-based chapters, the Balbonis examine the spiritual concomitants of the illness experience and the medical response that either elevate religious questions in care or dampen them. The subject matter is fresh and handled with aplomb. The arguments are always interesting and at times surprising. This fascinating book represents one very intriguing approach to this great borderland and gives the reader original research and ideas to ponder aplenty. I benefitted from it."

—**Arthur Kleinman, MD,** Author of *What Really Matters*

"In this provocative and ambitious new book, the Balbonis offer a brilliant analysis of medicine's spiritual crisis, how it is grounded in a spirituality of immanence that cuts medicine off from the spiritual resources it needs to sustain genuine care for the sick—and what we can do to overcome it."

—**Farr Curlin, MD,** Josiah C. Trent Professor of Medical Humanities,
Co-Director of Theology, Medicine, and Culture Initiative,
Duke University, Durham, NC

"This splendid book is a work of truly *practical* theology, combining extensive religious scholarship with clinical experience, empirical research, and pastoral wisdom. In readily accessible prose, the Balbonis argue that medicine, while in denial, really needs religion. It should be of great value to patients and their caregivers as well as physicians, nurses, chaplains, and other health care professionals."

—**Daniel Sulmasy, MD, PhD, MACP,**
André Hellegers Professor of Biomedical Ethics,
The Pellegrino Center for Clinical Bioethics,
Georgetown University, Washington, DC

"The Balbonis offer a needed and thorough exploration of the interface between religion and medicine. This is a must read for anyone who cares about the future of healthcare or the future of religion."

—**Elaine Howard Ecklund, PhD,** Author of *Religion vs. Science*,
Herbert S. Autrey Chair in Social Sciences,
Rice University, Houston, TX

Hostility to Hospitality

Spirituality and Professional Socialization within Medicine

BY MICHAEL J. BALBONI, PHD

Instructor, Harvard Medical School

Minister, Longwood Christian Community and Park Street Church

Boston, MA

TRACY A. BALBONI, MD

Associate Professor, Harvard Medical School

Boston, MA

OXFORD
UNIVERSITY PRESS

OXFORD
UNIVERSITY PRESS

Oxford University Press is a department of the University of Oxford. It furthers
the University's objective of excellence in research, scholarship, and education
by publishing worldwide. Oxford is a registered trade mark of Oxford University
Press in the UK and certain other countries.

Published in the United States of America by Oxford University Press
198 Madison Avenue, New York, NY 10016, United States of America.

© Oxford University Press 2019

All rights reserved. No part of this publication may be reproduced, stored in
a retrieval system, or transmitted, in any form or by any means, without the
prior permission in writing of Oxford University Press, or as expressly permitted
by law, by license, or under terms agreed with the appropriate reproduction
rights organization. Inquiries concerning reproduction outside the scope of the
above should be sent to the Rights Department, Oxford University Press, at the
address above.

You must not circulate this work in any other form
and you must impose this same condition on any acquirer.

Library of Congress Cataloging-in-Publication Data
Names: Balboni, Michael J., author. | Balboni, Tracy A., author.
Title: Hostility to hospitality : spirituality and professional socialization
within medicine / by Michael J. Balboni, Tracy A. Balboni.
Description: Oxford ; New York : Oxford University Press, [2019] |
Includes bibliographical references.
Identifiers: LCCN 2018011372 | ISBN 9780199325764 (pbk. : alk. paper)
Subjects: | MESH: Religion and Medicine | Physician-Patient Relations |
Spirituality | Terminal Care | United States
Classification: LCC R733 | NLM BL 65.M4 | DDC 610—dc23
LC record available at https://lccn.loc.gov/2018011372

1 3 5 7 9 8 6 4 2

Printed by Webcom, Inc., Canada

We dedicate this book to
Caleb Spencer, our son, a faithful and courageous steward
and
Eva Elizabeth, our daughter, full of life consecrated to God

CONTENTS

PREFACE

As a married couple engaged in the joys and struggles of life partnership, raising two delightful children, working together as academics in the field of medicine, and co-leading the Longwood Christian Community, a ministry to healthcare trainees in Boston, we have come to see our own marital experience as a metaphor of what remains possible for medicine and faith. Although there has been a long-term divorce of sorts between these spheres, our own experience gives us hope that, despite many differences, reconciliation and partnership remain possible.

We became aware of this possibility early in our marriage, while Tracy was in medical school and Michael in theological seminary. Tracy would share stories with Michael about the sick patients she was caring for at the hospital. Michael would discuss theological ideas with Tracy as he learned about the spiritual dimensions of suffering, illness, and caregiving. This launched us into an ongoing dialogue where we discovered how both spheres became more whole through the light shed from the other. Spirituality and theology had something transformative to say about the existential crisis of illness, suffering, and death for many patients, in contrast to the deafening silence offered by the often mechanistic, reductionist lens of medicine. Spirituality and theology can also speak into and rekindle clinicians' deep motivations to care, addressing growing burnout from practice conditions formed by healthcare delivery models increasingly based on the "bottom line" rather than on care and compassion. Likewise, scientific medicine had something powerful to say to theology by exemplifying how to focus on practical rather than merely theoretical human concerns, as well as how to evaluate theological claims through the employment of scientific study and analysis. Rather than being non-overlapping, as suggested by Stephen Jay Gould,[1] each sphere holds the possibility to interlock with one another for the benefit of seriously ill patients and all who care for the sick.

While in our conversations these seemed to fit well together, we saw how strangely divided our two worlds were from one another. The church had seemingly little to say to medicine beside "thank you" and a few bioethical "though shalt nots." On the other hand, medicine was eerily silent toward religion or even occasionally disparaging toward patients' spiritual expressions sometimes getting in the way of medical care. As a Protestant Congregational minister working with medical students,

Michael also witnessed how many medical students and young physicians entered medicine because they understood a "call" from God to care for the sick, but then, after getting into medical school, some expressed angst about how their faith was utterly suppressed or considered irrelevant. Some worried that it may be illegal to talk to their patients about spiritual matters because it violated legal statutes. Many medical students and residents who were quite religious themselves and needed no convincing of its importance felt that it was hard enough to learn the complexities of medical care, let alone swim against the mighty current silently demanding their unqualified separation from spirituality or religion.

Our own experience and intuition reinforced our understanding of both a real separation and also the possibility of partnership. Tracy grew up within a family heritage of scientists and clinicians, including her mother, a rheumatologist; her father, a critical care specialist; her step-dad, an emergency medicine physician; and her stepmother, a nurse. Also in her family heritage, Tracy's great uncle, Luther Terry, was the first Surgeon General of the United States to lead a controversial public health antismoking campaign against the tobacco industry in the 1960s. Tracy's scientific heritage played a role in her skepticism toward faith. But a number of experiences as an undergraduate at Stanford and then a medical student at Harvard transformed her spiritual views. Having become more aware of the role of faith, Tracy also saw how many of her patients approached their illnesses through a spiritual or religious lens. This led her down the path of empirical research in the field with an eye toward the practice of medicine.

In quite the opposite direction, Michael grew up with devout religious parents, having heard a divine call to ministry when he was 16 years old. Science and academia were often viewed suspiciously by those within his spiritual community. It was only after moving back to Boston for further ministerial preparation and attending Park Street Church in downtown Boston that he began to understand the possibility of real partnership and collaboration between science and religion. Yet it was only through partnership with Tracy that he began to see how the empirical sciences were not only compatible but necessary for theology and practice. This eventually led him to receive social-scientific training and research partnership with Tracy in order to understand how faith operates among the seriously ill and how religious communities are involved in the care of the sick.

Ironically, we both grew up in ways that socialized us (in opposite directions) to believe in a fundamental separation between science and medicine. Yet our career paths, informed by our own marriage, opened us to realize that this cultural disposition of animosity, carried forward especially for the past two centuries, gets it mostly wrong. Scientific medicine *needs* faith; without it science is *bereft of purpose* even to be pursued at all. Scientific medicine, so apt to forget that grounding purpose is requisite, can be blind to the purposes (and their profound ripple effects) that so quickly have filled the void left when traditional spiritualities are pushed out of that grounding role. Furthermore, spirituality and faith are *frail and disconnected from the realities of human suffering* without science and medicine. While we live in a culture that socializes us to think and act in ways based on dichotomies, divisions of labor, and separated spheres of power, there is also the way of integration, unity, and toward the weaving of a seamless garment. We experienced this firsthand in our own lives and believe together that we are called to stand in the gap, inviting both spheres to reconsider their broken partnership in the care of the sick.

Undergirding this book is not only our experience as a married couple but two supporting communities. One source of support has come from the Harvard Medical community, where we are currently on faculty, serving at Brigham and Women's Hospital and Dana-Farber Cancer Institute. Contrary to the biases we have alluded to, we have both received overwhelming support from institutional and faculty leaders at Harvard in pursing research in medicine and spirituality. This has included the launch of the Harvard Initiative in Health, Religion, and Spirituality. Multiple leaders at Harvard have gone out on a limb in providing guidance, financial support, and institutional protection, which has allowed us to pursue these controversial questions. Neither our research portfolio nor this book would have been possible without others clearing a pathway for us. We are grateful to each of them, including Drs. Jay Harris, Susan Block, David Silbersweig, Anthony D'Amico, Arthur Kleinman, Holly Prigerson, Howard Koh, and James Tulsky. We stand on the shoulders of giants, beneficiaries of these truly remarkable leaders at Harvard. By their own example, they clearly prize the pursuit of scientific truth rather than ideology, and they put patient care far above themselves.

A second source of support, not nearly as esteemed as Harvard, but with as much grit and passion, is the Longwood Christian Community, an intentional community of healthcare students living together in a "postmodern monastery." In regards to creed and practice, the community has drawn especially from Saint Benedict of Nursia[2] and Dietrich Bonhoeffer's *Life Together*[3] and has been guided by the "Mere Christianity" described by C. S. Lewis.[4] We include multiple families and many single adults, and, from the beginning, we have been a diverse racial/ethnic mix of black, brown, yellow, and white, representing many Christian traditions, including Charismatic, Reformed, Anglican, Roman Catholic, and nondenominational, to name a few. While community members have attended more than two dozen local parishes around the city, especially Park Street Church has held an invisible but critical role in enabling our community to spiritually thrive. Since its inception, about 200 young medical students, physicians, nurses, therapists, dentists, pharmacists, basic scientists, public health researchers, and others have lived together across the street from Harvard Medical School and the Harvard-Chan School of Public Health. We eat, pray, and play together, and we do science and patient care under a conviction that the health sciences and faith can be friends, both gifts from the same Ultimate Source. Among community alumni, there are many now working in health institutions, and there are also academic faculty at a host of teaching centers such as Duke, UNC, Baylor, University of Wisconsin, Vanderbilt, Harvard, University of Texas, Dartmouth, Boston University, Tufts, UCLA, John Hopkins, Penn, Brown, Gordon-Conwell, and Wheaton. Much of this book is the product of our participation within this community, among these friends for the past 16 years, fostered through many discussions, prayers, arguments, failures and victories, collaborative research, and an array of experiences consisting of a stew of the baked beans of science, medicine, and faith. Through the Longwood Christian Community, we not only stumbled onto a path that has stimulated key ideas, but we have personally seen some of these ideas working themselves in practice among those we have had the privilege to know and love through life together in community.

References

1. Stephen Jay Gould. *Rocks of ages: science and religion in the fullness of life*. 1st ed. New York: Ballantine; 1999.
2. Timothy Fry, ed. *The Rule of St. Benedict in English*. Collegeville, MN: The Liturgical Press; 1982.
3. Dietrich Bonhoeffer. *Life together*. 1st ed. New York: Harper; 1954.
4. C. S. Lewis. *Mere Christianity: a revised and enlarged edition, with a new introduction of the three books, the Case for Christianity, Christian Behaviour, and Beyond Personality*. New York: Macmillan; 1952.

ACKNOWLEDGMENTS

This project was also made possible by generous financial support from Harvard's Program on Integrative Knowledge and Human Flourishing, the Issachar Fund and the John Templeton Foundation. Kimon Sargeant, our program officer from Templeton, took a chance on us in writing this book, and, though its completion is several years later than anticipated, we are grateful for Templeton's support. We also acknowledge the late Dr. Jack Templeton, MD, who was president of the foundation and ultimately approved our funding request. He provided a valuable piece of advice in 2011, maintaining the importance for us to rework the book outline with the goal of having it published with a university press. We wish he were around to engage it today. It was also through the support of the Templeton Foundation that Michael gained critical mentorship from Farr Curlin, MD and Daniel Sulmasy, MD, PhD, who were at the time at the University of Chicago. Both have continued to be inspiring scholarly mentors and friends.

We also owe a special note of thanks to our editor and assistant editor at Oxford University Press, Marta Moldvai and Tiffany Lu. Marta moved heaven and high water to bring this project to final production. Thank you, Marta, for joining with us and making our argument more feasible for others to read and consider. You represent to us the kind of commitment operating in the world of publishing that is needed among clinicians within healthcare.

We are also grateful to John Yoon, MD and Daniel Kim, PhD candidate, both from the University of Chicago, who read Parts II and III and offered extremely valuable input on several key chapters. Likewise, thanks is due to John Braucher, a medical student who studied with us during the summer of 2017. He provided helpful edits on several chapters. We also thank Bridget Rector who read some early chapters in Part I and provided her editorial expertise as we were developing the project. Similarly, we thank Claire Wolfteich, a theologian at Boston University, and John Peteet, MD, our esteemed senior colleague at Harvard. They both served as the principal readers of Michael's doctoral dissertation, and their scholarly input from that earlier project from a decade ago has in several ways carried its way forward into this one. John is a giant in the spirituality and health field, and he has been a scholarly trail blazer at Harvard. We are also indebted to our former and current research assistants, Christine Mitchell, Rebecca Quinones, and Alexandra Nichipor. Since 2012 they have each played important roles within the Harvard Initiative on Health, Religion, and Spirituality; and each contributed in unique ways in supporting our research and finishing this manuscript.

In addition to these, we especially desire to mention two others who not only read many drafted chapters of this book, but who also have influenced us for the better.

First, we owe debts of inestimable gratitude to William Pearson, PhD, formerly an anatomy teacher and campus minister with Harvard Medical School and currently serving as an associate professor of anatomy at the Medical College of Georgia. He provided both of us with a unique level of spiritual mentorship for the past two decades. Bill pursued us like a shepherd seeking lost sheep. Only God knows all the people who have been touched by Bill's compassion and generous spirit, first as a minister, but also as a visionary who has the gift to see what few others will take time to note, let alone believe. Even so, many of the best ideas in this book emerged from countless conversations with Bill. He also took time to read key chapters in the book, providing extremely helpful input especially in Part III. Bill has always been about lifting up others around him, rarely receiving the recognition that we know he deserves. We cannot adequately give him enough tribute other than to alert readers that his influence overshadows not only this book but our lives as well.

We also owe a great debt to our colleague, Tyler VanderWeele, PhD, Professor of Epidemiology and Biostatistics at the Harvard-Chan School of Public Health, and who co-leads with us the Harvard Initiative on Health, Religion, and Spirituality. Tyler read and provided critical input on Parts II and III of the book. Tyler has brought enormous passion, optimism, humility, intellectual insight, and methodological rigor to all of our research since we started working together in 2009. We truly cannot imagine a better colleague or friend. Through him we have glimpsed the truth from the writer of Ecclesiastes: "Though one may be overpowered, two can defend themselves. A cord of three strands is not quickly broken."

While we received a great deal of insight and suggestions from all those mentioned, the book's faults are entirely our own. The book's title is taken from Henri Nouwen, a pastoral theologian, who describes our general need for a spiritual shift from hostility to hospitality in *Reaching Out*. As a co-authored work, segments from Chapters 2, 4, and 5 are based on previously published peer-review research overseen by Tracy as these reflect her disciplinary background. While a few tables, figures, and paragraphs are reproduced from prior reports, most of the information and data have been reformatted for this project. Additionally, some chapters in Parts II and III were principally written by Michael since they reflect his primary discipline of theology. All the major ideas and writing are shared by both of us, whereas some of the secondary material in Parts II and III generally reflect Michael's disciplinary perspectives. While we do not agree on all matters written here, the major substantive ideas and thoughts reflect our mutually shared views.

We thank the following publications for granting permission to reproduce excerpts from previously published articles.

The articles "The Relationship of Spiritual Concerns to the Quality of Life of Advanced Cancer Patients: Preliminary Findings"[i] and "'If God Wanted Me Yesterday, I Wouldn't Be Here Today': Religious and Spiritual Themes in Patients' Experiences of Advanced Cancer"[ii] were originally published by SAGE Publications.

The articles "'It Depends': Viewpoints of Patients, Physicians, and Nurses on Patient–Practitioner Prayer in the Setting of Advanced Cancer,"[iii] "Religion, Spirituality, and the Hidden Curriculum: Medical Student and Faculty Reflections,"[iv] and "Nurse and Physician Barriers to Spiritual Care Provision at the End of Life"[v] were originally published by Elsevier.

The articles "The Role of Spirituality and Religious Coping in the Quality of Life of Patients with Advanced Cancer Receiving Palliative Radiation Therapy"[vi] and "Why Is Spiritual Care Infrequent at the End of Life? Spiritual Care Perceptions among Patients, Nurses, and Physicians and the Role of Training"[vii] were originally published by the American Society of Clinical Oncology.

The article "Reintegrating Care for the Dying, Body and Soul. Harvard Theological Review" originally appeared in *Harvard Theological Review*.[viii]

Notes

i. S. R. Alcorn, Balboni M. J., Prigerson H. G., Reynolds A., Phelps A. C., Wright A. A., Block S. D., Peteet J. R., Kachnic L. A., Balboni T. A. The relationship of spiritual concerns to the quality of life of advanced cancer patients: preliminary findings. *J Palliat Med.* 2010;13(5):581–588.

ii. W. D. Winkelman, Lauderdale K., Balboni M. J., Phelps A. C., Peteet J. R., Block S. D., Kachnic L. A., VanderWeele T. J., Balboni T. A. 'If God wanted me yesterday, I wouldn't be here today': religious and spiritual themes in patients' experiences of advanced cancer. *J Palliat Med.* 2011;14(9):1022–1028.

iii. M. J. Balboni, Babar A., Dillinger J., Phelps A. C., George E., Block S. D., Kachnic L., Hunt J., Peteet J., Prigerson H. G., VanderWeele T. J., Balboni T. A. 'It depends': viewpoints of patients, physicians, and nurses on patient–practitioner prayer in the setting of advanced cancer. *J Pain Symptom Manage.* 2011;41(5):836–847.

iv. M. J. Balboni, Bandini J., Mitchell C., Epstein-Peterson Z. D., Amobi A., Cahill J., Enzinger A. C., Peteet J., Balboni T. Religion, spirituality, and the hidden curriculum: medical student and faculty reflections. *J Pain Symptom Manage.* 2015;50(4):507–515.

v. M. J. Balboni, Sullivan A., Enzinger A. C., Epstein-Peterson Z. D., Tseng Y. D., Mitchell C., Niska J., Zollfrank A., VanderWeele T. J., Balboni T. A. Nurse and physician barriers to spiritual care provision at the end of life. *J Pain Symptom Manage.* 2014;48(3):400–410.

vi. M. Vallurupalli, Lauderdale K., Balboni M. J., Phelps A. C., Block S. D., Ng A. K., Kachnic L. A., Vanderweele T. J., Balboni T. A. The role of spirituality and religious coping in the quality of life of patients with advanced cancer receiving palliative radiation therapy. *J Support Oncol.* 2012;10(2):81–87. Reprinted with permission. Copyright 2012–2013 American Society of Clinical Oncology. All rights reserved.

vii. M. J. Balboni, Sullivan A., Amobi A., Phelps A. C., Gorman D. P., Zollfrank A., Peteet J. R., Prigerson H. G., Vanderweele T. J., Balboni T. A. Why is spiritual care infrequent at the end of life? Spiritual care perceptions among patients, nurses, and physicians and the role of training. *J Clin Oncol.* 2013;31(4):461–467. Reprinted with permission. Copyright 2012–2013 American Society of Clinical Oncology. All rights reserved.

viii. Balboni, M., Balboni, T. Reintegrating care for the dying, body and soul. *Harvard Theological Review* 2010; published by Cambridge University Press, reproduced with permission.

Hostility to Hospitality

Introduction

A Rising Hostility in American Medicine

> The crisis in the doctor–patient relationship is part of the ominous, unhealthy, livid condition of human relations in our entire society, a spiritual malaria. . . . It is not true that the diagnosis or the treatment of a patient comes about in a way completely unaffected by religious and philosophical commitments. The doctor's commitments are as much a part of it as scientific knowledge and skill.[1] [pp. 235–237]
>
> —Rabbi Abraham Heschel, 1963

American medicine is spiritually sick. In describing what is at stake, Harvard historian Charles Rosenberg characterizes American medicine as suffering from a "chronic attitudinal malaise," where we hold enormous expectations from medicine yet also grieve in disappointment.[2] [p. 2] On the personal level, part of the complaint is that medicine often fails to heal despite its technological promises. Relatedly, our clinicians and hospitals too often seem reductionist, greedy, bureaucratic, and impersonal in their care. From a systems level, many understandably worry about medicine's increasing costs, lack of access to the most advanced therapies, and the multiple socioeconomic and racial inequities that plague America's health system. Yet beneath these individual and collective symptoms, Rabbi Heschel, speaking before the American Medical Association, suggested that medicine's sickness was primarily spiritual, rooted in the deepest commitments of clinicians.

This book extends Heschel's argument by offering a partial diagnosis of medicine's spiritual malaise. If you rank among the critics of spirituality or religion, perhaps our working premise has already lost you. Yet having trained and worked in Boston for more than two decades, our encounters with our colleagues throughout Harvard indicate that most clinicians do not dismiss the relationship between medicine and spirituality (or religion, for that matter), if for no other reason than because they see how important it is to many of their patients. If you are willing to give us a chance, we think we can make a reasonably strong case that there is something fundamentally spiritual at stake in the care of patients, and that, for their sake, it is critical that we collectively take a probing look at what ails medicine's soul. This book is written to those clinicians who work on the frontlines of serious illness and others with them— hospital chaplains, community clergy and theologians, health systems leaders, and interested patients and family members—who are willing to reexamine multiple layers of evidence pertaining to medicine and spirituality. Our primary intent, however, is to engage those who already have a suspicion that spirituality may have some role in the care of patients, especially those facing serious illness, and yet are still trying to gather how deep the rabbit hole goes between spirituality and all that ails today's medicine.

Part of the conundrum begins with definitions of spirituality and religion, which is less straightforward than some may initially reason. (Readers interested in this topic should see Chapter 8, where we provide an extended discussion of definitions for spirituality and religion.) In summary, we note two approaches, the substantive and functional, in how these terms may be conceptualized. The popular cultural view is to define religion from a substantive perspective, which pertains to the supernatural, transcendent, superhuman, or the gods.[3] Spirituality is typically associated with the immaterial realm and meaning-making. Contrastingly, the approach we lean toward is based on a functional understanding of spirituality and religion, first articulated by French sociologist Emile Durkheim[4] and then further championed by a variety of twentieth-century scholars such as anthropologists Clifford Geertz[5] and Robert Bellah,[6] Harvard theologian Paul Tillich,[7] and University of Chicago religious historian Martin Marty.[8] A functional understanding of spirituality and religion is less focused on the specific content that comprises religion (such as the superhuman or the gods) and instead concentrates on what is the ultimate concern or greatest love of said religion. From within this functional approach, spirituality and religion are closely related but not identical. Spirituality refers to the immaterial connection between the lover and the object chiefly loved. Religion concerns the external structures that support and enable an ultimate concern or greatest love. Clearly, both conceptual approaches hold scholarly legitimacy, but we have opted for a functional understanding of spirituality and religion in this volume primarily because it provides a broad lens for interpretation of the cultural dynamics that surround medicine and the care of the sick. As will become clearer in Part III, we find that a functional understanding of spirituality and religion opens new policy possibilities that offset what often appears to be a culture war between secular and religious perspectives. Functional understandings, unlike substantive definitions, open within an increasingly pluralistic society[9] innovative ways to interpret the relationship of spirituality and religion within medicine, so that traditional "religious," "spiritual but not religious," and deeply "secular" persons may uncover shared values and common ground in the care of the sick.

Growing Hostility in Patient–Clinician Relationship

During the latter half of the nineteenth century, a medical–religious partnership within Europe and the United States was common in both launching and managing hospitals[10,11] and in the moral and vocational framework of many nurses and physicians.[12,13] It was common to think of the physician as one called to a sacred profession.[13] There was a generally recognized spiritual connotation related to the practice of medicine as a vocation and sacredness in the care of the sick. But it was also during this time period, while the embers of Enlightenment burned hot, that cultural cynicism concerning physician compassion began to flourish. As religious partnership waned, signs of dissatisfaction with an increasingly impersonal medicine grew.

These changes are illustrated by highlighting three late nineteenth- and early twentieth-century paintings: *The Doctor* (Luke Fildes, 1890), *Science and Charity* (Pablo Picasso, 1897), and *Sentence of Death* (John Collier, 1908).[i]

Sir Luke Fildes's *The Doctor* was immediately considered a success upon its debut in London (Figure 1.1). It depicts a patient-centered physician at an all-night vigil in the home of a dying child, and, according to Fildes's biographer, the painting was based on the artist's own personal experience of the death of his one-year-old son, years earlier on Christmas morning. Fildes was especially moved by the character and compassion of Dr. Gustavus Murray, who stayed by the child throughout the night. While the artist's final portrait invented a new scene and characters, Fildes sought to memorialize the professional devotion that touched him during his own child's death.

The Doctor skillfully captures the physician's compassion and commitment to his patient. The setting is in the family home, and, judging from the make-shift bed and shabby carpet, the family comes from little means. At the center of the painting is the physician's face as it connects with the patient. A straight line can be drawn between the physician's gaze and the patient's face, and the clinician's body is fully leaning toward the child. The posture suggests an almost reverent genuflection toward the patient. In the background, the mother grieves and the father stares at the physician, perhaps finding some consolation in his careful attention. Medicine's role within this painting is on the side table, represented by a cup and a few simple tools, not immediately in the light of the lamp. Although the child is clearly ailing, there is little more that medicine can do. Despite the fact that medicine may be exhausted, the physician's presence, gaze, and posture depict a social ideal of patient-centered care. Spirituality

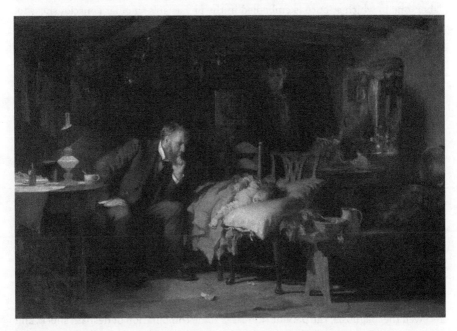

Figure 1.1 The Doctor, exhibited 1891, Sir Luke Fildes (1843–1927). Copyright, Tate, London 2017.

is integrated within and expressed by the physician. In this way, medicine and spirituality seem to be merged within the character of the doctor.

Seven years later, Pablo Picasso completed his painting *Science and Charity*, which contains notable elements that echo Fildes's painting but offer a starkly different story of the patient–clinician relationship. Readers can explore details of this work by following the link from the Picasso Museum in Barcelona (http://www.bcn. cat/museupicasso/en/exhibitions/science-and-charity.html).[ii] Painted at the age of 15, it is one of the few of his classical works. As with Fildes, Picasso's own painful experiences may have influenced this painting:[14] his beloved younger sister Conchita died at the age of seven from diphtheria in 1895. Picasso made a vow to God that he would never pick up a brush again if only God would heal Conchita of her illness.[15] After she died, however, Picasso threw himself into his work, finishing *Science and Charity* the next year.

The background is likely a religious hospital or monastic-hospice setting, suggested by the presence of the religious nurse (or nun) who serves the patient a warm drink and the ornate picture frame above the patient, which has some suggestion of a religious icon at the top of the frame. The center focus of the painting is the patient's face, her eyes focused on the child held by the nurse. Perhaps the most striking feature of the portrait is the contrast in gaze between the physician and nurse. While the nun's eyes are focused on the patient, the physician focuses on his watch.[iii] Just as striking, while the nurse reaches out toward the patient, the physician's bodily posture is erect and his face is turned away from the patient as he silently consults his watch to take her pulse. The patient's child, securely in the hands of the nun, finds feminine protection and care even as the mother appears seriously ill. The painting portrays a divided labor, one in which science is embodied in the physician's singular consciousness focused on bodily mechanisms, and human compassion is displayed through the nurse's eyes, gesture, and recognition of the patient's multiple needs, including support of her motherly burden. There is little doubt that Picasso's physician is concerned with a focus on bodily mechanisms, taking the patient's pulse, whereas spirituality emanates in and through the nurse. In this painting, medicine and spirituality are presented as separated by the role of the healthcare professional. There is little humanity or compassion presented within the physician's disposition, and yet the care of the patient seems to be held together by the presence of the nun and the larger spiritual context in which the patient receives her care.

In 1908, John Collier created *The Sentence of Death*,[iv] part of the Victorian genre of "problem pictures" that depict ambiguous scenes filled with irony, tension, and deliberate vagueness of meaning (Figure 1.2).[16] Collier's title is a critical clue ensuring that viewers understand that the physician has shared a devastating diagnosis to a relatively young and well-to-do patient who does not appear to be experiencing serious symptoms yet.

The setting for this portrait comes closest to the contemporary physician's professional office, which appears stately and suggests the physician's prosperity. The center of the painting is the patient's face and eyes, which gaze directly at viewers. Having received the diagnosis, the patient expresses some combination of despair, shock, and resignation. Most unsettlingly, the young man seems to stare directly at the viewer, pulling him or her into the room itself rather than allowing a comfortable distance.

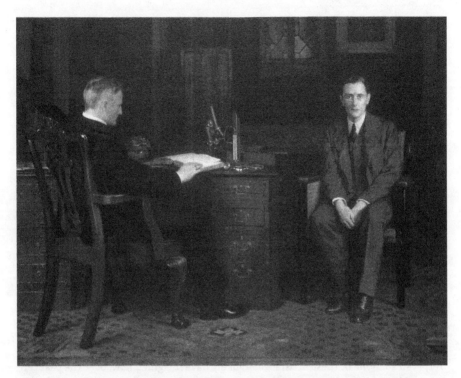

Figure 1.2 The Sentence of Death, 1908, John Collier (1850–1934). Reproduction by permission of Wolverhampton Art Gallery.

It is difficult not to empathize with the patient's shock and confusion. The patient's lonely state is further exacerbated by the physician, whose gaze remains fixed on the medical book that sits feebly on his desk. The physician's ineffectiveness is expressed by the way he slouches slightly in his chair, his desk creating distance from the patient, his eyes diverted, his whole bearing expressing the inability to offer comfort because medicine is powerless to undo the young man's death sentence. In Collier's depiction, spirituality and religion are visibly absent within the scene, with the exception of the patient's eyes, which seem full of fear as he stares at the reality of his own mortality. There is a vague suggestion of the unanswered existential questions that will plague the young man in the days ahead.

Each of these paintings narrate a changing story that includes an underlying hostility embedded within the medical profession toward spirituality and religion. Old medicine, represented by *The Doctor*, conveys the compassion of the physician but also a technologically feeble medical science, especially before the many major advances seen in the twentieth century. *Science and Charity* portrays the reductionist tendencies of a scientific medical profession that has lost personal connection with the patient. Yet it also shows how a division of labor may still uphold human compassion through the active presence of caregivers with strong religious commitments. In *The Sentence of Death*, we glimpse how a medical practice characterized by immanence (i.e., a focus on science, materialism, and the things of this world) is disjoined from traditional spirituality or religion, resulting in the abandonment of the patient. Unlike *The Doctor*, the patient is utterly alone in the revelation of his finitude. In contrast to *Science and Charity*, there is no person or institution to speak hope to him or to point to meaning. Produced over an 18-year span, these three paintings capture the transfer of spirituality and religion in the context of medicine from the caring physician himself (Fildes) to a religious representative and institutional context (Picasso), before showing the final collapse into its visible absence (Collier).[v]

Each portrait also captures hostilities that have increased over the past century. The impact of disease has been partially mitigated by the powers of scientific healing and palliative care. Yet, in all three paintings, the sting of death remains inescapably with us. So as contemporary medicine neglects or avoids spirituality and religion, it produces a significant void within the patient's experience. Medicine's retreat from spiritual partnership leaves many patients without important resources or the direction needed to navigate the experience of illness.

In a similar manner, medicine's forgotten relationship with spirituality and religion undermines personal caregiving as it attracts powerful social forces that are hostile to personal and compassionate care. Picasso and Collier depicted the loss of personal caregiving by portraying the physician as preoccupied with scientific and bodily matters, treating the patient as a diagnosis rather than as a whole person.[17] While the powers of science and technology have so obviously brought enormous human benefits, these developments have also undercut the significance of person-centered care in medicine. Yet, even so, none of these artists would likely have imagined how, over the past century, additional forces—economic, legal, and bureaucratic—combined with the scientific and technological, would intensify the challenge of offering human-centered, compassionate care. While the vast majority of our nurses and physicians today are extremely caring people, the structures of the medical system are increasingly hostile to such care (Figure 1.3).

This book will argue that these trends toward hostility are inexorably linked to spirituality and religion. Though clinicians desire to provide deep human care to the sick, the social forces around medicine are increasingly dominated by impersonal and mechanistic factors. At the same time, there are no clear institutions embedded within medicine that are able to advocate for the personal dimensions of human compassion. The separation of both religious institutions and spiritual rationalities from medicine leaves the social force of compassion to be worked out by individuals. Institutions that believe in human compassion, such as hospitals and the medical professions, are finding it increasingly difficult to maintain these essential human commitments when enormous institutional resources are expended toward the combination of research, growing bureaucratic controls, and the bottom-line of the market. We argue that there is no force that can resist and properly order the ominous powers of rationalization besides human compassion supported by spirituality and religion. Most clinicians are amazingly compassionate persons, but a separation of medicine from spiritual resources is now increasingly taking its toll on our social systems aimed to care for and heal the seriously ill. There is no clear sign of any power besides spirituality and religion strong enough to reorder the impersonal and hostile powers surrounding medicine or to heal the sickness that festers within the patient–clinician relationship.

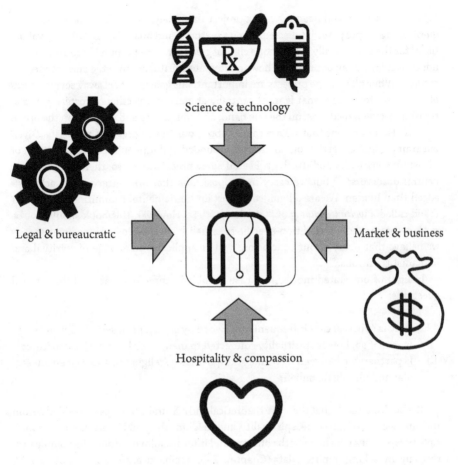

Figure 1.3 The four primary social forces informing the care of patients in American medicine.

We will conclude that new portraits are needed, painted not by artists, but discovered and lived out by clinicians themselves in this new century. Our argument is that hostility—toward the faith of individual patients or as embedded in larger social structures—can only be transformed into hospitality if medicine regains a newly envisioned partnership with spirituality and religion. In this book, we lay out how it is possible to heal American medicine.

Overview of Hostility to Hospitality

The central motive behind our book is to describe why spiritual care is avoided or neglected by clinicians within the context of serious illness and then consider the large-scale, cultural consequences of this divorce between medicine and spirituality/religion. Readers should be warned that this not a book on ethics. It is not an overview of the field of spirituality and health[18-20] or a project that analyzes the scientific evidence by questioning its purpose,[21,22] discrediting its methods and analysis,[23] or offering validation[24] for the field. Finally, this is not a clinical guide on "how to" provide spiritual care[25] nor does it lay out an approach in how to integrate spirituality into the current medical model.[26] While all of these projects are important, our goal is to peel away several layers of the onion to expose what is most centrally at stake in rejecting or fostering a relationship between medicine, on the one hand, and spirituality and religion, on the other.

It is also important that we are candid about our theological commitments. Given our training and expertise, our analysis is grounded and influenced by the tradition of Christian spirituality and theology. Even if some pretend to be so, there are no purely neutral observers[27,28] but we carry presuppositions that are better openly acknowledged than hidden. We are all guided by certain fundamental commitments, or what Freud called a *weltanschauung* or "worldview."[29 [p. 2]] However, this book should not be read as coming from a tradition-specific spirituality and theology of medicine [25-27] as we believe that many of our conclusions will be applicable to a range of spiritual and humanist traditions.[30,31]

In light of our stated motive, our case unfolds in three parts around three broad questions:

I. Why is spiritual care infrequently provided by clinicians in serious illness?
II. Is, and if so, how is spirituality connected to medicine's basic social structures?
III. Is partnership between medicine and spirituality/religion possible given our secular and pluralistic milieu?

The book contends that there are theoretical and cultural dynamics embedded within the intersection of medicine, spirituality, and religion. The problem itself requires multiple perspectives which are both coherent and interdisciplinary. Thus, the volume proceeds by unpacking empirical data (Chapters 2–5), sociological analysis (Chapters 6–7), theological considerations (Chapters 8–12), and future political policy and direction (Chapters 12–16). Although every chapter contributes to the book's thesis, the central argument of the book is carried forward in Chapters 2, 7, 10, 12, 13, 15, and 16.

Accordingly, in Part I, our analysis begins by evaluating empirical evidence drawn from our Religion and Spirituality and Cancer Care (RSCC) study, where we conducted surveys of seriously ill cancer patients as well as the nurses and physicians who cared for them. Yet the data presented in Chapters 2–5, can only be more clearly understood by contextualizing them within four deep cultural beliefs (what Peter Berger called "plausibility structures"[32]). Hence, Chapters 6–7 further expand on how and why a growing separation between medicine and traditional spirituality was defensible within our culture during the late-nineteenth and twentieth centuries. Together, these empirical and sociological viewpoints assist in explaining why spiritual care during serious illness is infrequently provided today by clinicians.

Beginning in Part II, our approach turns to theologically informed considerations since there are still lingering questions that neither our data nor sociological theory can adequately explain. For some, Part II will be the most unfamiliar, and, while our conclusions may disquiet, they are necessary to consider if we are going to accurately understand certain currents that flow beneath the surface. At the risk of oversimplification, the burden of our argument in Chapters 8–12 is that contemporary medicine functions or takes on a *religious-like* form within the underlying values and structures of the larger medical system. Contemporary medicine operates with an implicit understanding of personhood. From a certain view, the structures of medicine hold surprising correlations with religious ones. Likewise, some patients turn to medicine with a religious-like faith and hope. Similarly, clinicians and health organizations frequently infer that healing is the genius of their own making. In the absence of a formal spiritual or religious framework—mostly removed from medicine during the twentieth century—medicine in its underlying values and social structures appears itself religious-like. We argue that these cultural dynamics are unavoidable because serious illness is simply terrifying to most humans and raises basic existential questions. Thus, despite having largely removed traditional spirituality from our medical professions and organizations, spirituality itself does not altogether disappear, as secularization theorists once surmised, but reemerges, essentially divinizing medicine as our savior and our hospitals as contemporary temples of modernity. Thus, in response to our second question, we argue that the removal of spirituality and religion from medicine's values and structures led to the unintentional result of immanence itself taking on a religious-like energy. This seems to us to be completely unintended but also unavoidable when self-conscious spirituality and traditional religion are expunged within a context of the existential crisis of illness, pain, suffering, and confrontation with our mortality.

Accordingly, Part III takes this theological analysis and considers its practical implications for where American medicine has come in regard to spirituality and religion and some possible directions in which to go. In Chapter 13, we argue that these religious-like manifestations in contemporary medicine, or what we call a "spirituality of immanence," not only undermine the spiritual care of patients from within their own religious tradition, but it also has created conditions for impersonal social forces surrounding medicine to penetrate and take over. By blocking traditional religions from influencing medicine, extremely powerful social forces related to technology, the market, and law-bureaucracy have now arisen within medicine, ensuring that the care of patients will only increasingly become more impersonal. One irony is that while most nurses and physicians are amazingly caring individuals, their individual compassion is caught within a thick web of social powers that cannot be undone unless traditional moral and spiritual traditions are brought back into medicine. In response to our third question, therefore, we not only find that partnership is possible, but that it is inevitable. An equally important question is whether our society will favor one type of spirituality over another within medicine, or if it will opt for a truly level playing field. We describe in Chapter 15 how medicine can renew its partnership with traditional spiritualities supported by a policy approach termed *structural pluralism*. While this approach may hold long-term consequences for some of medicine's basic structures, we describe how this policy can be pursued in a democratic, scientific, and incremental manner. We conclude in Chapter 16 that, by being resocialized within the thick healing accounts of the world's great moral and religious traditions, clinicians will rediscover, as Heschel once suggested, their deepest commitments to hospitality and compassion in the care of the seriously ill. In rediscovering the riches of hospitality toward the sick, this partnership between medicine, and spirituality/religion will also lead toward the conditions needed for a professional unity that enables nurses and physicians to jointly stand against the hostile, impersonal forces threatening the care of patients.

Notes

i. We thank our research assistant Alexandra Nichipor, MTS, for conducting research on these paintings and artists, drafting portions of the following paragraphs, and providing suggestions for interpreting these works of art within their historical context.

ii. Copyright issues prevent us from reproducing *Science and Charity* in this volume.

iii. There are six existing sketches of the painting, each depicting different character positions of the physician and child. In several of the sketches, the physician is depicted more positively in either facing the patient directly or by playing with the child. Picasso clearly chose to portray an impersonal and distant relationship between the patient and physician. The painting and the sketches are available at the Picasso Museum in Barcelona, Spain, and can also be viewed online: http://www.bcn.cat/museupicasso/en/collection/mpb110-046.html

iv. Because the original painting is in poor condition, we have chosen to present a reproduction of Collier's painting in this volume. In Collier's original depiction of the scene, the physician's eyes appear to be looking down at his desk where a medical book and instruments rest. The reproduction, however, appears to shift the physician's gaze slightly more toward the patient, although it is difficult to be certain. We have chosen to reproduce the reproduction because the condition of the picture is of much higher quality. Our discussion, however, is a reflection of Collier's original rendition.

v. We do not intend to imply that these changes took place entirely during this 18-year period, but rather that they were gradual throughout the nineteenth and twentieth centuries. The medical profession changed gradually and only partly, since today there are still many compassionate physicians. The point here is that there were cultural shifts taking place throughout this time, with Fildes's representing the older ideal, Picasso capturing how some institutions managed a division of labor, and Collier seeing medical science as empty in its power to heal or provide hope within terminal illness. The paintings capture these general shifts in concept between the late nineteenth and early twentieth century.

References

1. David L. Freeman, Abrams Judith Z. *Illness and health in the Jewish tradition: writings from the Bible to today.* Philadelphia: Jewish Publication Society; 1999.

2. Charles E. Rosenberg. *Our present complaint: American medicine, then and now.* Baltimore: Johns Hopkins University Press; 2007.

3. Christian Smith. *Religion: what it is, how it works, and why it is still important.* Princeton: Princeton University Press; 2017.

4. Emile Durkheim, Cosman Carol, Cladis Mark Sydney. *The elementary forms of religious life.* Oxford/New York: Oxford University Press; 2001.

5. Clifford Geertz. Religion as a cultural system. In: Banton M, ed., *Anthropological approaches to the study of religion.* London: Tavistock Publications; 1965:1–46.

6. Robert Neelly Bellah. *Habits of the heart: individualism and commitment in American life.* Berkeley: University of California Press; 1985.

7. Paul Tillich. *Dynamics of faith.* New York: Harper; 1958.

8. Martin E. Marty, Moore Jonathan. *Politics, religion, and the common good: advancing a distinctly American conversation about religion's role in our shared life.* 1st ed. San Francisco: Jossey-Bass Publishers; 2000.

9. Diana L. Eck. *A new religious America: how a "Christian country" has now become the world's most religiously diverse nation.* 1st ed. San Francisco: Harper San Francisco; 2001.

10. Guenter B. Risse. *Mending bodies, saving souls: a history of hospitals.* New York: Oxford University Press; 1999.

11. Charles E. Rosenberg. *The care of strangers: the rise of America's hospital system.* New York: Basic Books; 1987.

12. Gary B. Ferngren. *Medicine and religion: a historical introduction.* Baltimore: Johns Hopkins University Press; 2014.

13. Jonathan B. Imber. *Trusting doctors: the decline of moral authority in American medicine.* Princeton: Princeton University Press; 2008.

14. J. J. Fins, Del Pozo R. Commentary: science and charity. *Medicine and the Arts.* 2013;88(4):476.

15. A. Huffington. Creator and destroyer. *The Atlantic Magazine.* June 1988.

16. Pamela M. Fletcher. *Narrating modernity: the British problem picture, 1895–1914.* Aldershot UK/Burlington, VT: Ashgate; 2003.

17. Eric J. Cassell. *The nature of suffering and the goals of medicine.* 2nd ed. New York: Oxford University Press; 2004.

18. Daniel P. Sulmasy. *The Rebirth of the clinic: An introduction to spirituality in health care.* Washington, DC: Georgetown University Press; 2006.

19. Michael J. Balboni, Peteet John R. *Spirituality and religion within the culture of medicine: from evidence to practice.* New York: Oxford University Press; 2017.

20. Mark Cobb, Puchalski Christina M., Rumbold Bruce D. *Oxford textbook of spirituality in health-care.* Oxford: Oxford University Press; 2012.

21. Joel James Shuman, Meador Keith G. *Heal thyself: spirituality, medicine, and the distortion of Christianity.* New York: Oxford University Press; 2003.

22. Jeffrey Paul Bishop. *The anticipatory corpse: medicine, power, and the care of the dying.* Notre Dame, IN: University of Notre Dame Press; 2011.

23. Richard P. Sloan. *Blind faith: the unholy alliance of religion and medicine.* 1st ed. New York: St. Martin's Press; 2006.

24. Harold G. Koenig, King Dana E., Carson Verna Benner. *Handbook of religion and health.* 2nd ed. New York: Oxford University Press; 2012.

25. Harold G. Koenig. *Spirituality in patient care: why, how, when, and what.* 3rd ed. West Conshohocken, PA: Templeton Press; 2013.

26. Christina M. Puchalski, Ferrell Betty. *Making health care whole: integrating spirituality into health care.* West Conshohocken, PA: Templeton Press; 2010.

27. Michael Polanyi. *Personal knowledge; towards a post-critical philosophy.* New York: Harper & Row; 1964.

28. Thomas Samuel Kuhn. *The structure of scientific revolutions.* 2d ed. Chicago: University of Chicago Press; 1970.

29. Armand M. Nicholi. *The question of God: C. S. Lewis and Sigmund Freud debate God, love, sex, and the meaning of life.* New York: Free Press; 2002.

30. John R. Peteet, D'Ambra Michael N. *The soul of medicine: spiritual perspectives and clinical practice.* Baltimore: Johns Hopkins University Press; 2011.

31. Mark Lazenby, McCorkle Ruth, Sulmasy Daniel P. *Safe passage: a global spiritual sourcebook for care at the end of life.* Oxford: Oxford University Press; 2014.

32. Peter L. Berger. *The sacred canopy: elements of a sociological theory of religion.* 1st ed. Garden City, NY: Doubleday; 1967.

PART I

EMPIRICAL AND SOCIOLOGICAL PERSPECTIVES ON THE SEPARATION OF MEDICINE AND SPIRITUALITY

2

The Spiritual Event of Serious Illness

"Illness is a spiritual event," suggests internist and philosopher, Daniel Sulmasy.[1] [p. 17] This claim deserves substantiation and debate. Is illness in fact a spiritual event? Is spirituality important to patients as they face serious illness? Do patients desire spiritual support and engagement from people within the medical system? This chapter's investigation of spirituality and medicine begins where all medicine should—with an in-depth account of patients' actions, experiences, and attitudes as they relate to spirituality within medicine. If spirituality is central to illness, then there should be evidence for this claim within patient research.[i]

We explore this claim through an in-depth examination of cancer patients at four Boston hospitals surveyed in our Religion and Spirituality in Cancer Care (RSCC) study. The results of this study provide a vivid and in-depth snapshot of patient attitudes and experiences as they journey through life-threatening illness.

Spirituality in Patients' Experience of Terminal Illness

The RSCC study is a survey-based, multisite, cross-sectional study of 75 advanced cancer patients (73% response rate) that explores how spirituality functions in the terminal cancer experience. We interviewed patients being cared for at academic teaching hospitals associated with Harvard and Boston Universities. The study also characterizes the spiritual concerns of advanced cancer patients and investigates the value that patients place on receiving spiritual care from within the medical system. The study was approved by Institutional Review Boards, and the original study findings focused on patients were published in peer-reviewed journals.[ii] Methods for the study protocol are available in those prior reports and briefly described in the endnotes.[iii]

Patient Demographic Information

Patient information is shown in Table 2.1. Consistent with the region, a majority of patients were white and had some college background. The most common cancers were lung, breast, and lymphoma. As rated by a physician performance evaluation (Karnofsky Performance Status), on average, patients were unable to work but able to live at home and care for most personal needs with varying amounts of assistance.

The RSCC study provides a snapshot of denominational characteristics in the Boston area, which, with some variation, reflect those of the United States. In the

Table 2.1 **Sample characteristics of terminally ill inpatients and outpatients consecutively selected from four Boston Hospitals**

Age, years, M (SD)	60.7 (11.9)
Male, n (%)	37 (54)
Married, n (%)[a]	40 (58)
Non-white race, n (%)	12 (17)
Education, years, M (SD)	15.3 (3.4)
Income, greater than $50,000, n (%)[b]	32 (46)
Karnofsky performance status, M (SD)[c]	68.2 (19.7)
Cancer type	
Lung, n (%)	23 (33)
Prostate, n (%)	5 (7)
Breast, n (%)	11 (16)
Colorectal, n (%)	6 (9)
Heme/Lymphoma, n (%)	11 (16)
Ovary, n (%)	1 (1)
Other, n (%)	12 (17)
Overall McGill quality of life, M (SD)[d]	104.9 (25.1)
Physical, M (SD)[d]	10.07 (4.1)
Psychological, M (SD)[d]	28.72 (9.6)
Existential, M (SD)[d]	42.97 (11.4)
Support, M (SD)[d]	16.82 (3.5)
Religious tradition	
Catholic, n (%)	32 (46)
Non-Catholic Christian, n (%)	22 (32)
Jewish, n (%)	5 (7)
Other, n (%)[e]	10 (15)
Religiousness	
Very religious, n (%)	14 (20)
Moderately religious, n (%)	25 (36)
Slightly religious, n (%)	17 (25)
Not at all religious, n (%)	13 (19)
Spirituality	
Very spiritual, n (%)	26 (38)
Moderately spiritual, n (%)	24 (35)

Table 2.1 **Continued**

Slightly spiritual, n (%)	14 (20)
Not at all spiritual, n (%)	5 (7)
Interaction of religiousness and spirituality	
Religious and spiritual	37 (53)
Spiritual not religious	13 (19)
Religious not spiritual	2 (3)
Neither religious nor spiritual	17 (25)
Religious service attendance	
1 time per year or less	25 (36.8)
2–5 times per year	11 (16.2)
6–11 times per year	7 (10.3)
1–3 times per month	0 (0)
1 time per week or more	25 (36.8)

Abbreviations: M—mean; SD—standard deviation

[a] Married patients include only patients who are currently married and excludes patients who are divorced or widowed.

[b] Three patients (4%) refused to answer information about their income and 2 patients (3%) did not know their income

[c] A measure of functional status that is predictive of survival, where 0 is dead and 100 is perfect health. 70 is "caring for self, not capable of performing normal activity or work."

[d] A validated measure of quality of life with four domains: physical well-being, psychological, existential, and social support. Overall McGill quality of life possible scores 0 to 160. Physical QOL possibly scores 0 to 20, psychological QOL possible scores 0 to 40, existential QOL possibly scores 0 to 60 and support QOL possible scores 0 to 20. The overall QOL includes additional items that are not included in any of the four listed subdomains.

[e] Protestant includes all other non-Catholic Christian denominations.

Of the patients with other religious traditions, 1 (1%) was Muslim, 3 (4%) were Buddhist, 2 (3%) professed no religious tradition, and 4 (6%) responded 'other.'

RSCC sample, 78% of patients identified with the Christian tradition, whereas 7% were Jewish, 4% were Buddhist, and 1% were Muslim. The RSCC patient sample had a higher number of Roman Catholics (46%) and lower number of Protestants (32%) compared to the general US population (24% Catholic and 51% Protestant), but rates are similar to regional expectations in the state of Massachusetts (43% Catholic and 28% Protestant). National surveys have indicated that 3–7% of the US population identify with non-Christian religious traditions.[2] Our findings also track with the US Religious Landscape Survey, which found that most US respondents identify with Christianity.[3,4] While religious demographics remain in flux,[5] it is necessary to avoid a tendency to overexaggerate religious diversity in America.[6] Currently, more than 70% of people in the United States identify with Christian traditions. Data indicate that the youngest generation of Americans (coined the "Nones"[7]) is less likely to identify with Christianity or any other traditional religious community. It is unclear if the

Nones will remain unaffiliated throughout their lives, or if, as psychological theories of aging and the life cycle predict,[8-10] there will be a gravitation toward religion and spirituality in the aging process,[11] one intensified within the experience of illness.[12]

A majority of RSCC patients reported being moderately to very religious (56%) and moderately to very spiritual (73%). After combining religious and spiritual characteristics, 53% of patients described themselves simultaneously as moderately to very religious and spiritual, 19% were spiritual but not religious, and 25% were neither spiritual nor religious. A majority of Boston patients indicated that they attended religious services less than once per month (63%) while 37% attended regularly. These findings were higher than expected since religiousness is considerably lower by region in the Northeastern part of the United States. Boston is not the buckle of the so-called Bible Belt.

There are three observations that may help place these findings into context. First, religiousness and spirituality increase with the onset of life-threatening illness.[11] Consequently, religious surveys of the general population will always underestimate the role of spirituality and religion in the serious illness context. There are no prospective data following people as they transition from relative health to serious illness, though, so the size of change cannot be estimated. There is limited evidence that suggests both that higher levels of stress are associated with increased religiousness and that patients experiencing advanced cancer report significant changes in daily spiritual activities (e.g., prayer) after diagnosis (47% before vs. 61% after, $p < 0.0001$).[12] In a study of 108 women with gynecologic malignancies, 49% reported becoming more religious after diagnosis, with none becoming less religious.[13] This has been termed the "foxhole" effect[14] (a reference to the adage that there are no atheists in war foxholes). Freud (1928) believed this shift emerges out of a direct confrontation or heightened awareness of one's fear of death or hope for immortality. This effect does not necessarily "explain" the origin of religion, as Freud believed,[15] but it is a dynamic that sheds light on why religion and spirituality become increasingly operational when physical health wanes.

Second, while religious service attendance is a powerful predictor for a number of health outcomes,[16] it is an imprecise proxy for spiritual commitment within serious illness. Several studies have found that religious service attendance decreases with the onset of illness and aging.[12,17,18] But while attendance wanes, there is a corresponding increase in private spiritual activities.[12] This likely reflects patients' decreasing physical mobility but deepening spiritual consciousness. Consequently, there should be caution in placing too much emphasis on religious service attendance.

Third, while religiousness and spirituality are affected by regional variation, US patients in the medical system as a whole identify with the Christian tradition and are fairly religious. A survey of 542 hospital patients in North Carolina found an extremely high endorsement of religious attitudes and practices, with 65% attending religious services at least a few times per month.[19] In another study of 100 terminally ill patients living in Houston, 80% of patients were Protestant, and these had remarkably high levels of self-reported spirituality and religiousness.[20] In a survey of 230 patients surveyed from multiple sites around the United States, religion was considered important by 68% of terminally ill patients,[12] with the highest rates among blacks (89%) and Latinos (79%). Finally, in a survey of cancer patients in New York City, 22% of patients attended religious services weekly, and 66% described themselves as spiritual but not religious.[21]

What we may conclude from these studies is that there is regional variation. Consider, for example, the contrast between Houston's largely Protestant and traditionally religious patient perspective versus New York City's large, Roman Catholic, and spiritual-not-religious patient population. In between these extremes, a majority of patients are affiliated with Christian denominations and are moderately religious in their self-description. The RSCC survey reflects this national reality, where 78% of patients were Christian, 73% were spiritual, and more than half considered themselves spiritual and religious.

Patient Experience of Religion and Spirituality

General questions about spirituality, religiousness, and religious service attendance may fail to capture the true levels of spiritual engagement by patients facing life-threatening illness. As we consider patients' overall experience within serious illness, better measurement tools reveal the depth to which spirituality penetrates the illness experience. In the RSCC data, we present four additional lines of evidence (in addition to cruder measures such as religious service attendance and self-ratings of religiousness) that reveal a surprisingly high prevalence of religious and theistic experiences within advanced illness. This evidence includes additional measures evaluating (1) the importance of religion/spirituality within illness and (2) patients' spiritual needs and concerns.

Importance of Religion/Spirituality

We asked patients to respond "yes" or "no" to the question: "Has religion or spirituality been important to your experience with your illness?" Most patients (78%) indicated that religion or spirituality had been important to their cancer experience. Approximately one-half of patients who had responded that they were slightly/not at all religious (44%) or spiritual (28%) did indicate that religion or spirituality was important to them. This may indicate that these patients were experiencing a spiritual transition. One such patient was Ms. F., a 74-year-old highly educated Roman Catholic widow diagnosed three months prior to the interview with metastatic lung cancer. She was attending Mass weekly but labeled herself as only "slightly religious" and "slightly spiritual." The interview revealed a number of unresolved spiritual issues. Although expressing confidence in God's forgiveness, she seldom forgave herself for things that she had done wrong, and she had been asking for forgiveness for her sins. Ms. F. said that she was angry with God but also seeking a closer connection to God. When asked how religion and spirituality (R/S) was important to her illness experience, she responded, "I'm praying a lot more. I'm receiving cards, which are mass cards, from family and friends. It's just incredible, incredible. It's been just important to me." She described her nearly 100-year-old mother as constantly praying for her. She described her mother's religious faithfulness as the bedrock for her own ability to cope with her illness. She said her mother "helped me to be more faithful and have more faith." We do not know if Ms. F. was able to experience further spiritual resolution. She died eight months after the interview. What is clear from her story is that her description of herself as slightly religious/spiritual only skimmed the surface of the powerful spiritual experiences at work in her life.

In the RSCC study, patients were asked: "How has religion or spirituality been important to your experience with your illness?" Patient responses were audio-taped and transcribed verbatim. Transcriptions were independently coded line by line by a theologian and physician and were then compiled into two preliminary coding schemes.

Table 2.2 **Qualitatively grounded religious/spiritual themes in patients' experiences of advanced cancer (n = 53 of 68)***

n (%)	Theme	Representative Quote
39 (74)	**Spiritual coping**	*I don't know if I will survive this cancer, but without God it is hard to stay sane sometimes. For me, religion and spirituality keeps me going.*
	Defined as patients' expressions of how religion/spirituality impacted their endurance of the cancer experience.	
31 (58)	**Spiritual practices**	*I pray a lot. It helps. You find yourself praying an awful lot. Not for myself, but for those you leave behind. There will be a lot more praying.*
	Defined as patients' descriptions of religious/spiritual practices important to their cancer experience.	
28 (53)	**Faith beliefs**	*It is God's will, not my will. My job is to do what I can to stay healthy—eat right, think positively, get to appointments on time, and also to do what I can to become healthy again like make sure that I have the best doctors to take care of me. After this, it is up to God.*
	Defined as patients' references to religious/spiritual beliefs important to their experience of cancer.	
20 (38)	**Spiritual transformation**	*Since I have an incurable disease that will shorten my life, it has made me focus on issues of mortality and sharpened my curiosity on religion/spirituality and what the various traditions have to say about that. I've spent a lot of time thinking about those issues, and it has enriched my psychological, intellectual, and spiritual experience of this time.*
	Defined as patients' expressions of transformation in religious/spiritual beliefs or participation resulting from the cancer experience.	
11 (21)	**Faith communities**	*Well, I depend a lot upon my faith community for support. It's proven incredibly helpful for me.*
	Defined as patients' referring to a religious/spiritual community (e.g., clergy or other spiritual supporters) as important to their cancer experience.	

*53 of 68 indicated religion or spirituality was important to their cancer experience.

Following principles of grounded theory,[22] a final set of themes and subthemes inductively emerged through an iterative process of constant comparison with input from two physicians, a theologian, and a sociologist. Transcripts were then recoded, with coders working independently and using the derived themes and subthemes. The interrater reliability score was high (kappa = 0.85).

Five primary themes were extracted from patients' open-ended descriptions of the importance of spirituality to their cancer experience: spiritual coping, spiritual practices, faith beliefs, spiritual transformation, and faith communities (Table 2.2).

Spiritual Coping

Spiritual coping was defined as patients' expressions of how spirituality impacted their endurance of the cancer experience. This was the most widely expressed theme within the open-ended interviews (identified by 39 respondents, or 74%). The most frequently cited way that spirituality facilitated coping was by extending longevity (10 of 39), exemplified by this statement by a participant: "You've got to have faith and a positive outlook because it is going to help you last longer." Other spiritual coping concepts mentioned by patients included a promise of a potential cure (9 of 39), source of strength (8 of 39), source of meaning (8 of 39), foundation of comfort (7 of 39), acceptance (6 of 39), and emotional stability (5 of 39). A 49-year-old African-American woman with metastatic lung cancer, who died five months after the interview, expressed her coping with a passionate faith:

> With the way the world is now, the only thing you see is what man wants you to see, and God wants you to see more than that. You can't always believe in man because man will deceive you in a minute. But with God, he's true. He's gone and bled for us, he going to bless us. You just have to put more faith in him, and he will make sure everything is alright. He has lifted all my burdens from me. Where the devil kept a door closed, God or Jesus Christ opened two doors for me. And I give him all the praise because at times I didn't think I was worthy. But he still loves me no matter how unworthy I am or feel that I am. He loves me for who I am. And that's my question. You just have to have that faith and belief when everything happens to me. I've never been sick. Eighteen years working hard and never been sick. When it happened to me, he said, "Time for you to take a little nap." Everybody thought that I had one foot in the grave, but Jesus said, "I have plans for you." And look at me now, I tell them all that I am one of Jesus Christ's blessed. Because when they thought that I was going to be in a nursing home and everything, just look at me. You have to have positivity and stay away from the negativity. You got to stay away from the shoulda, coulda, woulda. OK? You give your faith to God and the Lord Jesus Christ. And you have to stay positive and deal with your belief. And I believe in God. And he has been good to me ever since.

In similar fashion, a 46-year-old Roman Catholic science teacher and father of two elementary school–aged girls explained, in tears, the complexity of his own coping experience:

Since being diagnosed with cancer [seven years before interview], the way my wife and I pray together has become a lot more clear, and we have made our faith the absolute center of our lives with our children. If it weren't for my faith, I don't know how I would have kept my equilibrium through this process. It is definitely through grace. My natural state of anxiety and manic nature would have spiraled out of control by now if I wasn't being tempered by grace. It is profound. Some people say to me that I'm doing so well, but I can't take any credit for it. Whenever I'm at the hardest places in life, God just sends his Holy Spirit, and it just takes over, just like he said it would. That's been my experience [patient sobbing]. A lot of saints go through a dark night of the soul where they don't feel God's presence so intensely. That happens too. I think that Mother Teresa wrote about that in her book. Part of the process of going through this life as a human being has to do with being supportive and supporting yourself. There are certain periods that God puts you on your two feet and he says that you should try walking on your own a bit. That is part of it too.

Although these two patients are extremely different (gender, race, socioeconomic background), faith framed their cancer experience in remarkably similar ways. Neither

Table 2.3 **Prevalence of religious coping in patients receiving palliative radiation therapy (*n* = 68)**

Koenig's Religious Coping Index	n (%)
To what extent do your religious beliefs or activities help you cope with or handle your illness?	
Not at all	11 (16.4)
To a small extent	5 (7.5)
To a moderate extent	15 (22.4)
To a large extent	23 (34.3)
It is the most important thing that keeps you going	13 (19.4)
Pargament's RCOPE Index[a]	
I've been looking for a stronger connection with God.	56 (81)
I've been seeking God's love and care.	58 (84)
I've been seeking help from God in letting go of my anger.	33 (48)
I've been trying to see how God might be trying to strengthen me in this situation.	52 (75)
I've been focusing on religion to stop worrying about my problems.	41 (59)
I've been trying to put my plans into action together with God.	44 (64)
I've been asking for forgiveness for my sins.	46 (67)

[a] Responses on a 4-point scale (0–3) were considered affirmative if individuals answered prompts with one of the following categories: "Somewhat," "Quite a bit," or "A great deal."

turned to their faith with the intention of finding a means to cope, but nevertheless they each experienced an enormous power through their faith that provided meaning to endure their trial. In measuring religious coping[23,24] we found that a majority of patients (84%) indicated that they relied on their religious beliefs to cope with their illness, and most relied on at least one or more of the religious coping types in the RCOPE instrument (see Table 2.3). These findings depict that religious coping is pervasive among most patients and offers a powerful means to have peace and strength.

Spiritual Practices

The spiritual practices theme was defined as patients' descriptions of practices important to their cancer experience. This theme was raised by 58% of patients. The most frequently noted practice was prayer (27 of 31).[iv] Patients reported praying for themselves (21 of 27), praying more frequently (5 of 27), receiving prayer from others (4 of 27), praying with others (3 of 27), and praying for others (4 of 31). The most cited reason for prayer was to ask for strength (4 of 27), illustrated by a patient who shared, "I just say to God, 'Okay. You're going to give me something to deal with, just give me the strength to deal with it.'" A few patients indicated that they were praying for healing (3 of 27). This was often conceptualized in Christian language; for instance: "Jesus said that if you had belief the size of a mustard seed you could move mountains; and I find myself asking, 'Why not me? Why can't I be like the masses that were healed?'" A few patients conceptualized healing in terms of New Age spiritual practices: "I have a personal faith to heal that goes alongside Western treatments. This consists of believing in myself and my inner capacities to heal. I go and do my alternative therapies in order to finish healing, which the radiation was not able complete."

Less frequently perceived benefits derived from engaging in spiritual practices included guidance (1 of 27) and perseverance (1 of 27). Additional practice subthemes mentioned were religious service attendance (6 of 31), reading sacred writings (1 of 31), and meditation (1 of 31).

Faith Beliefs

The faith beliefs theme was defined as patients' references to spiritual beliefs important to their cancer experience. A majority of patients (53%) mentioned one or more beliefs as playing an important role. Several patients wanted to make it clear that spirituality had played a significant role in their life independent of and preceding cancer (13 of 28), making comments such as "religion has always played an important part of my life." Another frequently mentioned belief was trusting God's will (12 of 28). The centrality of this belief was expressed by a 35-year-old father who died from lymphoma three years after our interview. He described himself as a very religious and spiritual Protestant who attended church services weekly:

> I'm a Christian man, and I think that God doesn't randomly put people on a path to do strange things, or bless or curse them with one thing or another. So I think that I was given a certain number of days on this earth from day one, and I don't think that changes any with my diagnosis. So, that to

me is very important because it tells me that if God wanted me yesterday, I wouldn't be here today. And if he wants me to survive this twenty years without a cure, then that's His will also. . . . I thank God every day when I wake up because I still feel fine. I'm not symptomatic of anything, and I go to bed and I feel fine. And I thank God for my daughter, my wife and my little one that's on the way. We're four-and-a-half-months pregnant. And, um, so I just don't think it's a random occurrence. I think that, you know, for me religion and faith in God means that you have to follow the path that He puts you on. And, you know, that could be a long path or a short path, but I have to do with it what it is.

Additional faith belief subthemes included belief in an afterlife (7 of 28). For example, one patient indicated that, while she did not want to focus on dying, she knew that physical death was not the end: "I don't want to say that it is a future event, but I don't think that I'm just going to die and then just be nothing."

Finally, some patients explained that their faith beliefs were spiritual in nature but not religious (5 of 28). One 54-year-old female patient explained:

My spirituality is an energy form. A lot of people have offered to put me on their church prayer list or chapel or whatever. And I think if a friend or person believes in that, it is giving a gift to you as a cancer patient, which is something that they believe in. I do not necessarily believe in their form, but I think that it probably does do a heck of a lot of good to help me because when a person believes in what they are doing, even if it doesn't do me any good, certainly it will not do me any harm. It is a win-win for me; and if they believe in it, then it is a win for them also because it is a gift they are giving. I personally believe that spirituality is an energy that is beyond what we can understand. And I consider myself a spiritual person even though I would rarely sit in a chapel or church.

What this theme illustrates is that spirituality takes particular forms, not only in actions like prayer, but around faith beliefs concerning the nature of reality, the afterlife, and the meaning of illness. Such beliefs play a critical role in being able to respond to the existential questions that arise for many facing mortality.

Spiritual Transformation

The spiritual transformation theme, defined as patients' expressions of transformation in R/S beliefs or participation resulting from the cancer experience, was raised by 38% of patients. Several patients mentioned that their cancer engendered a new or deeper reflection on faith and mortality (10 of 20), reflected in statements such as "it's a transformative experience to have an illness such as this, and when you have that you have to reevaluate all you've done in life, who you are, and who you're going to be." Patients also expressed spiritual transformation through an enhanced personal faith (8 of 20), an increase in faith-based activities (8 of 20), a heightened sense of companionship with God or a higher power (7 of 20), and a greater appreciation for life and health (3 of 20). Two months before she passed away, a 54-year-old African-American Protestant woman spoke of her spiritual transformation:

> Well, you find out that you have fourth stage cancer and boom, everything is over. And then I turned to Christ again. The body might be gone, but I'm still alive and I know that there is a place for me afterward. I know that I have my family and I have faith, and it's going to be better for me when I go there. There's still a place for me to go, you know, I will be with my father and my mother, and all my siblings, and just meet up with everybody.

A 62-year-old Roman Catholic white male also reflected on his spiritual quest after diagnosis:

> It is funny that people wait till they have a threatening disease because then they seem to turn to God for help. Any belief in God or an inkling in a higher power is something you start researching because the unknown is very scary to everybody, and there are so many thoughts and philosophies on reincarnation and your soul and energy and going to a better place. You try to research this out in case your prognosis doesn't turn out the way that you want it to and you end up crossing over and dying. However, when you look for God, I found that in my own personal experience, the things that I feared the most, after I got diagnosed with cancer, I learned to accept, because for some reason asking God (who I think is my God) to stand by me, I have felt his presence on more than one occasion. It really has put a big grin on my face saying "Uh-huh." This has been my own personal experience, and not something that I just made up. It's something that happened through the intervention of whoever that greater power is outside of myself.

As cross-sectional data, the RSCC study cannot directly measure spiritual change over time, especially before and after illness. Only large, epidemiological studies could prospectively demonstrate a spiritual change by following healthy patients into terminal illness. But the RSCC data do suggest that many patients indicate spiritual changes, described primarily in constructive and integrating terms, and that it is the illness event itself that catalyzes spiritual change.

Faith Communities

The faith community theme, defined by patients referring to an R/S community (e.g., clergy or other spiritual supporters) as important to their cancer experience, was raised by 21% of patients. For example, a 48-year-old white Pentecostal woman with metastatic breast cancer described how her cancer reoccurrence had shifted her priorities toward serving in her church:

> God has always been number one. Church, church, church! But I had other things like family, work, and my job—a job I hated for 21 years at the phone company. After being diagnosed with cancer the first time, I went back to

work. After being diagnosed again, I will not be going back but hope to go on disability. I'm going to fight [going back to the phone company]. I don't belong there. I feel that I've gotten closer to God this time around. . . . I realize that there are other things that I should be doing with the church. I have a long road ahead of me, but I've also been through a lot. My husband passed away from cancer when he was 33, and I have a daughter. I kept working [at the phone company] because that was what I was supposed to do. Now I realize that the second time around that I was doing it not because I wanted it. I feel like God is saying, "OK, you've got cancer again and we've got to do something about it, and I want you to slow down and work for the church." I knew in my heart that I wasn't doing the right thing with work but it was good money. I love kids and I now have kids [from Sunday School] who are in their thirties coming to me telling me how much of a mentor I was for them. That's what was wrong [patient began sobbing].

Similarly, an African-American patient rediscovered the importance of her church after her diagnosis:

God has been preparing me for a while. And church, it was just in my bones. "I've got to go to church; I've got to go to church." June 4th was Pastor X Sunday, and I got blessed with the Holy Spirit. Six days after that, that's when everything came out. That is how good God is. And I still have him in my bones. "Got to go to church Sunday; got to go to church Sunday." I go to hear the Word, and it feels good. I might not be a member of my church, but I go to hear the Word. I was brought up on church as a little girl, and it feels good; it is in my bones and deep down in my soul now.

Religious communities can clearly hold a powerful social role in the life of patients facing life-threatening illness as it offers supportive relationships, pastoral support, and relational connection within a time of change and potential disintegration.[25] Yet studies also suggest that serious illness decreases patients' religious community participation and religious service attendance, likely because of less mobility and the difficulty in being among groups of people when feeling unwell.[12] This is likely a primary factor explaining why fewer patients endorsed it in comparison to other themes mentioned.

In summary, most patients in the study indicated that spirituality was important to their experience of life-threatening illness, with spirituality being manifested in five primary ways: coping, practices, beliefs, transformation, and community. Many of these themes were interrelated and mutually sustained one another. Three out of four patient interviews contained at least two themes, illustrating theme interrelationships. Recall Ms. F., who reported feeling comfort at receiving prayers and mass cards from her family and friends and found that this encouraged her own attempts to reconcile with God. Her experience demonstrates connections between spiritual practice (prayer), faith community (spiritual family and friends), and spiritual transformation (increased faith) in this patient's cancer experience.

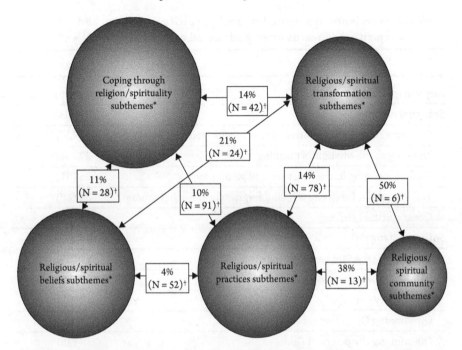

Figure 2.1 **Exploratory diagram of religious and spiritual subtheme interrelationships in patients' experiences of advanced cancer.** Proportion of subthemes that are significantly correlated to one another of the total potentially related subthemes (% of N). Exploratory analyses of subtheme relationships were performed utilizing Spearman correlations.
*The area of each theme's circle corresponds to the proportional theme frequency.
†Proportion of subthemes that are significantly correlated to one another of the total potentially related subthemes (N).

We created Figure 2.1 to better illustrate the interconnections among spiritual practice, faith community, and spiritual transformation.[v] The arrows and percentages represent the level of correlation existing between each of the five themes, suggesting how the themes track with one another based on patient responses.

Patients' Spiritual Concerns

In the RSCC study, religious and spiritual concerns encountered in the advanced cancer experience were assessed quantitatively and qualitatively using a 15-item needs checklist (Table 2.4) based on previous studies.[26-28] Methods of development are available in the endnotes.[vi]

Most participants (86%) identified one or more religious or spiritual concerns. The RSCC study assessed conceptual subcategories, which we termed "seeking" and "struggle." Spiritual seeking refers to the recognition of a spiritual deficit that engendered a search for existential and/or spiritual resources to fill a void. Most

Table 2.4 **Prevalence of spiritual struggles, spiritual seeking, and total spiritual concerns among advanced cancer patients (N = 69)**

	n (%)
Any spiritual concerns[a]	**59 (86)**
Spiritual seeking[b]	**57 (83)**
Seeking a closer connection with God or with your faith	37 (54)
Thinking about what gives meaning to life	37 (54)
Finding meaning in the experience of your cancer	35 (51)
Thinking about forgiveness (being forgiven or forgiving others)	33 (48)
Other spiritual seeking[c]	11 (16)
Spiritual struggle[d]	**40 (58)**
Wondering why God has allowed this to happen	21 (30)
Wondering whether God has abandoned me[e]	20 (29)
Being angry with God	17 (25)
Questioning God's love for me[e]	17 (25)
Questioning the power of God[e]	17 (25)
Feeling that cancer is God's way of punishing me for my sins and lack of devotion[e]	15 (22)
Wondering what I did for God to punish me like this[e]	15 (22)
Doubting your belief in God or in your faith	14 (20)
Wondering whether my church has abandoned me[e]	8 (12)
I've been thinking that the devil made this happen[e]	9 (13)
Other spiritual struggles[f]	2 (3)

[a] This includes all patients who reported at least one spiritual seeking or at least one spiritual struggle item.

[b] This includes all patients who reported at least one spiritual seeking item.

[c] Eleven patients expressed other forms of spiritual seeking. These included seeking greater religious practice (2), reflection on spiritual beliefs (3), seeking to live life to the fullest despite cancer (1), desiring to give to others less fortunate (1), praying for the well-being of oneself or others (2), and finding meaning and peace (2).

[d] This includes all patients who reported at least one spiritual struggle item.

[e] Pargament's negative religious coping items (Kenneth I. Pargament, 1997). Frequencies are based on patients indicating "somewhat," "quite a bit," or "a great deal."

[f] Two patients expressed spiritual struggles other than the choices offered, including anger at God for loss of control and asking "why."

patients (83%) indicated that they were spiritually seeking within their illness. The most common spiritual seeking items, endorsed by approximately half of patients, included "seeking a closer connection with God or one's faith," "finding meaning in the experience of your cancer," "what gives meaning to life," and "thinking about forgiveness."

Spiritual struggle refers to the presence of a spiritual tension or conflict over sacred issues and questions.[29] The most commonly endorsed struggle (named by 30% of patients) was "wondering why God has allowed this to happen." Notably, 43% of patients described experiencing one or more of the spiritual struggles defined by Pargament's negative religious coping items.[vii] The frequency of several of these struggles is notable, including the experience of divine abandonment (29%), questioning God's power and love (25%), and feelings related to divine punishment (22%). We were surprised to find patients in a cosmopolitan city endorsing these spiritual struggles at a relatively high rate.

We also analyzed the relationship between how patients responded to the importance of religion or spirituality and the number of spiritual concerns they expressed (Table 2.5). Contrary to our original study hypothesis, we found that younger age was

Table 2.5 **Number of spiritual concerns by importance of religion/ spirituality in patients' experiences of advanced cancer (*n* = 68)**

| | | Religion or Spirituality Important to the Cancer Experience | |
	All	Yes	No
Religious and spiritual concerns	N (%)		
No religious/spiritual concerns	10 (15)	5 (9)	5 (33)
1–3 religious/spiritual concerns	23 (34)	19 (36)	4 (27)
4 or more religious/spiritual concerns	35 (51)	29 (55)	6 (40)

Committed non-spiritual 7% (N = 5)

Spiritually at peace 7% (N = 5)

Spiritually ambivalent 15% (N = 10)

Spiritual & seeking 71% (N = 48)

one key factor associated with more spiritual concerns[viii] but that there was no statistically significant difference in the number of spiritual concerns when comparing
patients who said that religion/spirituality was important versus those who said it
was not important in their experience of advanced cancer (p =.12). This suggests that
even after asking patients if religion was important to their experience, there may be
more going on beneath the surface. Serious illness invokes very difficult questions of
life and meaning. Younger persons facing life-threatening illness are more prone to
face existential crises since few are conditioned to consider their own mortality,[30] and
youth are also more likely to put off serious consideration of spiritual questions.[11,31]
Some patients appear to be unconsciously or silently struggling over these issues, not
having fully identified that they are essentially wrestling over spiritual and religious
concerns, and perhaps younger patients lack some religious language and concepts to
navigate their questions.

Among the patients interviewed, four categories emerged. Those who identified as
"Committed nonspiritual" (7%) indicated that religion or spirituality was not important to them, and they reported no spiritual concerns. Those who were "spiritually at
peace" (7%) said that religion or spirituality was important to them but reported no
spiritual issues with which they were struggling. A third group, the "spiritually ambivalent" (15%), indicated that religion or spirituality was not important to their cancer
experience, yet all of these (10 of 68) reported at least one spiritual concern, and more
than half (6 of 10) reported four or more spiritual concerns. The largest group were
those who said that religion or spirituality was important and also reported one or
more spiritual concerns (71%).

This information highlights several practical considerations as they pertain to religion and spirituality in the experience of terminal illness.

Only 7% of patients expressed no need for spiritual care, and they did not value
spirituality in their own lives (identified as the "committed nonspiritual" group).
These patients were consistently nonreligious and nonspiritual. We were surprised
by how small a minority this was, especially in a Boston-based survey—a region consistently lower in religiosity and spirituality in comparison to many other parts of the
United States.[3]

By contrast, the vast majority of patients, irrespective of whether they identified
spirituality or religion as personally important (93%), had some thoughts, emotions,
and experiences pertaining to spirituality and terminal illness. Those categorized
within the "Spiritual and seeking" and the "Spiritually at peace" groups can be
identified through a variety of approaches including one-item screening questions[32]; a
screening checklist[33]; short, open-ended questions[34]; or active listening attuned to the
potential importance of spirituality.[35 [p. 30]]

We were also surprised to discover an additional classification, the "Spiritually ambivalent," those who seemed disinterested in spirituality and religion yet acknowledged their own spiritual concerns and struggles. This group reported that religion
or spirituality was not important to their cancer experience, but the 15-item spiritual
concerns checklist (Table 2.4) unearthed spiritual issues operating just under the surface. Two-thirds of patients who said that spirituality or religion was unimportant
simultaneously acknowledged spiritual concerns. Members of this group, on the one
hand, say that religion is unimportant but, on the other hand, are influenced by religious interpretations of their illness. While future research is necessary to better

understand the reasons for this ambivalence, we would imagine that a contributing factor is that persons in this category adhere to a theistic orientation of a contradictory and inconsistent god.[27 (p. 357)] In other words, some of these patients hold to partly formed religious concepts learned as a child in places like Sunday School or picked up within nominally religious families but then never receive the "adult versions" of those teachings, which contain nuance and qualification. This creates a deep ambivalence so that patients look back to an undeveloped understanding of religious teaching about God but then lack relational connections to those same faith communities where they might better develop a theologically nuanced understanding of God and how God is believed to relate to their condition. Without this nuance, many patients are left in a state of spiritual confusion, as was Ms F. as she tried to navigate the contradiction of her anger with God at the very same time she longed for a deeper connection with God.

Spiritual confusion is illustrated by one of the patients interviewed in the RSCC study. Ms. G. was a 39-year-old, never-married female suffering from metastatic colorectal cancer. During the initial part of the interview, she consistently indicated that spiritual care did not apply to her and that she was not at all spiritual or religious. As the interview continued, we learned that she grew up Roman Catholic but did not attend religious services and no longer knew what she believed. But she admitted that she felt punished by God and was questioning God's power. She had also been asking for forgiveness for her sins and trying to see how God might give her strength. She agreed that she was angry with God and doubting her belief in God. Throughout the interview, the patient expressed some anger and unresolved grief about her spiritual condition. Ms. G.'s spiritual ambivalence illustrates how religion and spirituality operate among some who say they are not religious or spiritual. Her example certainly illustrates limitations to a single-item question. Without additional probing or the employment of more sophisticated spiritual checklists, about 15% of Boston patients will likely be classified as uninterested in spirituality or religion when in fact there are multiple spiritual issues brooding under the surface and needing address.

Ms. G's state of spiritual ambivalence suggests that her unresolved religious and spiritual issues are what psychologist Kenneth Pargament described as a spiritual "fork in the road."[36] Spiritual concerns will either lead toward resolution or toward spiritual disintegration and decline. One well-designed prospective study that evaluated the relationship of spiritual concerns and several mental health indicators found that unresolved spiritual concerns were associated with worse quality of life and worse mental health outcomes.[37] The same study reported that struggling with the divine was associated with higher rates of mortality. In the RSCC study, we found that a greater increase in spiritual concerns was associated with worse psychological well-being.[38] Thus, spiritual concerns mark an area of tension and confusion that erode personal well-being.

Although we cannot state with certainty the frequency with which patients experience spiritual transformation, this would appear to be a key pathway that leads to spiritual resolution and peace. This highlights the importance of spiritual care, the role of chaplains, and the importance of religious communities in assisting and supporting the large majority of patients who face spiritual concerns in terminal illness.[37] Patients such as Ms. G. are especially at risk because of their spiritual struggles and disconnection from spiritual supporters. When we asked Ms. G. if it would be appropriate for medical staff to offer spiritual care, she indicated that it was occasionally appropriate to do so. She said, "To be asked means that it is not being pushed. Asking doesn't impose." She felt that if she had been approached by medical staff for prayer, she would personally find it supportive. While Ms. G. initially appeared to be categorically nonreligious or nonspiritual, additional probing unearthed spiritual concerns and a willingness to engage over these issues if offered sensitively. We do not know if Ms. G. resolved her spiritual concerns and ambivalence before her death 14 months after our interview.

Conclusion

We began this chapter by indicating that we would empirically test the claim that "Illness is a spiritual event."[1] [p. 17] The chapter explored patients' personal accounts of spirituality and illness and found that the majority of patients consider spirituality and religion as important to their illness experience and that an even greater majority have one or more spiritual concerns. Only 7% were consistently nonreligious or nonspiritual. The RSCC study also highlighted several interlocking themes that explain how religion and spirituality operate within a person's personal experience. One key theme, spiritual transformation, highlights a shift that takes place for many patients within illness. Almost all patients, as they are forced to stare at the reality of their own mortality, find that our cultural camouflage of death disappears,[30] and this serves as a catalyst for patients to directly consider and weigh spiritual issues. While our Boston-based study is not a large sample, what is notable about it is that it provides a "thick" account of patient experience, and it does so within a metro area that is far less religious than many other places in the United States. This suggests that if a similar study were performed in most other places in America (perhaps with the exception of New York City, San Francisco, Seattle, Portland, etc.), the intensity of spirituality and religion would be considerably higher. All told, these data confirm the claim that, for nearly all, illness emerges as a spiritual event of great importance.

Perhaps you think that this merely has to do with soft measures of patient experience. Does spirituality and religion effect hard outcomes within serious illness? Although we think it is problematic to think in categories of "soft" and "hard" outcomes, we assess the data that get at this question in the next chapter.

Notes

i. For those readers curious about a more robust distinction between spirituality and religion, please see Chapter 8.

ii. S. R. Alcorn, Balboni M. J., Prigerson H. G., Reynolds A., Phelps A. C., Wright A. A., Block S. D., Peteet J. R., Kachnic L. A., Balboni T. A. "If God wanted me yesterday, I wouldn't be here today": religious and spiritual themes in patients' experiences of advanced cancer. *J Palliat Med.* 2010;13(5):581–588; W. D. Winkelman, Lauderdale K., Balboni M. J., Phelps A. C., Peteet J. R., Block S. D., Kachnic L. A., VanderWeele T. J., Balboni T. A. The relationship of spiritual concerns to the quality of life of advanced cancer patients: preliminary findings. *J Palliat Med.* 2011;14(9):1022–1028; M. Vallurupalli, Lauderdale K., Balboni M. J., Phelps A. C., Block S. D., Ng A. K., Kachnic L. A., Vanderweele T. J., Balboni T. A. The role of spirituality and religious coping in the quality of life of patients with advanced cancer receiving palliative radiation therapy. *J Support Oncol.* 2012;10(2):81–87.

iii. Patients were enrolled in the study between 2006 and 2008. Eligibility criteria included diagnosis of an advanced, incurable cancer, active receipt of palliative radiation therapy, age greater than 21 years, and adequate stamina to undergo a 45-minute interview. We excluded patients who met criteria for delirium or dementia by neurocognitive examination and those not speaking English or Spanish.

All research staff underwent a one-day training session in the study protocol and the scripted, interviewer-administered questionnaire. Patients were recruited from four Boston, Massachusetts, hospitals affiliated with Harvard University and Boston University: Beth Israel Deaconess Medical Center, Boston University Medical Center, Brigham and Women's Hospital, and Dana-Farber Cancer Institute. Patients were consecutively selected from physician schedules, and all eligible patients were approached for participation. To mitigate selection bias, potential participants were told, "You do not have to be religious or spiritual to answer these questions. We want to hear from people with all types of points of view." Participants provided written, informed consent according to protocols approved by each site's human subjects committee. Definitions for religion and spirituality grounded the study's design and were provided to participants at the beginning of the interview, with spirituality defined as "a search for or a connection to what is divine or sacred" and religion defined as "a tradition of spiritual beliefs and practices shared by a group of people." Of 103 patients approached, 75 (73%) participated. Seven patients had missing data, five due to being too sick/fatigued to complete the interview (indicated by their lower average Karnofski performance status than other participants, 36.0 vs. 68.8, $p = 0.003$), yielding a total of 68 patients (91% of 75).

Assessment of Spiritual Care is a 17-item questionnaire assessing cancer patient's spiritual care perceptions and experiences as related to their oncology physicians. The frequency of spiritual care was assessed with (1) an adjectival scale to quantify overall perceived frequency of spiritual care and (2) a quantification of episodes and types of spiritual care received from oncology physicians. The impact of spiritual care experiences was also assessed using an adjectival scale and an open-ended question. Additionally, patients were given a series of spiritual care examples (the same list was also used in the practitioner survey, discussed in Chapter 5), and they assessed what practices (if any) should be performed to support (1) the spiritual needs of cancer patients in general and (2) their experienced spiritual needs. Additionally, patients assessed how regular spiritual care would impact cancer patients' experience of illness both quantitatively (adjectival scale) and qualitatively. They were also asked to assess the importance of oncology physicians considering cancer patients' spiritual needs quantitatively (adjectival scale) and qualitatively. Patients' spiritual care needs and the role that R/S played in the patient's experience of illness were also assessed both quantitatively and qualitatively. All qualitative portions of the instrument were tape-recorded and transcribed, and the study investigators assessed face validity.

The religiousness/spirituality of practitioners and patients was assessed using the NIA/Fetzer Brief Multidimensional Measure of R/S for Use in Health Research (MMRS). This instrument was chosen because of its rigorous psychometrics and the incorporation of multiple subdomains of religiousness and spirituality.

Religious coping was assessed with two questionnaires. Frequency of religious coping was assessed with Koenig's Religious Coping Index. Pargament's Brief Religious Coping Scale (RCOPE), a 14-item questionnaire that assesses positive and negative religious coping, was used to characterize religious coping. Positive religious coping includes seeking spiritual connection with God, seeking spiritual support from God, collaboration with God to solve problems, and experiencing forgiveness. Negative religious coping includes interpreting illness as either punishment from God or the work of demonic influence, questioning God's power or presence, and feeling abandoned by one's religious community. This instrument has demonstrated good construct validity and internal consistency in a healthcare setting. Two items from the MMRS that assess overall religiousness and spirituality were used to assess practitioner religiousness and spirituality. Both practitioners and patients were asked about their religious affiliation and frequency of participation in organized religious activities.

Other measured variables within the RSCC survey include demographic information, gender, patient disease variables, and health status information (obtained from the medical record at baseline and updated for survival information only every six months for one year after study entry). In addition, a brief assessment of the interview was performed by the interviewer.

iv. Since these data are qualitatively derived, they are not considered generalizable. Here we do not provide percentages (%) because we do not want to confuse readers in thinking that these are generalizable percentages. Rather, we have indicated how many patients responded in an open-ended fashion to the question without being directly prompted to do so. This also means that the percentages most likely underreport the total number of patients who would endorse the concept if they were asked directly in a typical survey question.

v. We would like to especially thank Dr. Sara Alcorn of Johns Hopkins University who originally conceived of this figure and created it while working with us as a Harvard Medical student. While the authors further developed the figure in partnership with Dr. Alcorn, special credit is due to her for Figure 2.1.

vi. Patients were asked, "What spiritual issues have you had as you have been dealing with your illness?" Response options were created by an expert panel and were consistent with prior studies of religious and spiritual concerns in the setting of advanced illness. Pargament's validated negative religious coping items were incorporated into the quantitative assessment because they assess religious struggles. Responses to negative religious coping items options were "not at all," "somewhat," "quite a bit," and "a great deal," with the spiritual struggle considered present when patients answered "somewhat" or greater. Patients were also asked, in an open-ended manner, "What other spiritual issues have you experienced?" Responses were transcribed verbatim.

vii. The seven questions targeted to identify negative religious coping are: "Wondered whether God had abandoned me," "felt punished by God for my lack of devotion," "wondered what I did for God to punish me," "questioned God's love for me," "wondered whether my church had abandoned me," "decided the devil made this happen," and "questioned the power of God." For more information, see Pargament et al., "The Brief RCOPE," 2011.

viii. Potential predictors of spiritual concerns were examined by simple linear regression (continuous, ordinal, and dichotomous variables) and ANOVA (categorical variables). Predictors of greater religious and spiritual concerns included younger age ($\beta = -0.11, p < 0.001$), increasing religiousness ($\beta = 0.83, p = 0.03$), and increasing spirituality ($\beta = 0.89, p = 0.04$). Gender, race, education, performance status, religious affiliation, and importance of religion and spirituality to the cancer experience were not associated with frequency of spiritual concerns.

References

1. Daniel P. Sulmasy. *The rebirth of the clinic: an introduction to spirituality in health care.* Washington, DC: Georgetown University Press; 2006.
2. Association of Religion Data Archives. www.thearda.com. Accessed December 1, 2013.
3. US Religions Landscape Survey. 2008; http://religions.pewforum.org/maps. Accessed August 1, 2011.
4. Pew Research Center. Religious Landscape Study. 2015; http://www.pewforum.org/religious-landscape-study/. Accessed October 1, 2016.
5. Diana L. Eck. *A new religious America: how a "Christian country" has now become the world's most religiously diverse nation.* 1st ed. San Francisco: Harper San Francisco; 2001.
6. Larry Dossey. *Prayer is good medicine: how to reap the healing benefits of prayer.* 1st ed. San Francisco, CA: Harper San Francisco; 1996.
7. Robert D. Putnam, Campbell David E. *American grace: how religion divides and unites us.* 1st Simon & Schuster hardcover ed. New York: Simon & Schuster; 2010.
8. Erik H. Erikson. *Childhood and society.* 2d ed. New York: Norton; 1964.

9. Harry R. Moody, Carroll David. *The five stages of the soul: charting the spiritual passages that shape our lives.* 1st Anchor Books ed. New York: Anchor Books; 1997.

10. James W. Fowler, Nipkow Karl Ernst, Schweitzer Friedrich. *Stages of faith and religious development: implications for church, education, and society.* New York: Crossroad; 1991.

11. Robert C. Atchley. *Spirituality and aging.* Baltimore: Johns Hopkins University Press; 2009.

12. T. A. Balboni, Vanderwerker L. C., Block S. D., Paulk M. E., Lathan C. S., Peteet J. R., Prigerson H. G. Religiousness and spiritual support among advanced cancer patients and associations with end-of-life treatment preferences and quality of life. *J Clin Oncol.* 2007;25(5):555–560.

13. J. A. Roberts, Brown D., Elkins T., Larson D. B. Factors influencing views of patients with gynecologic cancer about end-of-life decisions. *Am J Obstet Gynecol.* 1997;176(1 Pt 1): 166–172.

14. J. Halberstadt, Jong J., Bluemke M. Foxhole atheism, revisited: the effects of mortality salience on explicit and implicit religious belief. *J Exp Social Psychol.* 2012;48(5):983–989.

15. Peter L. Berger. *A rumor of angels: modern society and the rediscovery of the supernatural.* Exp., with a new introduction by the author. ed. New York: Anchor Books; 1990.

16. Tyler J. Vanderweele. Religion and health: a synthesis. In: Michael Balboni and John Peteet, ed. *Spirituality and religion within the culture of medicine.* New York: Oxford University Press; 2017:357–401.

17. M. R. Benjamins, Musick M. A., Gold D. T., George L. K. Age-related declines in activity level: the relationship between chronic illness and religious activities. *J Gerontol, Series B, Psychol Sci Social Sci.* 2003;58(6):S377–385.

18. H. G. Koenig, Pargament K. I., Nielsen J. Religious coping and health status in medically ill hospitalized older adults. *J Nerv Ment Dis.* 1998;186(9):513–521.

19. H. G. Koenig. Religious attitudes and practices of hospitalized medically ill older adults. *Int J Geriatr Psychiatry.* 1998;13(4):213–224.

20. M. O. Delgado-Guay, Hui D., Parsons H. A., Govan K., De la Cruz M., Thorney S., Bruera E. Spirituality, religiosity, and spiritual pain in advanced cancer patients. *J Pain Symptom Manage.* 2011;41(6):986–994.

21. A. B. Astrow, Wexler A., Texeira K., He M. K., Sulmasy D. P. Is failure to meet spiritual needs associated with cancer patients' perceptions of quality of care and their satisfaction with care? *J Clin Oncol.* 2007;25(36):5753–5757.

22. Juliet M. Corbin, Strauss Anselm L. *Basics of qualitative research: techniques and procedures for developing grounded theory.* 3rd ed. Los Angeles: SAGE; 2008.

23. H. G. Koenig, Cohen H. J., Blazer D. G., Pieper C., Meador K. G., Shelp F., Goli V., DiPasquale B. Religious coping and depression among elderly, hospitalized medically ill men. *Am J Psychiatry.* 1992;149(12):1693–1700.

24. K. I. Pargament, Koenig H. G., Perez L. M. The many methods of religious coping: development and initial validation of the RCOPE. *J Clin Psychol.* 2000;56(4):519–543.

25. M. J. Balboni, Sullivan A., Enzinger A. C., Smith P. T., Mitchell C., Peteet J. R., Tulsky J. A., VanderWeele T., Balboni T. A. US clergy religious values and relationships to end-of-life discussions and care. *J Pain Symptom Manage.* 2017;53(6):999–1009.

26. A. Moadel, Morgan C., Fatone A., Grennan J., Carter J., Laruffa G., Skummy A., Dutcher J. Seeking meaning and hope: self-reported spiritual and existential needs among an ethnically-diverse cancer patient population. *Psychooncology.* 1999;8(5):378–385.

27. Kenneth I. Pargament. *The psychology of religion and coping: theory, research, practice.* New York: Guilford Press; 1997.

28. K. I. Pargament, Feuille M., Burdzy D. The Brief RCOPE: current psychometric status of a short measure of religious coping. *Religions.* 2011;2:51–76.

29. A. L. Ai, Pargament K. I., Appel H. B., Kronfol Z. Depression following open-heart surgery: a path model involving interleukin-6, spiritual struggle, and hope under preoperative distress. *J Clin Psychol.* 2010;66(10):1057–1075.

30. Ernest Becker. *The denial of death.* New York: Free Press; 1973.

31. Christian Smith, Snell Patricia. *Souls in transition: the religious and spiritual lives of emerging adults.* Oxford/New York: Oxford University Press; 2009.

32. G. Fitchett, Risk J. L. Screening for spiritual struggle. *J Pastoral Care Counsel.* 2009;63(1–2):1–12.

33. R. K. Sharma, Astrow A. B., Texeira K., Sulmasy D. P. The Spiritual Needs Assessment for Patients (SNAP): development and validation of a comprehensive instrument to assess unmet spiritual needs. *J Pain Symptom Manage.* 2012;44(1):44–51.

34. C. M. Puchalski. Spirituality and end-of-life care: a time for listening and caring. *J Palliat Med.* 2002;5(2):289–294.

35. John R. Peteet, D'Ambra Michael N. *The soul of medicine: spiritual perspectives and clinical practice.* Baltimore: Johns Hopkins University Press; 2011.

36. K. I. Pargament. Spiritual struggles as a fork in the road to growth or decline. *PlainViews.* 2008;4(23). http://plainviews.healthcarechaplaincy.org/Default.aspx. Accessed October 1, 2016

37. K. I. Pargament, Koenig H. G., Tarakeshwar N., Hahn J. Religious coping methods as predictors of psychological, physical and spiritual outcomes among medically ill elderly patients: a two-year longitudinal study. *J Health Psychol.* 2004;9(6):713–730.

38. W. D. Winkelman, Lauderdale K., Balboni M. J., Phelps A. C., Peteet J. R., Block S. D., Kachnic L. A., VanderWeele T. J., Balboni T. A. The relationship of spiritual concerns to the quality of life of advanced cancer patients: preliminary findings. *J Palliat Med.* 2011;14(9):1022–1028.

3

Spirituality and End-of-Life Outcomes

We found in the prior chapter that most patients experience serious illness within a framework related to spirituality and religion. Illness, spirituality, and religion are difficult to separate within the patients' experience. In this chapter, we will show that this experience impacts outcome measurements from quality of life, to medical utilization, to costs. Spirituality and religion cannot be privatized to experience alone but they have a large-scale, systems-level impact. Medical outcomes data are important because a system-level impact associated with patient spirituality is relevant no matter if one is a skeptic or believer. Skeptics and believers may interpret the normative meaning of the data in a radically distinct manner, but both should generally agree that it is impactful and should at a minimum be engaged since spirituality has a measurable ripple effect across care of the seriously ill.

Hence, this chapter will outline some key research in the field especially within serious illness and end of life and then briefly outline how this research has begun to influence national guidelines pertaining to spiritual care. But, before engaging this, we begin with a brief response to those who object in principle to doing outcomes research on spirituality and religion.

A Response to Objections to Outcomes Research

Measuring spirituality and religion using scientific methods does not make sense to everyone. There are two constituencies who have raised serious objections to spirituality and health research: advocates of religion and religious skeptics. For those deeply committed to protecting faith, there has been a concern among some that a focus on spirituality within medicine leads to an instrumental use of religion within healthcare. In other words, this research assumes that the "spirit" serves the "body."[1] Functional approaches to religion reverse foundational assumptions embedded in most religious traditions concerning the proper ordering of human aims. Most religions suggest that the body serves the spirit, rather than that the soul can be a tool for bodily health. Thus, it is reasonable to see why there have been many religious objections to scientific studies examining the health benefits of religion.[1] People should not "get religion" for primarily health reasons.

While we acknowledge that some may take an instrumental approach to spirituality and religion, we alternatively argue that the motivation to do outcomes research is not inherently based on an instrumental use of religion for bodily health. For those who uphold the intrinsic value of spiritual traditions, as we do, outcomes research is employed not to prove that religion is a human good, but as a constructive tool providing vital information to those traditions. For example, Balboni et al.'s finding that religious community spiritual support leads to more aggressive care at the end of life allows religious communities to ask the important question of whether they conceive of this as fitting with their tradition's conception of a good death.[2] Based on these data, we subsequently studied this issue further and found that many congregational leaders do not believe that receiving aggressive care at the end of life is part of a good dying,[3,4] and many are unaware that their spiritual support leads to these outcomes.[5] This is an example in how empirical research can partner with spirituality and further the ends of a religious tradition that are consistent with itself. Religious critics need to differentiate between research driven by instrumental goals of religion versus research consistent with the intrinsic goals or religious rationality. These are not all the same.

Outcomes research can describe a phenomena but cannot provide normative or ethical judgments about that phenomena.[6] Once it becomes clear that empirical research is a description of what "is" and not what "ought to be,"[7] then apologetic agendas proving or disproving religion through research are properly seen as non sequiturs. However, empirical research can become a critical tool that assists religious communities in accomplishing their mission and evaluating the impact of a theological position or spiritual practice.[8] In this way, outcomes research is "converted" as a critical tool that serves a spiritual tradition's mission to be faithful.[9] This motivation not only avoids a charge of instrumentalizing religion, but understands the social sciences and outcomes research as a partner employed on behalf of religious traditions.[10]

On the other side of the argument, many skeptics have raised objections to employing scientific methods in the study of religion and medicine out of a concern that this valorizes religion when the proper social position should be the "separation of church and medicine."[11] A number of ethical and practical criticisms have been raised, with opponents calling the integration of spirituality and medicine "an unholy alliance"[12] and "a witches' brew."[13] These provocative dismissals do not acknowledge the complex relationship between religion and medicine, the history that we[14] and others have discussed at length.[15,16] Additionally, many of the criticisms by Sloan and others, while having some justification at the time of their writing in the early 2000s,[17,18] appear extremely dismissive, thus raising the legitimate concern that their conclusions were based on preconceived opinions and assumptions about the place of religion, rather than on an unbiased and open-minded evaluation of the scientific evidence. VanderWeele and others have demonstrated that there is now compelling evidence of a sufficiently high quality that supports the association between religion and public health.[8,19]

Outcomes research on terminal illness over the past decade or so has indicated that spirituality is an influential social construct that shapes worldviews and social practices within medicine. These studies have highlighted how religion has a powerful impact on adherent perceptions, activities, and decision-making, and, as Max Weber recognized long ago, religion constrains and influences large-scale economic systems.[20] Religions act as informal institutions that impose constraints affecting social, political, and economic relationships. This reality sharply contrasts with Richard Sloan's quip that spirituality is a private matter that is no more relevant to the concerns of health professionals than a patient's interest in NASCAR.[12 (p. 191)] Such disdain holds little empirical validity since it dismisses powerful sociological and economic forces operating at the intersection of serious illness, spirituality, and religion.

While we agree with Sloan that research in spirituality and medicine is fraught with methodological and ethical challenges,[12] later in this chapter we highlight how a growing body of empirical evidence demands heightened attention from researchers, clinicians, and healthcare policy makers as patients face life-threatening illness. Even if combining medicine and religion creates a dangerous "witches' brew,"[13] this does not negate how spirituality shapes medical decisions and costs—factors central to the healthcare system as a whole. Thus, even if one is a deep skeptic of religion, thinking it is akin to a witches' brew, it is a self-defeating position to ignore the influence of spirituality in medicine. Calling for a separation of religion and medicine considering a growing body of outcomes research is tantamount to placing our heads in the sand.[i]

Patient Spirituality and Medical Outcomes in Serious Illness

In light of this rationale, we turn now to more recent data linking spirituality and religion with three important outcomes. Studies have suggested that spirituality in the medical setting is associated with both positive and negative medical outcomes among patients with life-threatening illness related to (1) quality-of-life, (2) treatment preferences and medical decisions, and (3) medical utilization and costs. Outcomes research remains a key determinant in identifying national and international standards of caring for patients with life-threatening illness.[21-23]

Quality of Life

Several studies have found notable linkages between spirituality and quality of life among patients with advanced illness, demonstrating the importance of the spiritual domain in this context.[24,25] Brady et al. carried out a multisite, cross-sectional study of 1,610 cancer patients that found higher patient spirituality to be associated with improved quality of life after controlling for other predictors of quality of life. Patients with higher spiritual well-being reported enjoying life more even in the midst of pain and fatigue.

As internationally renowned Cornell medical sociologist, Dr. Holly Prigerson, has more recently shown in the *Coping with Cancer* study—an ongoing, multisite, prospective cohort study of advanced cancer patients followed through death and funded by the National Institutes of Health and National Cancer Institute (NIH/ NCI)—that patients who reported high support of their spiritual needs by religious communities or the medical team at baseline had better quality of life near death.[26] This association with quality of life remained even after controlling for various other known related factors. Similarly, when patients reported to have received spiritual care from the medical team, spiritual care was prospectively found to be associated with better patient quality of life when assessed by a family caregiver after death. Quality of life scores increased 28% on average among patients receiving either pastoral care services or spiritual support from the medical team, in comparison with those receiving no spiritual care. This notable statistical association remained in multivariate regression models that adjusted for race, baseline quality of life, trust within the patient–physician relationship, the patient's end-of-life treatment preferences, if the patient received advanced care planning, and if the patient received an end-of-life discussion from their clinician. Even after adjusting for all these confounders, quality of life was still strongly associated with spiritual care from the medical team. This finding is also supported by Steinhauser et al. (2000), who asked a random national sample of 340 patients with advanced illness to rank what factors they considered most important as they neared death. Of the nine attributes ranked by patients (e.g., presence of pain, dying at home), being at peace with God was second in importance, with pain control ranking only marginally higher. This suggests that one of the most important components to quality of life is spirituality and religion. When adequately engaged and addressed, spiritual considerations positively alter the patient's experience of serious illness and the end of life.

Similarly, in a randomized, controlled trial of a multidisciplinary intervention in advanced cancer patients that included a spiritual component, researchers found that patients receiving the intervention had prospectively improved quality of life in comparison with controls.[27] In addition, Kristeller et al. alternately assigned cancer patients to a short, semi-structured exploration of spiritual concerns by their oncologist and prospectively found a statistically significant improvement in depressive symptoms and quality-of-life ratings.[28] Conversely, other studies have found associations between spiritual pain and adverse physical and emotional symptoms, including increased depression, anxiety, and anorexia.[29]

Each of these studies provides evidence that as physical health worsens, spiritual health holds a central role in determining patient well-being. Spirituality may enable patients to endure the suffering that comes with advanced illness and dying. In the words of one patient from our Religion and Spirituality and Cancer Care (RSCC) study, "I don't know if I will survive this cancer, but without God it is hard to stay sane sometimes. For me, religion and spirituality keeps me going."[30 [p. 4]] In addition, spiritual support provided by an array of sources (e.g., religious communities, the medical system, pastoral visitation) may allow patients to both express and explore the spiritual dimensions of approaching the end of life, ultimately leading to spiritual peace.[31] Spiritual support may enable patients to meet the degrading physical decline accompanied with dying with the strength and peace provided by spirituality. As another dying Boston patient expressed to us, "[Spiritual care] would help lift the patient up, give him joy, a sense of meaning, and realize they are not alone, and you're never alone but God is there with you."[32 [p. 2542]] These studies illuminate why patient spirituality and spiritual care are associated with quality-of-life measures and need to factor into medical care standards.

Treatment Preferences and Medical Decisions

Several studies have found associations between spirituality, treatment preferences, and medical decision-making. In a study of lung cancer patients, respondents cited faith in God as the second most important factor influencing their medical decisions, behind only pain control.[33] A cross-sectional study by True et al. of 68 patients with advanced cancer found that patient spirituality provided a strategy for facing disease.[34] "When I first got cancer, I said 'Lord, I don't know nothing about this, I'm just turning it over to you, and you take care of it.' And so that's what I'm letting Him do."[34 [p. 177]] As expressed by this patient, faith can provide tremendous reassurance within the unknowns of medical decision making. However, research has also now shown how religion may have a negative impact when it comes to how patients make some treatment decisions. For example, True's et al. study found that patients who turn to and rely on divine support were more likely—even after adjusting for ethnicity—to not have a living will or a durable power of attorney.[34] Patients who relied on spirituality to cope with illness were also more likely to prefer to be hospitalized even when in a near-death condition and to receive life-supportive measures such as CPR. Similarly, in a multiregional study of 230 advanced cancer patients across the United States, multivariate analysis revealed that patient religiousness was associated with wanting all possible measures to extend life.[26] In additional analysis of these data, it was reported that high religious coping patients had a sixfold higher likelihood of preferring life-prolonging measures in the final week of life.[35] These patients were less likely to have a living will, a healthcare proxy, or a do-not-resuscitate order.

Why may spirituality mediate medical preferences and decision-making? One emerging answer comes from our development of an instrument called the *Life-Prolonging Religious Values in End-of-Life* instrument, which is a seven-item assessment of religious beliefs about end-of-life care.[ii] The scale evaluates four theological beliefs: (1) reliance on divine sovereignty, (2) belief in miracles,[iii] (3) pursuit of the sanctity of life, and (4) physical pain as part of redemptive suffering (see Figure 3.1).

Consider, for example, the concept of a reliance on God's sovereignty. The belief in divine sovereignty—that God is in control—may enable some patients to avoid thinking about medical decisions. Among US clergy we found that 28% of ministers are theologically sympathetic to patients who may defer medical decisions because they trust that God is in control of the future.[5] Since patients often experience a lack of control within the illness, they may want to defer to a sovereign power who they believe actively influences the future.[iv] Passive deferral to a sovereign God can be a response to the fear and anxiety engendered by the uncertainty associated with illness and can enable patients to cope with the overwhelming nature of medical decisions. Passive deferment of medical decisions is perceived as a morally faithful approach based on the belief in God's active presence and guidance throughout illness. This belief is interpreted as faithful rather than irresponsibly avoidant.

Another example pertinent to decision-making is a religious belief in divine miracles. Two-thirds of patients in pilot data from a follow-up study of Coping with Cancer also strongly endorsed a belief that God would heal them through a miracle.[36] Similarly, among US clergy, 86% agreed at least "a little" with congregants that God "will cure me" of this cancer despite a terminal diagnosis.[5] On the psychological level,

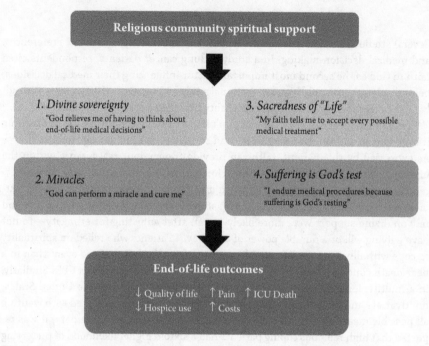

Figure 3.1 A proposed model of how religious community spiritual support is mediated by life-prolonging religious values, leading to more aggressive medical care at the end of life.

trusting for a miracle—"seeking control indirectly by pleading to God for a miracle or divine intercession"[37 [p. 522]]—is understood as a coping mechanism. Pleading for a divine intervention may signal that patients or family members have not yet accepted a terminal diagnosis as the last word—since the power of God can alter even the most impossible circumstances.[v] Consequently, though perhaps counterintuitively, trusting in a miracle may lead patients to interpret pursuit of aggressive care as a more consistent path—since a decision to enter hospice is seen as conceding that physical healing is no longer likely.[38 [p. 53]] They want to avoid "giving up on God before God has given up on them."[39 [p. 1390]] In contrast, pursuing aggressive therapies may be understood as an act of faith—taking every opportunity to allow healing to be given by God.[39,vi]

Racial and ethnic healthcare disparities in the United States are typically characterized by lower rates of medical care among minority groups; however, at life's end, this relationship reverses, with minorities experiencing more aggressive medical interventions.[31,40] This remains a critical healthcare disparity because greater medical care intensity at the end of life results in poorer patient quality of life near death and worse caregiver bereavement.[41,42] Reasons for these end-of-life disparities are not completely understood, but one emerging factor is how patient spirituality at the end of life impacts decision-making.[38] Data suggest that patient spirituality can conflict with the adoption of palliative care[43,44] and ultimately lead to more aggressive medical care, particularly for black and Latino patients.[35,38,44,45]

Strong religious beliefs about end-of-life care are more often held by racial and ethnic minority patients. Based on pilot data from a follow-up study in Coping with Cancer, investigators examined factors influencing racial and ethnic end-of-life disparities among patients with advanced cancer.[36] In a cross-sectional analysis from this database, blacks preferred aggressive end-of-life care more often than whites. However, when race and religious beliefs were placed simultaneously into the statistical model, race was no longer significant, whereas higher religious belief scores predicted greater preference for aggressive care. Latinos' treatment preferences did not differ significantly from whites'. What these data suggest is that it is not race or ethnicity primarily driving more aggressive care but the role of religious values.

What we learn from these data is that religious values hold a significant place within the religious and psychological experience of illness for many patients. It is also not surprising that spiritual beliefs are associated with patient preferences for aggressive care and medical decision-making. The composite score indicates that there is a compounding effect—certain religious beliefs reinforce one another in the medical decision-making process. Preliminary data suggest that these beliefs mediate the relationship between religious coping, race/ethnicity, and end-of-life treatment preferences and medical decisions. As research continues to expand at the intersection of spirituality and outcomes, a granular focus leads to greater understanding of the causal chain between spirituality and outcomes.

Medical Utilization

Three prominent studies within the Coping with Cancer study have found a prospective association between spiritual measures and medical utilization. First, Phelps et al. examined the impact of positive religious coping on medical care received by terminal cancer patients at the end of life.[35] Positive religious coping in a health context refers to how patients' reliance on religious beliefs and practices influences how they engage with illness. Religious coping was measured using Pargament's Brief RCOPE, a 14-item, validated questionnaire comprised of positive (e.g., "seeking God's love and care") and negative (e.g., "wondering whether God has abandoned me") coping strategies.[46] Other psychological factors were also measured, including demographic information, reception of an end-of-life conversation, and preferences for end-of-life care. Researchers completed a postmortem assessment gathering medical usage in a patient's last seven days. Patients whose religious coping scores were below the median were considered low religious copers, and those above the median (50% of the sample) were classified as high religious copers. The study found that positive religious copers were three times more likely to receive intensive life-prolonging care such as receipt of resuscitation and two times more likely to die in an intensive care unit. These findings adjusted for known confounders including age, ethnicity, performance status, psychosocial variables, acknowledgement of terminal illness, and treatment preferences reported at baseline. What made this study especially intriguing (perhaps leading to its substantial press coverage) was that it was the first study to find a prospective association between a religious factor and actual higher medical usage.

Two additional studies from Coping with Cancer examined correlations between support of terminal cancer patients' spiritual needs by the medical system[47] and religious communities.[2] Of the 343 patients studied, those whose spiritual needs were largely or completely supported by the medical team (26% of the sample) had three times higher odds to enter hospice than patients who did not receive adequate spiritual support from the medical system. In addition, the study reported that high religious coping patients whose spiritual needs were largely or completely supported by the medical system were five times more likely to receive hospice care in the last week of life and five times less likely to receive aggressive medical care. These findings persisted after accounting for multiple medical, psychological, and religious confounders in the statistical analyses.

In an additional study, we evaluated the influence of religious community spiritual care at the end of life.[2] This study found that patients who were well-supported by their religious communities (43% of the sample) were approximately three times less likely to receive hospice, two-and-half times more likely to receive aggressive measures in the last week of life, and six times more likely to die in the intensive care unit. Table 3.1 provides a comparison between patients who were spiritually well-supported by the medical team and patients who were well-supported by their religious communities.

Religious community spiritual support of high religious coping patients led to even more pronounced aggressive outcomes: these patients were 11 times more likely to receive aggressive care and had 22-times higher odds of dying in the intensive care unit.[2] Such findings translate into higher costs for the medical system. In unpublished analysis, similar results were found in the association between higher religious community spiritual support and significantly higher costs in the final week of life.[vii] Aggressive medical usage was found to be most common among patients with a predilection to cope with advanced illness through religion (often combined with ethnicity). Further reinforcement by faith community spiritual support leads to greater medical utilization and higher costs.

Nevertheless, spiritual support from the medical system—including physicians, nurses, and chaplains—was reported to reverse this association between aggressive medical usage and high religious copers who received religious community spiritual support.[2] This suggests that medical system spiritual support is an essential component that lessens futile medical treatment near life's end. Those medical professionals who are proficiently "fluent" in engaging religious beliefs may be better able to influence patients in making medical decisions. Nurses and physicians who are simultaneously familiar with the limits of medicine and the underlying theology accepted by a patient (as illustrated in Figure 3.1) can assist their patients in navigating the complex medical decision-making process with spiritual sensitivity.[48] Since clinicians are aware of medicine's limitations in advanced illness, they may be able to more sensitively emphasize how medical options such as palliative care and hospice might be best aligned with spiritual preparation at the end of life. In contrast, nonmedical professionals, including clergy and members of religious communities, may overestimate medicine's capacity to cure or extend life. Studies suggest that clergy are less familiar with signs of advancing illness and lack fluency with the language and context of medicine.[4] Such differences in medical knowledge and personal experience may

Table 3.1 **Comparison of spiritual support from the medical system versus religious communities in their association with the receipt of hospice in the final week of life**

	Unadjusted Odds Ratio [95% CI]	p	Adjusted Odds Ratio [95% CI]	p
Predictor for Hospice Care in Last Week of Life				
Religious/Spiritual support from the medical team	1.65 [0.92–2.96]	0.09	2.99 [1.45–6.17]	**0.003**
Religious/Spiritual support from religious communities	0.53 [0.33–0.86]	**0.01**	0.38 [0.20–0.72]	**0.003**
Predictor for Aggressive Care in Last Week of Life				
Religious/Spiritual support from the medical team	0.67 [0.21–1.45]	0.31	0.38 [0.15–0.98]	**0.04**
Religious/Spiritual Support from religious communities	1.63 [0.87–3.05]	0.13	2.55 [1.10–5.93]	**0.03**
Predictor for Dying in the Intensive Care Unit				
Religious/Spiritual support from the medical team	0.69 [0.25–1.88]	0.46	0.23 [0.06–0.85]	**0.03**
Religious/Spiritual support from religious communities	3.77 [1.53–9.28]	**0.004**	5.73 [1.74–18.93]	**0.004**

Data comparison based on prior publications including T. A. Balboni et al., Provision of spiritual care to patients with advanced cancer: associations with medical care and quality of life near death. *J Clin Oncol.* 2010;28(3):445–452, and T. A. Balboni et al., Provision of spiritual support to patients with advanced cancer by religious communities and associations with medical care at the end of life. *JAMA Intern Med.* 2013;173(12):1109–1117.

explain why spiritual care provision leads to opposite utilization decisions by patients. These differences do not necessarily reflect distinct theological positions between religious communities and medical professionals but instead differing applications that follow from contrasting interpretations of the patient's context. Consequently, when patients receive spiritual care from medical professionals, they are more likely to choose less aggressive medical options even if clergy and religious communities are involved. Congregant choices toward less aggressive medical care are also more aligned with clergy goals of care.[3,4]

The importance of spiritual support from medical professionals can also be measured in regards to costs to the healthcare system. In Balboni et al.'s subsequent report[49] associating spiritual care with end-of-life medical care it was found to impact end-of-life medical costs in adjusted analysis. Costs were higher when patients reported that their spiritual needs were inadequately supported ($4947 vs. $2833,

$p = 0.03$), particularly among minorities ($6,533 vs. $2,276, $p = 0.02$) and high religious copers ($6,344 vs. $2,431, $p = 0.005$). Thus, medical care for patients whose spiritual needs were poorly supported by the medical system cost on average $2,441 more than medical care for patients who were spiritually well-supported by the medical team. The study estimated that inadequate spiritual care for cancer patients therefore accounts for approximately $1.2 billion in higher costs per year, an estimate that would be significantly higher if the scope of the study included noncancer patients or if the time frame expanded beyond outcomes in the last week of life.

In light of our earlier discussion pertaining to the instrumental use of spirituality, we caution against seeing these data within an instrumental framework that subjugates spirituality to market forces. By contrast, our primary motive in examining this association is based on Weber's economic recognition that spirituality and the markets are deeply interrelated.[50,51] The hypothesis operating within our analysis is that failure to provide spiritual care within serious illness leads to several unwanted outcomes, beginning with poorer spiritual peace, but additionally including systemic considerations including overutilization of medical technologies and higher costs at the end of life. These outcomes represent distortions within patient-centered practice since an essential part of care of the seriously ill includes spiritual care. It should not be surprising that when an essential component is absent, costs increase. When medicine fails to engage central issues of meaning and purpose expressed in patient spirituality, then there is a measurable effect across the social system.[viii] We do not follow those who might conclude that providing spiritual care brands healthcare cheaper. Rather, when what is intrinsic and essential to patient care is missing, a variety of distortions take place—in this case, leading to higher costs at the end of life.

A Case Example

To place these research findings in a practical context, consider the following factual case (alias names used) drawn from the RSCC study.[48,ix]

Mr. R is a 46-year-old married male with metastatic (incurable) cancer, the father of two elementary-school-age daughters, and a highly religious Roman Catholic layman. He is well-educated and articulate. He works as a public high school science teacher. After his initial diagnosis two years prior to our interview, he received surgery, chemotherapy, and radiation therapy with the aim of curing his disease. Twelve months later his cancer recurred, and, despite further aggressive chemotherapy, his cancer did not respond. Over the past month, the cancer progressed to the point of causing pain and difficulty with swallowing. His medical oncologist offered an experimental drug aimed at reducing but not curing the progression of his cancer, and Mr. R is strongly considering this clinical trial. He was advised first to undergo palliative radiation therapy to reduce his pain and difficulty with swallowing. The radiation oncologist explains to Mr. R that two weeks of "palliative radiation" should give him some relief from these symptoms. Mr. R then asks, "What does 'palliative' mean?" His physician explains that palliative radiation treatment aims to relieve symptoms of the cancer but will not cure the cancer itself. Upon hearing this explanation, Mr. R becomes angry, and states, "I don't like your attitude, doctor. We're going to kick this thing and I expect you to be on my team—or let's find another doctor who will be."

The day after this conversation took place, one of the authors interviewed Mr. R. During the interview, he told the story of his powerful religious conversion when he was 30 years old, after which he found his spiritual home in a Roman Catholic parish. This congregation formed a strong spiritual community that nurtured his faith as he struggled with cancer. He said that after his cancer diagnosis, both he and his wife became closer in their marriage and they made Christ the "absolute center" of their lives. Not surprisingly, he scored very highly on the positive religious coping scale.

During the interviewer-administered spirituality survey, Mr. R spontaneously recounted the aforementioned conversation with his physician. The fact that Mr. R naturally linked this conversation with his physician regarding his cancer prognosis with topics of spirituality is in and of itself telling of the fluidity between spiritual and bodily matters in this man's experience of his illness. However, his subsequent exchange with the interviewer further underscores the seamlessness of this interconnection. After Mr. R described the conversation with his physician, the interviewer asked him why it was so important for him to get better. "Because of my two daughters," Mr. R said. "God has given them to me as my responsibility, and I have to be around at least until they are grown." One of his daughters has a more severe form of autism.

Mr. R has been powerfully formed by his religious identity, and his own words illustrate the findings of Phelps et al. regarding how this may lead to an aggressive course of medical care at the end of life and result in a poorer death.[35] However, supporting a dying person in grappling with the spiritual realities of struggling with terminal illness may help that individual to undergo a transformation in their spiritual understanding of themselves and of their illness that ultimately can facilitate peace and acceptance.[47] How might Mr. R's clinicians provide this support? First, medical caregivers should be aware of their patient's faith and how it functions in the experience of illness. This can be achieved through a few basic questions included as part of a general assessment at the time of initial consultation, such as the FICA questionnaire proposed by Puchalski and Romer.[52,x] With the understanding gained from this initial assessment, Mr. R's clinicians would likely have been more aware of his need for spiritual support. While medical decisions are ultimately the patient's to make, they need not be made alone or with spiritual motivations that have not been fully disclosed and discerned by trusted advisors. Furthermore, aware of the important role of Mr. R's religious community, a clinician might consider inviting Mr. R to bring spiritual supporters to his appointments to facilitate an integrated discussion and understanding of his illness and the implications of any medical interventions. These supporters might include hospital chaplains, many of whom have considerable training and experience in the context of illness, or might also include the patient's pastor, an appropriate congregational member, or another spiritual friend. These examples of facilitating integration of religion and medical practice, such as taking spiritual histories and referring patients to chaplains, require minimal training and are easily performed by any medical caregiver regardless of faith background. However, nurses and physicians might also consider more deeply engaging the spiritual issues that are affecting patients' experiences of illness and medical care, particularly if these medical caregivers are specifically trained in such engagement or when the patient and clinician share similar faith perspectives.

Returning to Mr. R's case, a key spiritual issue involves Mr. R's religious sense of vocation as a father and provider. He says, "*If I were an older guy I think I would have much less attachment to survival. [But we each] have a certain work that you have to do on earth, and you want to complete that work which you feel responsible for. Raising my daughters is something that I have a big responsibility for.*" It appears to be this responsibility to see his children reach adulthood that drives Mr. R. to especially seek cure. Mr. R. believes that cure may come spontaneously through prayer or through the means of medicine. "*I believe that God does intervene in our affairs and that God will use whatever means at his disposal to effect a cure.*" Then he reflects on himself: "*Jesus said that if you had belief the size of a mustard seed you could move mountains. I find myself asking, 'Why not me? Why can't I be like the masses that were healed?'*" Clearly, Mr. R. feels the heavy burden to be present for his daughters, especially since one has a chronic disease.

While considerations of time and level of familiarity may limit a doctor's or nurse's ability to engage with the spiritual concerns of a patient such as Mr. R, a certain level of spiritual counseling is both appropriate and necessary. While Mr. R's cancer cannot be cured by contemporary medicine, it is a slow-growing cancer that can be potentially managed for years: 2.5 years elapsed between the time of our initial interview and Mr. R's death. During that course of time, Mr. R. had become close with one male nurse practitioner who was similar in age and was also Catholic. This became a pivotal relationship near the end of Mr. R's life.

Nurse Patrick had been part of Mr. R's care for several years. Mr. R. especially began to trust Patrick after one spiritual conversation that they shared in the exam room. Mr. R. told Patrick how he had been previously hospitalized with pneumonia and intubated. The medical team was gravely concerned that Mr. R. would die. But while lying in the ICU, Mr. R revealed to Patrick that God came to him in a voice and said, "It is not time for you yet." Shortly thereafter, Mr. R. experienced rapid improvement and scans showed that the pneumonia had dissolved. Mr. R. told Patrick that the clinicians in attendance could barely believe his miraculous recovery, which had no medical explanation. In hearing this story, Patrick expressed curiosity, asked many questions, and expressed amazement. After this encounter, the bond between Mr. R. and Nurse Patrick began to grow. Mr. R. was in and out of the hospital because of various complications, including a bone fracture and multiple lesions requiring palliative radiation. With the exception of Patrick, Mr. R's relationship with most of his other clinicians was uncomfortable as he was constantly questioning and challenging them in a way that they perceived as arrogant. During his hospital visits, Mr. R. and Patrick would share prayers together, sometimes holding hands silently, and sometimes they would recite the "Our Father" prayer together. These become frequent encounters, and a strong spiritual connection flourished between the two of them.

In the last month of Mr. R's life, he experienced recurrent spine metastasis, which led to most of the medical team encouraging Mr. R. to consider hospice care. One surgeon argued for spine surgery. Nurse Patrick called for a family meeting that included Mr. R's wife and seven other nurses and physicians. However, the meeting was going poorly because Mr. R. was belligerent, angry, and pushing the team away.

Then Patrick stopped the meeting saying, "Mr. R., can you and I talk for a moment? Would you all mind if you stepped out of the room for a few minutes?"

Mr. R. agreed, "Okay. Sure."

His wife asked, "Me too?"

"Yes, I think that would be better," replied Nurse Patrick.

Patrick sat on the edge of the bed, leaning against the window waiting until the room was clear and the door was closed. Then Patrick looked Mr. R. in the eye and said in slow, clear words: "What the f . . . are you doing? These people are trying to help you. The way you are acting and talking is not who you really are. This is not the way you want to be."

Then Patrick continued, "I think you feel scared and out of control, and I know it feels scary because you are the type of person who needs to be in control. We have that in common, so I understand."

Mr. R. was taken back by Patrick's strong words, but, after a long pause, he replied, "Yes, you are right. That is how I feel. My body is not cooperating. Nothing is cooperating. I'm frightened. And my family?"

Patrick answered, "You have to entrust your wife and kids to God. God loves them even more than you do. And you need to let these people help you. Mr. R., I want you to listen to me very clearly: I think His time for you has come."

After this exchange, they agreed to call everyone back into the hospital room. The dynamics of the meeting now felt more like a partnership. Mr. R. was no longer belligerent. The anger in his face had disappeared. After asking multiple questions, he and his wife agreed that further surgery was senseless, and they opted for home hospice care. From home a few days later, Mr. R. composed an email to Patrick indicating that he was grateful for Patrick's words as they were exactly what he needed to hear. He said that he realized he needed to be humbler. He also wrote that he knew and was accepting that he was not going to get better.

Twenty-five days after that family meeting, Mr. R. died at home without readmission to the hospital. A few days before his death, Patrick spoke with Mr. R's wife on the phone. She put the phone up to Mr. R's ear and Patrick spoke a few words and closed with a familiar prayer. Though too weak to speak, Mr. R. moaned an "Amen." This was the last word that Patrick heard Mr. R. speak.[xi]

This case exemplifies several points recounted in the research covered in this chapter. Patients with strong religious values have strong inclinations of belief driving them to pursue aggressive medical treatments.[35] These beliefs are often reinforced by a surrounding faith community who pray for a cure.[2,53] Approximately half of American patients facing the end of life are influenced by these religious dynamics. This is not a small portion of the population. Mr. R. was fortunate enough to have formed a strong spiritual bond with a nurse sharing similar age, ethnicity (Irish), and concordance of beliefs. While salty language does not fall within normal professional speech (!), Nurse Patrick felt that it was exactly what the moment required during the family meeting. Because of a prior spiritual bond shared between patient and clinician, and because of the insight and courage to tell the patient that his time had come, Mr. R. died in home hospice. Spiritual care from the nurse altered the pattern of aggressive care too frequently experienced by religious patients.[47] Many agree that a less aggressive form of medical dying is far more consistent with a religiously informed good death.[3] Nurse

Patrick's spiritual intervention came just in time to facilitate spiritual peace and acceptance for Mr. R.

National Guidelines on Spiritual Care

These research findings demonstrate that spirituality and spiritual care influence important medical outcomes, including quality-of-life, patient treatment preferences, medical-decision making, medical care utilization, and costs at the end of life. These studies demonstrate that patients' spirituality and the provision of spiritual care are not peripheral to the medical experience, but rather have a cascading effect measurable within other domains of medicine. Outcome studies highlight the importance of the inclusion of spiritual care as a key component of palliative care and point to the need for a comprehensive approach to spiritual care as part of palliative care of patients.

In light of a growing body of research[54,55] and lobbying attempts,[56,57] the Joint Commission, an independent accrediting and certifying agency of healthcare organizations in the United States, includes recognition of patient spirituality as part of end-of-life care.[21] The Joint Commission requires that "the social, spiritual, and cultural variables that influence the patient's and family members' perception of grief" (PC .01.02.01) be assessed at the end of life. Current policies also mandate that prioritization of end-of-life comfort and dignity requires that staff receive education in care that addresses spiritual needs (PC .02.02.13). Standards require that hospitals accommodate a patient's right to religious and other spiritual services (RI.01.01.01). These standards have increased in specificity over the past generation but do not currently require employment of hospital chaplains.[56 [pp. 37-38]] While the Joint Commission requires assessment and accommodation of patient spirituality, there remains significant latitude on *who* engages patients' spirituality, *how* it is administered, or the degree to which those standards are measured and enforced.

The National Consensus Project for Quality Palliative Care, a task force of the National Coalition of Hospice and Palliative Care, aims to identify and disseminate clinical practice guidelines that improve the quality of palliative care in the United States.[22] Currently in its third edition, the task force has identified the spiritual, religious, and existential aspects of care as one of eight domains for quality palliative care.[22] The guidelines are based on the consensus of leading clinicians and the existing evidence base[58 [p. 386]] and include recommendations from a 2009 consensus conference on spirituality and palliative care.[59] The guidelines require that an interdisciplinary team assess and address spiritual, religious, and existential dimensions of care and indicate that spiritual care professionals be incorporated into palliative care teams. In addition, assessments ideally use standardized forms and are documented in the patient's record. Addressing religious and spiritual needs must be consistent with the patient's and family's values. Likewise, quality palliative care will facilitate religious or spiritual expressions and rituals of the patient and family.

Both the Joint Commission and the National Consensus Project for Quality Palliative Care have provided recommendations and requirements concerning the medical system's responsibility to assess, accommodate, and address patients' religion or spirituality. Guideline specificity has been clearest among key stakeholders, such as in the consensus conference on spiritual care within palliative care.[59] A recent edition of the National Consensus Project partially incorporates recommendations from the 2009 consensus conference on quality spiritual care.

In contrast, the Joint Commission's standards remain ambiguous and insufficiently define institutional compliance. Thus, it appears that as organizational authority increases, there is less willingness to provide clear regulations on patient spirituality. For example, the Joint Commission mentions spirituality or religion three times in its regulations on end-of-life care. Part of the framing of patient spirituality is under the rubric of patients' rights (RI.01.01.01). The rubric measures hospital performance according to the following standard: "To the extent possible the hospital provides care and services that accommodates the patient's and his or her family's . . . spiritual end-of-life needs" (PC .02.02.13). The phrase "to the extent possible" is a significant concession since it provides hospitals a plausible claim that it is not reasonable to achieve the standard's aim. Similarly, the term "accommodates" requires healthcare organizations to "fit in with" (Latin for *accommodore*) the spiritual wishes, requests, or needs of patients and their family members. However, the language of "accommodation" may enable institutions to become passive agents as they willingly adjust to spirituality as part of patients' rights but do not actively incorporate the spiritual dimension of illness as part of their core institutional mission.

Is there compelling evidence that an agency such as the Joint Commission should transition from conceptualizing spirituality as a patient's right that requires institutional accommodation, to mandating hospitals to prioritize illness as a spiritual event? While that evidence was weaker 15–20 years ago, there is now a growing body of empirical literature revealing important substantiation beginning at the end of life, but also including a widening scope of outcomes from hospitalization,[60] to the surgical context, the intensive care unit, psychiatry, and OBGYN.[61]

Conclusion

Given this evidence, it is reasonable to expect that today's medicine would be permeated by spirituality and religion considering patient experience of illness, outcomes data, and at least some recognition of the importance of spirituality and spiritual care in national guidelines. We should expect to find that spiritual and religious symbols, language, and faith representatives would be ubiquitous in care of the seriously ill. We might expect to find that patients' spiritual experiences were carefully considered and engaged by nurses and physicians—those on the frontlines caring for the seriously ill. Though these might be reasonable expectations, we will discover, however, that the topic of spirituality and religion rarely surfaces in the patient–clinician relationship. We examine this issue next.

Notes

i. For an extended rationale defending the reasons to pursue spirituality and health research, we recommend that readers engage Tyler VanderWeele's "Religion and health: a synthesis."[8]

ii. Part of our Harvard team consisting of Andrea (Phelps) Enzinger, MD, Tyler VanderWeele, PhD, and the co-authors developed this measure in response to the *Coping with Cancer* findings. At the time of this book's publication, the measure is undergoing psychometric testing and has been employed in a new patient database not yet available for publication and also in the National Clergy Project in End-of-Life Care. The instrument is accessible in Balboni et al. (in table 2).[5]

iii. Several helpful articles on the relationship of medicine and miracles are available in the *Southern Medical Journal* 2007;(100)12.

iv. Pargament has categorized religious coping in three forms: self-directing, deferring, and collaborative. In this taxonomy, a belief in God's sovereignty functions as the religious justification for coping by following a passive religious deferral. This is defined as "passive waiting on God to control the situation" (see Pargament et al.[37]).

v. An interesting biblical example from the Hebrew Scriptures (2 Kings 20; Isaiah 38) is King Hezekiah who was "diagnosed" by the prophet Isaiah with a terminal illness (2 Kings 20.1: "you will not recover"). His pleading with God for a divine intervention led to the Lord changing Hezekiah's prognosis: "I have heard your prayer and seen your tears; I will add fifteen years to your life" (Isaiah 38.5).

vi. Sulmasy suggests that some patients who hold the belief in a divine miracle may not equate this belief with a pursuit of aggressive medical treatments; see Sulmasy.[39] A patient can choose to enter hospice and receive divine healing in that context. More empirical evidence is needed to ascertain those factors that influence patients to interpret a hope in a divine miracle and aggressive care. It is unclear why one patient interprets a belief in miracles with a spiritual responsibility to accept aggressive therapies and another patient with the same hope chooses comfort measures only.

vii. In unpublished analysis, it was found that patients who were well supported by their religious communities cost $2,299 (p < 0.001) more than patients who reported to not be well supported by religious communities. Among ethnic minority patients and high religious coping patients, the differences were even greater [$5650, p < 0.001 and $4,403, p < 0.001, respectively].

viii. In performing a cost analysis of spiritual care, our research team followed sociologist Max Weber, who long ago recognized the significant impact that religion has on an economic system In addition, we were also sensitive to the reality that we were seemingly monetizing spiritual care. It may have the appearance of a utilitarian and instrumental view of the importance of spiritual care ("Spiritual care is important because the healthcare system will save money"). As the team leaders on this analysis, we, the authors, would reject an instrumental approach to spirituality and spiritual care precisely because spiritual care is inherently worthwhile irrespective of costs. For this reason, we presented the data in this analysis not according to what would be saved if spiritual care were present, but according to the higher costs in light of the absence of spiritual care from medical professionals. If spiritual care is conceived first and foremost as an essential element in patient-centered care, then the issue isn't about justifying the cost of spiritual care but about realizing the various costs that may follow from its absence.

ix. We first reported on this case in the *Harvard Theological Review*.[48]

x. Suggested questions for healthcare workers include (1) Do you have spiritual beliefs that help you cope with stress? (2) What importance does your faith or belief have in your life? (3) Are you part of a spiritual or religious community? (4) How would you like me, your healthcare provider, to address these issues in your healthcare? See Puchalski (2000).

xi. Upon reflecting on these encounters, Nurse Patrick recounted to us in an interview: "These are the moments when I feel God works through me as a mouth piece. I get a joy and deep sense of calling, and it is the time I feel most connected to God. My consolation as a nurse is that there is more than just this earth, and it gives me comfort and joy that I'll see Mr. R. again" (phone interview with Michael Balboni, November 2017).

References

1. Joel James Shuman, Meador Keith G. *Heal thyself: spirituality, medicine, and the distortion of Christianity.* New York: Oxford University Press; 2003.
2. T. A. Balboni, Balboni M., Enzinger A. C., Gallivan K., Paulk M. E., Wright A., Steinhauser K., VanderWeele T. J., Prigerson H. G. Provision of spiritual support to patients with advanced cancer by religious communities and associations with medical care at the end of life. *JAMA Intern Med.* 2013;173(12):1109–1117.
3. V. T. LeBaron, Cooke A., Resmini J., Garinther A., Chow V., Quinones R., Noveroske S., Baccari A., Smith P. T., Peteet J., Balboni T. A., Balboni M. J. Clergy views on a good versus a poor death: ministry to the terminally ill. *J Palliat Med.* 2015;18(12):1000–1007.
4. J. J. Sanders, Chow V., Enzinger A. C., Lam T. C., Smith P. T., Quinones R., Baccari A., Philbrick S., White-Hammond G., Peteet J., Balboni T. A., Balboni M. J. Seeking and accepting: US clergy theological and moral perspectives informing decision making at the end of life. *J Palliat Med.* 2017;20(10):1059–1067.
5. M. J. Balboni, Sullivan A., Enzinger A. C., Smith P. T., Mitchell C., Peteet J. R., Tulsky J. A., VanderWeele T., Balboni T. A. US clergy religious values and relationships to end-of-life discussions and care. *J Pain Symptom Manage.* 2017;53(6):999–1009.
6. Jeremy Sugarman, Sulmasy Daniel P. *Methods in medical ethics.* 2nd ed. Washington, DC: Georgetown University Press; 2010.
7. R. E. Lawrence, Curlin F. A. The rise of empirical research in medical ethics: a MacIntyrean critique and proposal. *J Med Philos.* 2011;36(2):206–216.
8. Tyler J. Vanderweele. Religion and health: a synthesis. In: Balboni Michael, John Peteet, eds. *Spirituality and religion within the culture of medicine.* New York: Oxford University Press; 2017:357–401.
9. John Swinton, Mowatt Harriet. *Practical theology and qualitative research.* London: SCM; 2006.
10. John Milbank. *Theology and social theory: beyond secular reason.* Cambridge, MA: Blackwell; 1990.
11. N. Scheurich. Reconsidering spirituality and medicine. *Acad Med.* 2003;78(4):356–360.
12. Richard P. Sloan. *Blind faith: the unholy alliance of religion and medicine.* 1st ed. New York: St. Martin's Press; 2006.
13. R. J. Lawrence. The witches' brew of spirituality and medicine. *Ann Behav Med.* 2002;24(1):74–76.
14. M. J. Balboni, T. A. Balboni. Medicine and spirituality in historical perspective. In: John Peteet, D'Ambra Michael, eds. *The soul of medicine: spirituality and world view in clinical practice.* Baltimore: Johns Hopkins University Press; 2011:3–22.
15. Gary B. Ferngren. *Medicine and religion: a historical introduction.* Baltimore: Johns Hopkins University Press; 2014.
16. Gary B. Ferngren. Medicine and spirituality: a historical perspective. In: Balboni Michael, John Peteet, eds. *Spirituality and religion within the culture of medicine.* New York: Oxford University Press; 2017:305–323.
17. R. P. Sloan, Bagiella E. Spirituality and medical practice: a look at the evidence. *Am Fam Physician.* 2001;63(1):33–34.
18. R. P. Sloan, Bagiella E., Powell T. Religion, spirituality, and medicine. *Lancet.* 1999;353(9153):664–667.
19. T. J. VanderWeele, Balboni T. A., Koh H. K. Health and spirituality. *JAMA.* 2017;318(6):519–520.
20. Max Weber, Baehr P. R., Wells Gordon C. *The Protestant ethic and the "spirit" of capitalism and other writings.* New York: Penguin Books; 2002.
21. Joint Commission. 3.7.0.0 ed: E-dition; 2013:PC.02.02.13.
22. NCP Clinical Practice Guidelines for Quality Palliative Care. National Consensus Project. 2013; 3rd Edition: http://ww.nationalconsensusproject.org/guideline.pdf. Accessed March 28, 2013.
23. T. Borneman, Ferrell B., Puchalski C. M. Evaluation of the FICA tool for spiritual assessment. *J Pain Symptom Manage.* 40(2):163–173.

24. C. J. Nelson, Rosenfeld B., Breitbart W., Galietta M. Spirituality, religion, and depression in the terminally ill. *Psychosomatics.* 2002;43(3):213–220.

25. M. J. Brady, Peterman A. H., Fitchett G., Mo M., Cella D. A case for including spirituality in quality of life measurement in oncology. *Psychooncology.* 1999;8(5):417–428.

26. T. A. Balboni, Vanderwerker L. C., Block S. D., Paulk M. E., Lathan C. S., Peteet J. R., Prigerson H. G. Religiousness and spiritual support among advanced cancer patients and associations with end-of-life treatment preferences and quality of life. *J Clin Oncol.* 2007;25(5):555–560.

27. T. A. Rummans, Clark M. M., Sloan J. A., Frost M. H., Bostwick J. M., Atherton P. J., Johnson M. E., Gamble G., Richardson J., Brown P., Martensen J., Miller J., Piderman K., Huschka M., Girardi J., Hanson J. Impacting quality of life for patients with advanced cancer with a structured multidisciplinary intervention: a randomized controlled trial. *J Clin Oncol.* 2006;24(4):635–642.

28. J. L. Kristeller, Rhodes M., Cripe L. D., Sheets V. Oncologist Assisted Spiritual Intervention Study (OASIS): patient acceptability and initial evidence of effects. *Int J Psychiatry Med.* 2005;35(4):329–347.

29. M. O. Delgado-Guay, Hui D., Parsons H. A., Govan K., De la Cruz M., Thorney S., Bruera E. Spirituality, religiosity, and spiritual pain in advanced cancer patients. *J Pain Symptom Manage.* 2011;41(6):986–994.

30. S. R. Alcorn, Balboni M. J., Prigerson H. G., Reynolds A., Phelps A. C., Wright A. A., Block S. D., Peteet J. R., Kachnic L. A., Balboni T. A. "If God wanted me yesterday, I wouldn't be here today": religious and spiritual themes in patients' experiences of advanced cancer. *J Palliat Med.* 2010;13(5):581–588.

31. K. E. Steinhauser, Christakis N. A., Clipp E. C., McNeilly M., McIntyre L., Tulsky J. A. Factors considered important at the end of life by patients, family, physicians, and other care providers. *JAMA.* 2000;284(19):2476–2482.

32. A. C. Phelps, Lauderdale K. E., Alcorn S., Dillinger J., Balboni M. T., Van Wert M., Vanderweele T. J., Balboni T. A. Addressing spirituality within the care of patients at the end of life: perspectives of patients with advanced cancer, oncologists, and oncology nurses. *J Clin Oncol.* 2012;30(20):2538–2544.

33. G. A. Silvestri, Knittig S., Zoller J. S., Nietert P. J. Importance of faith on medical decisions regarding cancer care. *J Clin Oncol.* 2003;21(7):1379–1382.

34. G. True, Phipps E. J., Braitman L. E., Harralson T., Harris D., Tester W. Treatment preferences and advance care planning at end of life: the role of ethnicity and spiritual coping in cancer patients. *Ann Behav Med.* 2005;30(2):174–179.

35. A. C. Phelps, Maciejewski P. K., Nilsson M., Balboni T. A., Wright A. A., Paulk M. E., Trice E., Schrag D., Peteet J. R., Block S. D., Prigerson H. G. Religious coping and use of intensive life-prolonging care near death in patients with advanced cancer. *JAMA.* 2009;301(11):1140–1147.

36. T. A. Balboni, Maciejewski P. K., Balboni M. J., et al. Racial/ethnic differences in end-of-life treatment preferences: the role of religious beliefs about care, Abstract 6529. *J Clin Oncol.* 2013;31.

37. K. I. Pargament, Koenig H. G., Perez L. M. The many methods of religious coping: development and initial validation of the RCOPE. *J Clin Psychol.* 2000;56(4):519–543.

38. C. P. Wicher, Meeker M. A. What influences African American end-of-life preferences? *J Health Care Poor Underserved.* 2012;23(1):28–58.

39. D. P. Sulmasy. Spiritual issues in the care of dying patients: ". . . it's okay between me and god." *JAMA.* 2006;296(11):1385–1392.

40. A. Hanchate, Kronman A. C., Young-Xu Y., Ash A. S., Emanuel E. Racial and ethnic differences in end-of-life costs: why do minorities cost more than whites? *Arch Intern Med.* 2009;169(5):493–501.

41. A. A. Wright, Keating N. L., Balboni T. A., Matulonis U. A., Block S. D., Prigerson H. G. Place of death: correlations with quality of life of patients with cancer and predictors of bereaved caregivers' mental health. *J Clin Oncol.* 2010;28(29):4457–4464.

42. A. A. Wright, Zhang B., Ray A., Mack J. W., Trice E., Balboni T., Mitchell S. L., Jackson V. A., Block S. D., Maciejewski P. K., Prigerson H. G. Associations between end-of-life discussions,

patient mental health, medical care near death, and caregiver bereavement adjustment. *JAMA*. 2008;300(14):1665–1673.

43. P. Rosenfeld, Dennis J., Hanen S., Henriquez E., Schwartz T. M., Correoso L., Murtaugh C. M., Fleishman A. Are there racial differences in attitudes toward hospice care? A study of hospice-eligible patients at the Visiting Nurse Service of New York. *Am J Hosp Palliat Care*. 2007;24(5):408–416.

44. K. S. Johnson, Elbert-Avila K. I., Tulsky J. A. The influence of spiritual beliefs and practices on the treatment preferences of African Americans: a review of the literature. *J Am Geriatr Soc*. 2005;53(4):711–719.

45. L. Crawley, Payne R., Bolden J., Payne T., Washington P., Williams S. Palliative and end-of-life care in the African American community. *JAMA*. 2000;284(19):2518–2521.

46. K. I. Feuille, Pargament, M., Burdzy D. The Brief RCOPE: current psychometric status of a short measure of religious coping. *Religions*. 2011;2:51–76.

47. T. A. Balboni, Paulk M. E., Balboni M. J., Phelps A. C., Loggers E. T., Wright A. A., Block S. D., Lewis E. F., Peteet J. R., Prigerson H. G. Provision of spiritual care to patients with advanced cancer: associations with medical care and quality of life near death. *J Clin Oncol*. 2010;28(3):445–452.

48. M. J. Balboni, Balboni T. A. Reintegrating care for the dying, body and soul. *Harv Theol Rev*. 2010;103(3):351–364.

49. T. Balboni, Balboni M., Paulk M. E., Phelps A., Wright A., Peteet J., Block S., Lathan C., Vanderweele T., Prigerson H. Support of cancer patients' spiritual needs and associations with medical care costs at the end of life. *Cancer*. 2011;117(23):5383–5391.

50. Max Weber. *The Protestant ethic and the spirit of capitalism*. New York: Scribner; 1976.

51. Rachel M. McCleary. *The Oxford handbook of the economics of religion*. New York: Oxford University Press; 2011.

52. C. Puchalski, Romer A. L. Taking a spiritual history allows clinicians to understand patients more fully. *J Palliat Med*. 2000;3(1):129–137.

53. M. J. Balboni, Sullivan A., Smith P. T., Zaidi D., Mitchell C., Tulsky J. A., Sulmasy D., VanderWeele T. J., Balboni T. A. The views of clergy regarding ethical controversies in care at the end of life. *J Pain Symptom Manage*. 2017;55(1):65–74.

54. J. R. Peteet, Balboni M. J. Spirituality and religion in oncology. *CA Cancer J Clin*. 2013;63(4):280–289.

55. N. M. El Nawawi, Balboni M. J., Balboni T. A. Palliative care and spiritual care: the crucial role of spiritual care in the care of patients with advanced illness. *Curr Opin Support Palliat Care*. 2012;6(2):269–274.

56. Wendy Cadge. *Paging God: religion in the halls of medicine*. Chicago/London: University of Chicago Press; 2012.

57. Bonnie Miller-McLemore. Revisiting the living human web: theological education and the role of clinical pastoral education. *J Pastoral Care Counsel*. 2008;62(1-2):3–17.

58. Mark Cobb, Puchalski Christina M., Rumbold Bruce D. *Oxford textbook of spirituality in healthcare*. Oxford: Oxford University Press; 2012.

59. C. Puchalski, Ferrell B., Virani R., Otis-Green S., Baird P., Bull J., Chochinov H., Handzo G., Nelson-Becker H., Prince-Paul M., Pugliese K., Sulmasy D. Improving the quality of spiritual care as a dimension of palliative care: the report of the Consensus Conference. *J Palliat Med*. 2009;12(10):885–904.

60. J. A. Williams, Meltzer D., Arora V., Chung G., Curlin F. A. Attention to inpatients' religious and spiritual concerns: predictors and association with patient satisfaction. *J Gen Intern Med*. 2011;26(11): 1265–1271.

61. Michael J. Balboni, Peteet John R. *Spirituality and religion within the culture of medicine: from evidence to practice*. New York: Oxford University Press; 2017.

4

The Frequency of Spiritual Care
at the End of Life

Evidence from Chapters 2 and 3 suggests that spiritual care is important for most patients and strongly correlated with a variety of medical outcomes, especially interconnected with medical decision-making. With the presence of some national guidelines requiring attention to patients' spiritual needs, an outsider might suppose that patient spirituality is a domain that receives serious attention within the medical system. However, those familiar with the practice of medicine know first-hand that this is not the case. This chapter continues to explore the empirical evidence from the Religion and Spirituality and Cancer Care (RSCC) study, but with a shift in focus from patients to the perspective of nurses and physicians. The chapter establishes that spiritual care is infrequently provided by clinicians. This chapter explores potential explanations for the considerable gap between the spiritual experience of patients on one side and contemporary medical practice on the other.

RSCC Survey

The RSCC study also included a survey of 339 nurses and physicians (60% response rate) who care for patients facing life-threatening illness located at four Boston teaching hospitals affiliated with Harvard and Boston University. Details of the survey methodology have been published previously in peer-reviewed journals, and a short account is available in the endnotes.[i]

Survey Measures

Practitioner demographic information (age, gender, race, field of oncology, and years of practice) was self-reported. Practitioners reported religiousness and spirituality using items from the validated Multidimensional Measure of Religiousness and Spirituality.[1] Also assessed were religious affiliation, religious service attendance,[1] and intrinsic religiosity.[ii,2] The Perceptions and Practices of spiritual care questionnaires were developed by an expert panel and piloted with advanced cancer patients and oncology nurses and physicians until no further survey modifications were made after three consecutive implementations. The survey included eight spiritual care examples based on the literature (e.g., taking a spiritual history, chaplaincy referrals).[3,4] In addition to these, the survey assessed patient and clinician perceptions of the appropriateness of clinicians providing eight types of spiritual care,[iii] views concerning patient–clinician prayer,[iv] perceived barriers to spiritual care,[v] and receipt of spiritual care training.[vi] Results of the study are described here and in Chapter 5 based within rigorous statistical analysis[vii] and qualitative methods.[viii]

Demographic Characteristics

Sample characteristics of the RSCC study are reported in Table 4.1. Patients, nurses, and physicians differed in multiple spiritual and religious characteristics, including spiritual tradition and self-ratings of spirituality and religiousness. Patients (47%) and nurses' (63%) denominational affiliation reflected the predominance of Roman Catholics living in the Boston metropolitan area. In contrast, the largest spiritual tradition represented among Boston physicians was Judaism (26%), followed by Roman Catholicism (24%) and Protestant groups (23%).

The study also used self-rating measures for religiousness and spirituality (Table 4.1). In general, respondents were more likely to rate themselves as moderately to very spiritual (64% of all respondents) in comparison to religious (40%). Detailed analysis highlights important differences between patients and medical professionals (Table 4.2).

Patients were the most likely to rate themselves as "moderately" or "very" religious and spiritual (53%), in contrast to nurses and physicians (38% and 32% respectively, $p < 0.001$). Nurses were the most likely to rate themselves as "moderately" or "very" spiritual and "not at all" or "slightly" religious (42%) in contrast to patients and physicians (19% and 25% respectively, $p < 0.001$). Physicians were the most likely to rate themselves as "not at all" or "slightly" religious and spiritual (39%), in contrast to patients and nurses (25% and 17% respectively, $p < 0.001$).

This pattern reveals that subgroups relate to religion and spirituality with differing perspectives. While Ammerman has argued that religion and spirituality are concepts with considerable overlap in American usage, her research suggests a three-part taxonomy in how Americans conceptualize spirituality: theistic spirituality, extratheistic spirituality, and ethical spirituality.[5]

These three spirituality types identified by Ammerman help decipher how patients, nurses, and physicians broadly position themselves within this matrix. A majority of patients interviewed make a direct link between spirituality and religion, conceptualizing both as pointing to a theistic orientation of beliefs, practices, and the mysterious experiences that occur among those open to God.[5 [p. 266]] According to this account, religious community participation makes a difference in the construction of spirituality; those connected to religious communities tend to produce and maintain theistic overtones within spirituality. Ammerman's view is supported by our data, which revealed that patients were more likely to attend religious services on a regular basis in comparison to medical professionals (Table 4.1). Consequently, there is a significant group of patients who, when they approach spirituality and spiritual care, connect these within a theistic framework interwoven with traditional religions.

Table 4.1 **Sample characteristics of advanced cancer patients, oncology nurses, and oncology physicians, N = 391**

	Patients N = 69	Nurses N = 118	Physicians N = 204	P^a
Female gender, n (%)	32 (46)	116 (98)	88 (42)	**<0.001**
Age, M (SD)	61(11.9)	46 (9.1)	41(9.8)	**<0.001**
Race/ethnicity, n (%)[b,c]				
White	57 (85)	108 (94)	154 (77)	
Black	8 (10)	2 (2)	4 (2)	
Asian, Indian, Pacific Islander	1 (1)	2 (2)	35 (17)	
Hispanic	1 (1)	1 (1)	3 (2)	
Other	1 (1)	1 (1)	5 (2)	**<0.001**
Field of Oncology, n (%)	NA			
Medical oncology		91 (77)	113 (54)	
Radiation oncology		13 (11)	46 (22)	
Surgical oncology		9 (8)	34 (16)	
Palliative Care		5 (4)	16 (8)	**<0.001**
Years in Practice, n (%)[b]	NA			
Resident or fellow		–	67 (33)	
1–5 years		24 (20)	38 (17)	
6–10 years		24 (20)	35 (17)	
11–15 years		15 (13)	23 (11)	
16–20 years		12 (10)	20 (10)	
21+ years		43 (36)	26 (12)	**<0.001**
Education, M (SD)	15 (3)	NA	NA	NA
Religiousness, n (%)[b]				
Not at all religious	13 (19)	29 (26)	62 (31)	
Slightly religious	17 (25)	33 (30)	66 (33)	
Moderately religious	25 (37)	43 (38)	54 (27)	
Very religious	13 (19)	7 (6)	17 (9)	**0.02**
Spirituality, n (%)[b]				
Not at all spiritual	5 (7)	6 (5)	30 (15)	
Slightly spiritual	14 (21)	18 (16)	57 (29)	
Moderately spiritual	24 (35)	58 (52)	75 (38)	

Table 4.1 **Continued**

	Patients N = 69	Nurses N = 118	Physicians N = 204	P[a]
Very spiritual	25 (37)	30 (27)	37 (19)	**<0.001**
Religious Service Attendance, n (%)				
<1 × per year	25 (36%)	33 (30%)	66 (33%)	
2–5 times per year	11 (16%)	28 (25%)	61 (31%)	
6–11 × per year	7 (10%)	24 (12%)	24 (12%)	
Weekly	25 (36%)	48 (24%)	48 (24%)	
Spiritual Tradition, n (%)[b]				
Catholic	32 (47)	70 (63)	47 (24)	
Protestant	22 (32)	17 (15)	45 (23)	
Jewish	5 (7)	6 (5)	51 (26)	
Muslim	1 (1)	0 (0)	2 (1)	
Hindu	0 (0)	2 (2)	11 (6)	
Buddhist	2 (3)	0 (0)	3 (2)	
No religious tradition	2 (3)	6 (5)	22 (11)	
Other	4 (6)	11 (10)	18 (9)	**<0.001**
Intrinsic Religiosity, n (%)				
Strongly disagree	–	31 (28)	51 (26)	
Somewhat disagree		11 (10)	22 (11)	
Neutral		26 (23)	45 (23)	
Somewhat agree		30 (27)	47 (24)	
Strongly agree		14 (12)	34 (17)	**0.83**

Abbreviations: NA—not assessed.

[a] *p* values based on chi-square test for categorical data. Age based on F statistic from ANOVA.

[b] Categories missing ≤5% of responses. Category percentages not adding to 100 are due to rounding.

[c] Refused to answer: 1 patient, 2 nurses, and 5 physicians.

The connection between spirituality and traditional religions among a majority of patients conditions their expectations about the substantive content of spiritual care. In other words, patients are most likely to view spirituality to be in relationship to a transcendent deity and beliefs and practices connected to that deity.

In contrast to patients, medical professional demographics suggest that they are more likely to favor nontheistic frameworks. Nurses were especially likely to report a

Table 4.2 **Comparison of spirituality and religion among patients, nurses, and physicians**

	Patients N = 69	Nurses N = 118	Physicians N = 204	p
Religious and Spiritual	53%*	38%	32%	<.001
Spiritual not Religious	19%	42%*	25%	<.001
Neither Religious nor Spiritual	25%	17%	39%*	<.001

*Largest representation within each subgroup.

spiritual but not religious identity (Table 4.2). Again using Ammerman's taxonomy, a majority of nurses appear to conceptualize spirituality in terms that are "extratheistic," defined as having a sense of something bigger than and outside one's self.[5] [p. 268] In her qualitative study, Ammerman found that two groups were especially likely to describe themselves in this way. Both the unaffiliated and Roman Catholics were comfortable using spirituality language either in exclusion of theism (the unaffiliated) or in addition to theistic spiritualities (Roman Catholics). In relation to the RSCC study, Roman Catholics comprised 63% of the nurses interviewed in Boston, and they appear to fit the description of being "conversant with the spiritual language of their traditions, but they also see spirituality in experiences beyond those traditions."[5] [p. 271] Preference for an extratheistic interpretation of spirituality may condition nurses' preferences of substantive spiritual care in terms of meaning-making and human interconnectedness rather than in reference to God. Among these nurses, spirituality was not defined in contrast to religion, but in addition to it.

The RSCC data are also compared to regional and national statistics pertaining to religious affiliation. Table 4.3 displays a comparison of physicians. In contrast to patients and nurses, physicians were most likely to be Jewish (26%) and describe themselves as neither spiritual nor religious. As we will suggest later in the chapter, it is likely that physicians as a group may lean toward what Ammerman terms an "ethical spirituality," which prioritizes human development in terms of a compassionate and virtuous person. In other words, physicians may tend to think of themselves in humanistic terms in contrast to traditionally religious concepts found among their patients or transcendent terms as seen among nurses. Differences in religious affiliation may also partially explain variations of perceived frequency of spiritual care discussed in the next section.

These differences in definition and self-identity likely hold an important role in shaping how patients and clinicians think about spiritual care. Thus, the religious and spiritual demographic makeups of the respondent subgroups are likely playing a key underlying role in the ways religion, spirituality, and spiritual care are conceptualized. We reason that these differences in belief influence the remaining data, including the frequency of spiritual care, its overall benefit, and its appropriateness.

Table 4.3 **Comparison of spiritual tradition among physicians, US population and Massachusetts population**

%	Boston Physicans[a]	US Physicians[b]	US Population[c]	Massachusetts Population[c]
Catholic	24.1	21.7	23.9	43
Protestant	26.1	38.8	51.3	28
Jewish	26.6	14.1	1.7	3
Unaffiliated	15.1	10.6	16.1	17
Hindu	5.5	5.3	0.4	0.5

[a] N = 204.

[b] Data from Curlin et al. Religious characteristics of US physicians, *JGIM*, 2005.

[c] Data from US Religious Landscape Survey.

Frequency of Spiritual Care

The RSCC survey measured perceived frequency of spiritual care using quantitative and qualitative response options (Table 4.4). Quantitative assessment of spiritual care frequency was determined by participants' reports of actual spiritual care receipt/provision experiences. After reviewing the eight examples of spiritual care, patients indicated those oncology nurses and physicians involved in their care and which practitioners provided any spiritual care during the course of their relationship. Similarly, after reviewing the spiritual care examples, nurses and physicians reported—for the last three advanced cancer patients seen in clinic—if they had provided any spiritual care at any point during each patient's care. Patients and practitioners also provided descriptive assessments of the frequency of spiritual care in advanced cancer care on a seven-point scale from "never" to "always." Practitioners were also asked: "How often do you *desire* to offer any type of spiritual care to advanced, incurable cancer patients?"

Using qualitative response options from "never" (given the value of 1.0) to "always" (given the value of 7.0) (see Figure 4.1), there were significant differences in perception of spiritual care frequency between patients and nurses (mean 1.78 versus 3.81, $p < 0.0001$) and between patients and physicians (mean 1.46 versus 3.19, $p < 0.0001$). Patients perceived the frequency of nurse-provided spiritual care to be "rarely" offered and physician-provided spiritual care to be between "never" and "rarely." In contrast, nurses indicated that, on average, they "occasionally" provided spiritual care, and physicians said they provided it "seldom."

In quantitative assessments of patient receipt of spiritual care from oncology practitioners, 12% (8 of 68) of patients indicated that they had received spiritual care from at least one nurse or physician at some point in their cancer experience. After asking patients to identify all their oncology nurses and physicians, patients were then asked to indicate whether each of their professional caregivers had offered any type of spiritual care at any point previously. Patients indicated that 13% of

Table 4.4 RSCC spiritual care frequency questions to patients, nurses, and physicians

---

Frequency of Spiritual Care Received or Provided

Patients:

In your experience with cancer, how often do your cancer DOCTORS perform ANY type of spiritual care?	Never Rarely
In your experience with cancer, how often do your cancer NURSES perform ANY type of spiritual care?	Seldom Occasionally
Nurses and Physicians:	Frequently Almost Always
How often do you offer any type of spiritual care during the course of your relationship with an advanced, incurable cancer patient?	Always
How often do you DESIRE to offer any type of spiritual care to advanced, incurable cancer patients?"	

Patients:

Who are the primary cancer DOCTORS actively involved in your cancer care right now? (indicate all that apply)	Medical oncologist Medical oncology fellow Radiation oncologist Radiation oncology Resident Other (please specify)

Which cancer DOCTORS, if any, have provided spiritual care at some time during the course of your relationship with them? (indicate all that apply)	Medical oncologist Medical oncology fellow Radiation oncologist Radiation oncology Resident Other (please specify) No doctors have provided spiritual care

---

Who are the primary cancer NURSES actively involved in your cancer care right now?	Medical oncology nurse Radiation oncology nurse Other (please specify)

Which cancer NURSES, if any, have provided spiritual care at some time during the course of your relationship with them?	Medical oncology nurse Radiation oncology nurse Other (please specify) No nurses have provided spiritual care

---

Nurses and Physicians:

Think back to the past 3 advanced, incurable cancer patients you saw. To how many of those patients have you provided ANY type of spiritual care during the course of their treatment?	None 1 patient 2 patients 3 patients

---

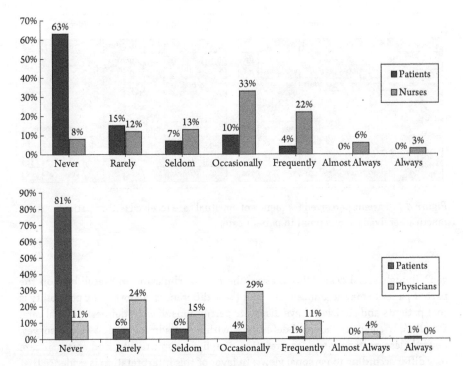

Figure 4.1 Advanced cancer patients (*N* = 68), oncology nurses (*N* = 114)*, and oncology physicians (*N* = 204) report of the frequency of receipt/provision of spiritual care. Patients, responding separately concerning nurses and physicians, were asked: "In your experience with cancer, how often do your cancer [nurses or doctors] perform ANY type of spiritual care?" Nurses and physicians were asked: "How often do you offer any type of spiritual care during the course of your relationship with an advanced, incurable cancer patient?"* Sample size reduced from 118 with four respondents with missing data.

patient–nurse relationships and 6% of patient–physician relationships included spiritual care (Figure 4.2). Patients' perceived difference in spiritual care frequency between nurses and physicians was statistically significant (*p* = 0.04).

Additionally, in assessments of spiritual care provision by clinicians, nurses reported to have provided spiritual care within 31% of their palliative care cancer patient relationships, and physicians reported to have provided spiritual care in the context of 24% of their palliative care cancer patient relationships.

These study findings corroborate other reports that spiritual care is infrequently provided by clinicians within serious illness.[6-8] Both qualitative and quantitative measures of frequency assessment yield an initial observation and conclusion regarding what may lie behind the differences in perception between patients and clinicians. The observation is that there are clear differences in how frequently spiritual care occurs as perceived by patients versus clinicians. Patients think they receive spiritual care *less frequently* than how often clinicians think they provide it. What accounts for this

Patient-nurse relationships									
no	no	no	no	no	no	no	no	no	no
no	no	no	no	no	no	no	no	no	no
no	no	no	no	no	no	no	no	no	no
no	no	no	no	no	no	no	no	no	no
no	no	no	no	no	no	no	no	no	no
no	no	no	no	no	no	no	no	no	no
no	no	no	no	no	no	no	no	no	yes
no	no	no	no	no	no	yes	yes	yes	yes
no	no	no	no	no	no	yes	yes	yes	yes
no	no	no	no	no	no	yes	yes	yes	yes

Patient-physician relationships									
no	no	no	no	no	no	no	no	no	no
no	no	no	no	no	no	no	no	no	no
no	no	no	no	no	no	no	no	no	no
no	no	no	no	no	no	no	no	no	no
no	no	no	no	no	no	no	no	no	no
no	no	no	no	no	no	no	no	no	no
no	no	no	no	no	no	no	no	no	no
no	no	no	no	no	no	no	no	no	no
no	no	no	no	no	no	no	yes	yes	yes
no	no	no	no	no	no	no	yes	yes	yes

Figure 4.2 Patient perceived frequency of spiritual care received within patient–practitioner dyads at any point in patient care.

gap? Though social desirability bias on the part of clinicians and recall bias on the part of patients may account for some of these differences, a more likely possibility is that patients and clinicians have disparate perceptions of what defines spiritual care. Despite our clear provision of definitions within the administration of the survey, nevertheless participants' interpretation of religion, spirituality, and spiritual care may differ according to personal views. In favor of this interpretation is evidence that many advanced cancer patients tend to be more religious and spiritual than clinicians (Table 4.2), consequently associating spiritual care with particular theistic beliefs, practices, and communities.[9] If religious beliefs are not discussed or traditional practices like prayer are not present, then a majority of patients do not consider "spiritual care" to have taken place. Contrastingly, clinicians conceptualized spiritual care primarily in nonreligious categories emphasizing an intentional human presence and partnership. A study of physician perspectives pertaining to spiritual care confirms this view.[10] Thus, when a clinician spends extra time listening to the deep concerns of a patient, or if there is a moment in which the clinician holds the hand of the patient, a majority of clinicians believe that these actions qualify as spiritual care.

Our initial conclusion is therefore that patients' more theistic-oriented understanding of spiritual care versus practitioners' more nonreligious, humanistic understandings may underlie differences in perceived frequency of spiritual care provision. For example, if patients view spiritual care in more religiously oriented terms than do clinicians, they would understandably view spiritual care as occurring less frequently than do clinicians who conceptualize spiritual care in extratheistic categories relating to compassionate humanistic care (e.g., human presence). Theistic-focused spiritual care is rarer, whereas humanistic or extratheistic spiritual care is more common. These different operating definitions may explain at least some of the perceived frequency differences between patients and clinicians regarding spiritual care.

Further substantiating this view, the RSCC study measured the frequency of eight spiritual care examples when patients or clinicians reported being part of a spiritual care interaction. Table 4.5 illustrates the frequency of spiritual care within

Table 4.5 **Frequency of spiritual care types, among all patient–provider relationships**

Type of Spiritual Care	Nurse Provision of Spiritual Care		Physician Provision of Spiritual Care	
	Patient-Reported[a]	Nurse-Reported[b]	Patient-Reported[a]	Physician-Reported[b]
Spiritual History	7%	3%	4%	3%
Encourage/Affirm Beliefs	10%	8%	4%	6%
Asked about Spiritual Issues	9%	5%	3%	3%
Invited Spiritual Conversation	4%	6%	4%	4%
Chaplain Referral	4%	7%	1%	5%
Asked About Spiritual Supporters	3%	5%	3%	3%
Invited/initiated joint prayer	0%	1%	0%	1%
Offer of Prayer	13%	2%	3%	2%
p^*	0.002	0.19	0.44	0.63

*All p values compare relative frequency across SC types.

[a] Percentage of patients; for example, 4% of patients reported spiritual history-taking by their physician, 7% by their nurse; N = 75 patients.

[b] Percentage of practitioner-provider relationships in which each type of spiritual care was ever performed, assessed among the last three patients with incurable cancer seen by the practitioner in clinic; hence each provider has three possible provider–patient relationships assessed: for nurses, N = 114 participants × 3 relationships = 342 total nurse–patient relationships; for physicians, N = 204 physicians × 3 relationships = 612 total physician–patient relationships.

patient–clinician relationships, demonstrating low frequencies of the eight types of spiritual care as perceived by patients, nurses, and physicians. For example, 3% of both doctors and nurses reported taking a spiritual history within all patient encounters. Similarly, patients recalled a spiritual history taking place within 7% of patient–nurse relationships and 4% of patient–physician relationships. Low chaplaincy referrals were also found in all dyadic relationships. These findings are generally consistent with the hypothesis that medical professionals interpreted "spiritual care" in generally humanistic terms and therefore perceived a higher frequency of spiritual care interactions. However, when asked specifically about theistic-oriented examples of spiritual care, perceived frequency among medical professionals aligns with patient perceptions.

Conclusion

In conclusion, the data suggest that clinicians infrequently provide spiritual care within life-threatening illness, at least within the perspective of patients' accounts. Nurses and physicians perceive spiritual care to be slightly more frequent. The gap that exists may partially be due to underlying religious demographic differences among patients, nurses, and physicians (Tables 4.2 and 4.3). Hence, while most patients experience illness as a spiritual event (Chapter 2), and there are notable medical outcomes and growing national guidelines calling for clinician spiritual care (Chapter 3), by most accounts, including nurses and physicians, it seldom occurs. Questions therefore arise regarding why clinicians neglect or avoid providing spiritual care in life-threatening illness. In the next chapter, we will begin exploring some possible hypotheses for its infrequency based within the RSCC data.

Notes

i. We first performed patient interviews in order to avoid prompting of spiritual care by the medical professional questionnaire (i.e., practitioners might be reminded to do spiritual care by filling out the survey). Oncology physicians and nurses were eligible if they cared for incurable cancer patients. Nurses and physicians were identified through information collected from departmental databases, and all practitioners were invited to participate via an email that contained a link to an online survey. Email invitations stated that the survey focused on spirituality and cancer care and highlighted that, "You do not have to be religious or spiritual to answer these questions. We want to hear from people with all points of view." Enrollment ran between October 2008 and January 2009. Practitioners were recruited from the same four Boston, Massachusetts, sites where patient interviews had been conducted: Beth Israel Deaconess Medical Center, Boston University Medical Center, Brigham and Women's Hospital, and Dana-Farber Cancer Institute.

Participants provided implied consent (given all elements of consent included in the survey) according to protocols approved by each site's human subjects committee. In order to enhance recruitment, respondents received a $10 gift card for participation. Of 537 nurses and physicians contacted, 339 responded (response rate = 63%; 59% among physicians, 72% among nurses). Eight of these practitioners did not provide care to incurable cancer patients, and nine did not finish the questionnaire, yielding 322 respondents (95% of 339, 204 physicians and 118 nurses). These response rates are similar to other higher-quality surveys of medical professionals on religion and spirituality.

All participants were provided the same definitions of religion, spirituality, and spiritual care throughout each survey. Predetermined definitions of spirituality and religion grounded the study design and were used to maximize response comparisons between patients, nurses, and physicians. Participants were given the following definitions:

Definition of Spirituality: Spirituality is a search for and/or a connection to what is divine or sacred (for example, God or a higher power).

Definition of Religion: Religion is a tradition of spiritual beliefs and practices shared by a group of people.

Definition of Spiritual Care: Spiritual care from doctors or nurses is care that supports a patient's spiritual health.

ii. Intrinsic Religiosity is the degree to which one's religiousness permeates one's daily life, including one's vocation. It was assessed based on a question from a national study of physicians[2]: "Please indicate the degree to which you agree with the following statement: My religious/spiritual beliefs influence my practice of medicine," and was measured on a 5-point scale from "strongly agree" to "strongly disagree" and within analyses dichotomized to "strongly agree/somewhat agree" versus "neutral/somewhat disagree/strongly disagree."

iii. Appropriateness of Spiritual Care. All participants rated the appropriateness of the eight spiritual care examples on a 6-point scale from "not at all" to "always appropriate." Item ratings were summed to generate an overall spiritual care appropriateness score (possible scores ranged from 6 to 48). Patients who had received spiritual care from nurses or physicians were asked, "How positive or negative was the spiritual care experience for you?" Practitioners who reported providing spiritual care to recently seen advanced cancer patients were asked, "Overall, how positively or negatively did the spiritual care experience affect your relationship with this patient?" Response options were on a 7-point scale from "very negative" to "very positive."

iv. Perceptions of Patient-Practitioner Prayer. Participants responded to two prayer scenarios—patient-initiated prayer and practitioner-initiated prayer. Participants rated (on a 6-point scale) their perceptions of the appropriateness of prayer in each setting and then provided open-ended explanations of their answers (recorded verbatim). Patients then rated how spiritually supportive patient–practitioner prayer would be for them (on a 4-point scale).

v. Barriers to Spiritual Care. Items assessing 11 spiritual care barriers were developed by an expert panel and piloted among oncology nurses and physicians. Participants were asked: "Below is a list of reasons spiritual care might not be performed even when ideally it would be performed. How significant are each of the following factors in limiting you from providing spiritual care?" Response options included "not significant," "slightly significant," "moderately significant," and "very significant." In exploratory analysis, item ratings were summed to generate an overall spiritual care barrier score (ranging between 11 and 44) measuring a cumulative effect of the 11 barriers.

vi. Spiritual Care Training. Practitioners answered "yes/no" to the following questions related to spiritual care training: (1) "Have you ever received training in providing any type of spiritual care?" and (2) "Would you desire further training in how to appropriately provide spiritual care to your patients?" Practitioners answered "yes/no" to this question as well: "Would you desire further training in how to appropriately provide spiritual care to your patients?"

vii. Chi-square tests were used to compare demographic information between patients, nurses, and physicians. Chi-square tests were also used to compare patient, nurse, and physician perceptions of the appropriateness of each spiritual care type, the importance of spiritual care, perceived spiritual care frequency, and perceived impact of spiritual care. When relevant, responses were dichotomized as "never/rarely" versus "occasionally/frequently/almost always/always." Chi-square tests using all seven categories without dichotomization gave similar results. Chi-square tests were used to compare nurse and physician responses to questions regarding spiritual care training.

Univariate (UVA) and multivariate (MVA) linear and logistic regression analyses were used to identify predictors of overall spiritual care appropriateness ratings for patients, nurses, and physicians and predictors of actual spiritual care provision for nurses and physicians. MVAs included demographic characteristics, patient Karnofsky Performance status, nurse/physician professional characteristics, religiousness/spirituality variables (religiousness, spirituality, affiliation, religious service attendance, and intrinsic religiosity), and spiritual care time and training. All reported p-values are two-sided and considered significant when $p < 0.05$. Statistical analyses were performed with R (version 2.13.1).

viii. Qualitative analysis. The analysis followed rigorous qualitative methodology— triangulated analysis, employment of multidisciplinary perspectives (medicine, chaplaincy, theology, sociology), and the use of reflexive narratives—aimed to maximize the transferability of interview data. Transcriptions were independently coded line-by-line by two researchers and were then compiled into two preliminary coding schemes. Following principles of grounded theory, a final set of themes and subcodes inductively emerged through an iterative process of constant comparison with input from researchers trained in multiple disciplinary perspectives including medicine, chaplaincy, sociology, social work, and theology. Transcripts were then recoded based on the final coding scheme by two researchers, each working independently.

The interrater reliability score was strong for the prayer data (kappa = 0.79) and global opinion responses (kappa = 0.9). Frequency of themes endorsed by patients, physicians, and nurses were compared using chi-squared or Fisher's exact test.

References

1. Fetzer Institute. *Multidimensional measurement of religiousness/spirituality for use in health research: a report of the Fetzer Institute/ National Institute on Aging Working Group.* Fetzer Institute, Kalamazoo, MI. 2003. See: http://fetzer.org/resources/multidimensional-measurement-religiousnessspirituality-use-health-research. Accessed May 7, 2018.
2. F. A. Curlin, Lantos J. D., Roach C. J., Sellergren S. A., Chin M. H. Religious characteristics of US physicians: a national survey. *J Gen Intern Med.* 2005;20(7):629–634.
3. NCP Clinical Practice Guidelines for Quality Palliative Care. National Consensus Project. 2013; 3rd Edition: http://ww.nationalconsensusproject.org/guideline.pdf. Accessed March 28, 2013.
4. B. Lo, Kates L. W., Ruston D., Arnold R. M., Cohen C. B., Puchalski C. M., Pantilat S. Z., Rabow M. W., Schreiber R. S., Tulsky J. A. Responding to requests regarding prayer and religious ceremonies by patients near the end of life and their families. *J Palliat Med.* 2003;6(3):409–415.
5. Nancy T. Ammerman. Spiritual but not religious? Beyond binary choices in the study of religion. *J Sci Study Religion.* 2013;52(2):258–278.
6. A. B. Astrow, Wexler A., Texeira K., He M. K., Sulmasy D. P. Is failure to meet spiritual needs associated with cancer patients' perceptions of quality of care and their satisfaction with care? *J Clin Oncol.* 2007;25(36):5753–5757.
7. J. W. Ehman, Ott B. B., Short T. H., Ciampa R. C., Hansen-Flaschen J. Do patients want physicians to inquire about their spiritual or religious beliefs if they become gravely ill? *Arch Intern Med.* 1999;159(15):1803–1806.
8. T. A. Balboni, Vanderwerker L. C., Block S. D., Paulk M. E., Lathan C. S., Peteet J. R., Prigerson H. G. Religiousness and spiritual support among advanced cancer patients and associations with end-of-life treatment preferences and quality of life. *J Clin Oncol.* 2007;25(5):555–560.
9. S. R. Alcorn, Balboni M. J., Prigerson H. G., Reynolds A., Phelps A. C., Wright A. A., Block S. D., Peteet J. R., Kachnic L. A., Balboni T. A. "If God wanted me yesterday, I wouldn't be here today": religious and spiritual themes in patients' experiences of advanced cancer. *J Palliat Med.* 2010;13(5):581–588.
10. T. P. Daaleman, Usher B. M., Williams S. W., Rawlings J., Hanson L. C. An exploratory study of spiritual care at the end of life. *Ann Fam Med.* 2008;6(5):406–411.

5

What Hinders Spiritual Care?

Empirical Explanations

As noted in the previous chapter, perceptions of spiritual care differ between patients and clinicians. But both patients and clinicians agree that spiritual care occurs infrequently. The Religion and Spirituality and Cancer Care (RSCC) study was designed to test six hypotheses about what factors hinder spiritual care provision, including (1) spiritual care is considered unimportant, (2) medical professionals do not desire to provide spiritual care, (3) it is considered inappropriate for medical professionals to provide spiritual care, (4) spiritual care by medical professionals negatively impacts the patient–clinician relationship, (5) medical professionals are impeded by perceived barriers, and (6) medical professionals are not adequately trained. After exploring these six hypotheses, we draw a conclusion about how the provision of spiritual care might be encouraged and enhanced in accordance with the desires of seriously ill patients.

Six Hypotheses in What Hinders Spiritual Care by Clinicians

Hypothesis One: Spiritual Care Is Considered Unimportant

Our first hypothesis was that spiritual care may be infrequent because it is considered unimportant by patients or medical professionals. The importance of spiritual care was measured using three distinct questions. First, patients rated the importance of nurses and physicians providing spiritual care on a 4-point scale from "not at all" to "very important" in response to the question, "How important is it for cancer nurses [or physicians] to consider the religious/spiritual needs of cancer patients?" Second, on 7-point Likert scales, nurses and physicians were asked, "How often do you think cancer nurses or physicians *should* include any type of spiritual care at some point during the course of care of advanced cancer patients?" Response options were on a 7-point scale from "never" to "always." Third, all participants were asked, "What if cancer doctors and nurses regularly provided spiritual care? Assume the spiritual care is done in an appropriate, sensitive way. For example, for a patient who is not religious or spiritual, the only spiritual care that might be given is the doctor or nurse asking about their religious/spiritual background. In a patient who is very religious/spiritual, the doctor or nurse might frequently provide spiritual care over the course of the relationship. How positive or negative do you think this would be for cancer patients?" Responses ranged from 1 (very negative) to 7 (very positive) on a 7-point Likert scale.

Most patients indicated that it was "moderately" to "very important" for physicians and nurses to consider patients' religious/spiritual needs as part of cancer care (58% of nurses and 62% of physicians); at least "slightly important," 86% and 87% respectively). Patients did not distinguish in importance between nurse-provided versus physician-provided spiritual care. A minority of cancer patients said that it was not at all important for nurses (13%) or physicians (14%) to consider the religious/spiritual needs of cancer patients.

Most nurses and physicians (87% and 80%) thought spiritual care should at least "occasionally" be provided during the course of care of advanced cancer patients. Nurses were more likely than physicians to indicate that spiritual care should be provided.[i]

In addition, the majority of patients (80%), physicians (72%), and nurses (85%) reported that regular provision of spiritual care by doctors or nurses would be at least slightly positive for patients (Figure 5.1). Although majorities in all three groups believed spiritual care to be positive, physician perceptions were more negative as compared to patients and nurses. Notably, a proportion of patients (18%), physicians (16%), and nurses (7%) did think that routine spiritual care would negatively impact patients. Previous receipt of spiritual care was significantly associated with a favorable patient perception of routine spiritual care ($p = 0.012$).[ii] In multivariable physician models, younger age (adjusted odds ratio [AOR], 1.06; 95% confidence interval [CI] 1.03–1.09; $p < 0.0001$) and spirituality (AOR, 5.39; 95% CI 2.89–10.08; $p < 0.0001$)

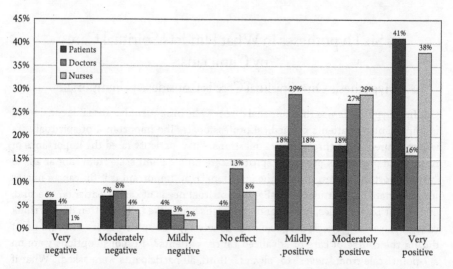

Figure 5.1 Attitudes toward spiritual care among patients with cancer, oncology nurses, and physicians. Differences between responses were tested with the Kruskal-Wallis test, yielding $p < 0.001$. There were differences between patients and nurses ($p < 0.001$) and patients and physicians ($p = 0.01$).

were associated with positive perceptions of spiritual care. No nurse characteristics were significantly associated with perceptions of spiritual care.

So, do patients and medical professionals consider spiritual care unimportant? These data suggest that a small minority of patients and medical professionals conceptualize religious and spiritual provision as unimportant, but large majorities perceive medical professional spiritual care in a positive light. This suggests that the infrequency of spiritual care is not well explained by the hypothesis that patients and clinicians dismiss spiritual care as unimportant.

Hypothesis Two: Medical Professionals Do Not Desire to Provide Spiritual Care

The RSCC study also hypothesized that the infrequency of spiritual care among medical professionals may be explained by a lack of desire to provide it. Perhaps medical professionals feel obligated to provide spiritual care based on recent palliative care guidelines but do not in fact want to comply. Hence, medical professionals were asked, "How often do you *desire* to offer any type of spiritual care during the course of your relationship with an advanced, incurable cancer patient?" Response options were on a 7-point scale from "never" to "always." A majority of Boston nurses (74%) and physicians (60%) desire to at least occasionally provide spiritual care.[iii]

Figure 5.2 compares nurses' and physicians' desire to provide spiritual care compared with the frequency that they reportedly provide it (shown in Figure 4.3). A large minority of nurses and physicians provided spiritual care less frequently than desired, whereas a small minority provided it more frequently than desired. There were significant differences between desire to provide spiritual care versus reported provision among nurses ($p < 0.001$) and physicians ($p < 0.001$).

Therefore, a large number of nurses and physicians desire to provide spiritual care more frequently than they actually do. This suggests that lack of desire in providing spiritual care is not a reason that explains its infrequent provision. A majority of clinicians desire to provide spiritual care, and a large minority want to provide spiritual care more frequently than they do in their current practice.

Hypothesis Three: It Is Inappropriate to Provide Spiritual Care

A third hypothesis that may explain the infrequency of spiritual care is that it is considered inappropriate by patients and medical professionals. In order to measure this, the RSCC study asked all participants to rate the appropriateness of the eight spiritual care examples on a 6-point scale from "not at all" to "always appropriate." The eight types of spiritual care that were assessed were those contained in National Consensus Project guidelines and other types of spiritual care reported previously in the literature.[1,2] The types of spiritual care examined ranged from the noncontroversial (e.g., asking the patient about her or his religious or spiritual background to see if it is important) to the debatable (e.g., a religious or spiritual medical professional initiating an offer to pray for the patient).[3]

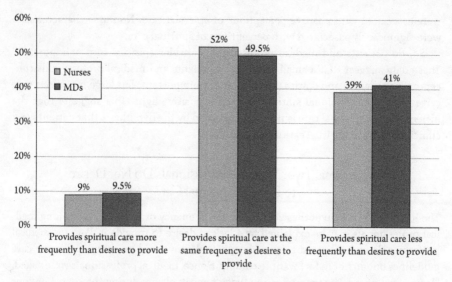

Figure 5.2 Comparison of nurses' (*N* = 113) and physicians' (*N* = 200) desire to provide spiritual care and self-reported frequency of spiritual care provision. On 7-point Likert scales, medical professionals were asked, "How often do you *desire* to offer any type of spiritual care during the course of your relationship with an advanced, incurable cancer patient?" Nurses and physicians were also asked, "How often do you offer any type of spiritual care during the course of your relationship with an advanced, incurable cancer patient?" Respondents were put in the left category when actual provision (e.g., rarely) was higher than desire (e.g., "never"); the middle category when their responses matched (e.g., "occasionally" and "occasionally"); and the right category if actual provision (e.g., "rarely") was lower than desire (e.g., "occasionally").

As Table 5.1 demonstrates, majorities of patients (62–90%), nurses (76–99%), and physicians (60–98%) rated each of the eight spiritual care examples as at least "occasionally appropriate" in the advanced cancer setting. The six spiritual care types were overwhelmingly endorsed as at least occasionally appropriate by nurses (95–99%) and physicians (91–98%). Patient endorsement of the appropriateness of the six spiritual care types were lower as compared to medical professionals but still represented significant majorities (72–90%).

Characteristics of Those Who Perceive Spiritual Care to Be Inappropriate

The study also examines the characteristics of those respondents who perceived spiritual care as less appropriate in the patient–clinician relationship. Item ratings were summed to generate an overall spiritual care appropriateness score (possible scores ranging from 6 to 48, with lower scores indicating less perceived appropriateness). Multivariate analysis assessed predictors of overall perceptions of spiritual care appropriateness at the end of life. In multivariate analysis of patient assessment of appropriateness of nurse-provided and physician-provided spiritual care, only male gender among patients significantly predicted reduced appropriateness scores ($\beta = -5.5$,

Table 5.1 Patient (N = 68), nurse (N = 114),* and physician (N = 204) perceptions of the appropriateness of the provision of spiritual care by oncology providers to advanced cancer patients

Spiritual Care Types	Appropriateness of Nurse Provision of Spiritual Care[a]			Appropriateness of Physician Provision of Spiritual Care[a]		
	Nurse-rated Appropriateness n (%)	Patient-rated Appropriateness n (%)	p[b]	Physician-rated Appropriateness n (%)	Patient-rated Appropriateness n (%)	p[b]
1. Asking about R/S background	111 (97)	55 (80)	<.001	192 (94)	57 (83)	.007
2. Encouraging spiritual activities or beliefs	113 (99)	50 (72)	<.001	198 (97)	50 (72)	<.001
3. Inviting patients to talk about R/S	113 (99)	58 (84)	<.001	189 (93)	57 (83)	.03
4. Asking how patients' R/S affects treatment decisions	108 (95)	53 (77)	.001	185 (91)	55 (80)	.05
5. Referral to a chaplain	112 (98)	62 (90)	.06	200 (98)	60 (87)	.002
6. Asking if patient wants R/S supporters in their care	113 (99)	59 (86)	.001	194 (95)	60 (87)	.09

* Sample size reduced from 118 with four respondents with missing data.
[a] Responses dichotomized to inappropriate (never/rarely appropriate) versus appropriate (occasionally/frequently/almost always/always appropriate).
[b] p values based on X^2 test.

$p = 0.03$ and $\beta = -5.0$, $p = 0.046$, respectively). In multivariate analysis assessing nurse perceptions of spiritual care, only lower intrinsic religiosity predicted reduced ratings of spiritual care appropriateness ($\beta = -3.47$, $p = 0.02$). In multivariate analysis assessing physician perceptions of spiritual care, only lower physician spirituality was significantly related to diminished ratings of spiritual care appropriateness ($\beta = -4.64$, $p = 0.001$). Despite these important variations, the larger story remains the same: the clear majority of those surveyed in the end-of-life setting feel that spiritual care by medical professionals is occasionally appropriate, and this hypothesis therefore does not explain why spiritual care is infrequent.

Is Prayer Inappropriate in the Patient–Clinician Relationship?

The most controversial type of spiritual care that the RSCC study evaluated was patient–clinician prayer. Participants responded to two prayer scenarios: patient-initiated prayer and clinician-initiated prayer. Who initiates prayer has previously been considered an important factor in determining the appropriateness of prayer in the patient–clinician relationship.[3,4] Participants rated (on a 6-point scale) their perceptions of the appropriateness of prayer in each setting. Patients also rated how spiritually supportive patient–clinician prayer would be for them (on a 4-point scale).

The majority of respondents indicated that patient-initiated prayer and clinician-initiated prayer were at least occasionally appropriate in the cancer setting. Though viewed as less frequently appropriate than patient-initiated prayer, the majority of respondents viewed clinician-initiated prayer as at least occasionally appropriate (Figure 5.3).

The RSCC findings are consistent with prior reports indicating that patient–clinician prayer is more frequently considered appropriate in end-of-life settings as compared to other settings.[1,5] But these findings stand in contrast to assertions that prayer should only be patient-initiated.[3,6] The RSCC data indicated that nurses were significantly more likely than physicians to view both forms of patient–clinician prayer as at least occasionally appropriate. When comparing participants' views of patient- versus clinician-initiated prayer, patients ($p = 0.03$), nurses ($p < 0.001$), and physicians ($p < 0.001$) more

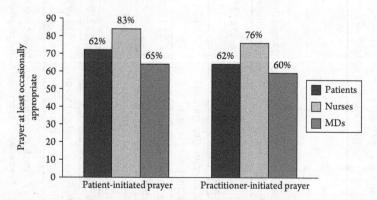

Figure 5.3 Respondents who indicated that patient–clinician prayer was at least "occasionally appropriate" according to initiation by patients and by clinicians.

frequently rated patient-initiated prayer as at least occasionally appropriate. Among patients who would potentially request prayer, most (86.0%) indicated receiving prayer in that setting as at least mildly supportive (62.8% classified it as moderately to very supportive). Most patients (80.0%) rated a clinician offering prayer as at least mildly supportive (55.7% described it as moderately to very supportive).

Analyses that predict perceptions of the role of prayer in the advanced cancer clinical setting are shown in Table 5.2. In analyses not controlling for other factors, respondents were more likely to view patient-initiated prayer and clinician-initiated

Table 5.2 **Univariable and multivariable predictors of viewing patient and clinician-initiated prayer as at least occasionally appropriate in the clinical care of advanced cancer patients, n = 379***

Patient-Initiated Prayer	OR (95% CI)	*p*	AOR (95% CI)	*p*
Respondent type				
Nurse	Ref		Ref	
Patient	0.70 (0.49–1.01)	.05	0.85 (0.37–1.96)	.75
Physician	0.36 (0.20–0.64)	<.001	0.90 (0.44–2.84)	.93
Catholic religious tradition[†]	2.67 (1.62–4.41)	<.001	1.90 (1.07–3.38)	.03
Female gender	3.13 (1.99–4.92)	<.001	2.14 (1.19–3.83)	.01
Spirituality	2.06 (1.59–2.66)	<.001	1.78 (1.28–2.47)	<.001
Religiousness	1.46 (1.15–1.86)	.002	0.99 (0.72–1.37)	.95
Clinician–Initiated Prayer	**OR (95% CI)**	*p*	**AOR (95% CI)**	*p*
Respondent type				
Nurse	Ref		Ref	
Patient	0.76 (0.55–1.05)	.10	0.63 (0.30–1.29)	.30
Physician	0.47 (0.28–0.78)	.003	0.73 (0.39–1.35)	.74
Catholic religious tradition[†]	2.75 (1.73–4.39)	<.001	2.27 (1.36–3.79)	.002
Female gender	1.67 (1.09–2.54)	.02	1.05 (0.62–1.78)	.86
Spirituality	1.40 (1.11–1.76)	.004	1.21 (0.90–1.63)	.20
Religiousness	1.35 (1.08–1.69)	.009	1.10 (0.83–1.47)	.50

Abbreviations: OR, odds ratio; AOR, adjusted odds ratio; CI, confidence interval, Ref, reference category.

*Sample reduced from 391 due to missing data.

[†]Catholic versus all others (other religious traditions and no religious tradition). Proportion viewing prayer as at least occasionally appropriate according to religious traditions: Catholics (77.9%), Protestants (54.8%), Jews (59.7%), Buddhists (57.1%), Hindus (63.6%), other religious traditions (57.6%), and no religious tradition (50.0%).

prayer as at least occasionally appropriate if they were female, more spiritual, and more religious. Perceptions of patient–clinician prayer were also influenced by religious affiliation, with Catholics being the most likely to perceive patient–clinician prayer as at least occasionally appropriate. Age, race, years of practice, and field of oncology were not predictive of perceptions of clinician-initiated prayer. In multivariable analyses, Catholic religious tradition, female gender, and increasing spirituality were significant predictors of viewing patient-initiated prayer as at least occasionally appropriate, whereas Catholic religious tradition was the only factor that remained a significant predictor of viewing clinician-initiated prayer as at least occasionally appropriate. Notably, in multivariable analyses, respondent type (patient, physician, or nurse) no longer predicted perceptions of patient–clinician prayer.

This analysis highlights variations among respondents as they conceptualize the appropriateness of engaging in patient-clinician prayer. Non-Catholics perceived prayer as less appropriate than Roman Catholics. This may be because prayer is emphasized as a central spiritual practice within the Roman Catholic tradition and is therefore perceived to be inherent and inseparable from spiritual care provision. It is not surprising that attitudes about the appropriateness of prayer are conditioned by respondents' own religious and spiritual commitments. What is surprising in this analysis is that personal faith commitments among respondents did not have a larger impact in shaping perceived appropriateness. Hence, most patients, nurses, and physicians endorsed the occasional appropriateness of even clinician-initiated prayer. What we gather from these data is that spiritual care interactions, even practices like shared prayer that are commonly viewed as highly controversial, are perceived to be far less problematic by the patients and clinicians who are involved.

Hypothesis Four: Spiritual Care Negatively Impacts the Patient–Clinician Relationship

Patients who had received spiritual care from nurses or physicians were asked, "How positive or negative was the spiritual care experience for you?" Clinicians who reported recently providing spiritual care to advanced cancer patients were asked, "Overall, how positively or negatively did the spiritual care experience affect your relationship with this patient?" Response options were on a 7-point scale from "very negative" to "very positive."

Table 5.3 shows participant assessments of the impact of spiritual care experiences. Large majorities of patients, nurses, and physicians rated their spiritual care experiences positively, and no participants indicated that spiritual care had a negative impact. However, physicians rated spiritual care experiences less positively than did patients ($p = 0.02$) and nurses ($p < 0.0001$).

This question measured patients and medical professionals who indicated when they had received or provided spiritual care within actual relationships. It is notable that no one reported a negatively interpreted experience. This does not imply, however, that spiritual care will always be a positive or neutral experience. What the RSCC study indicates is that when spiritual care is provided, it is often given in nonoffensive and constructively received ways. It suggests that clinicians are cautious in their

Table 5.3 **Patient, nurse, and physician assessment of the impact of actual spiritual care experiences as part of the patient–clinician relationship**

	Patient–Nurse Relationship[b]			Patient–Physician Relationship[b]		
	Patient Response	Nurse Response	p^a	Patient Response	Physician Response	p^a
Very Positive	67%	41%		72%	20%	
Moderately Positive	17%	29%		16%	29%	
Mildly Positive	17%	24%		8%	33%	
No Effect	0%	6%		4%	17%	
Mildly Negative	0%	0%		0%	0%	
Moderately Negative	0%	0%		0%	0%	
Very Negative	0%	0%	**0.20**	0%	0%	**0.02**

[a] Pairwise t-test *p*-values, adjustment method Holm (scaled ratings).

[b] The average appraisal scores based on a scale of 1 (very negative) to 7 (very positive) were 6.50 for patients, 5.05 for nurses, and 4.53 for physicians.

spiritual care interactions and perhaps require a high level of certainty that the care is desired and appreciated by patients. Nurses and physicians appear to accurately identify those patients who would find spiritual care offensive and avoid providing spiritual care to those patients. Thus, the measure partly disproves the original hypothesis since it shows that negative experiences of spiritual care are rare. It may still be the case, though, that medical professionals are extremely cautious because they are aware of the possibility of patient offense. If spiritual care became more frequent, we would expect to see an increase in negative assessments, but it seems unlikely that there would be a dramatic increase in negative assessments. Whatever the case, there is little evidence that negative experiences are common, and there is no evidence supporting hypothesis four that prior negative interactions have reduced the frequency of spiritual care.

Hypothesis Five: Spiritual Care Is Impeded by Perceived Barriers

We also hypothesized that there were a number of perceived barriers to the provision of spiritual care by nurses and physicians. In order to test this question, the RSCC project identified items assessing 11 spiritual care barriers developed by an expert panel and piloted among oncology nurses and physicians. Participants were asked: "Below is a list of reasons spiritual care might NOT be performed even when IDEALLY it would be performed. How significant are each of the following factors in limiting you from providing spiritual care?" Response options included "not significant," "slightly significant," "moderately significant," and "very significant."

Table 5.4 provides nurse and physician perceptions regarding barriers to providing spiritual care to advanced cancer patients. When nurse and physician responses are combined, the most frequently endorsed barriers (considered "moderately" or "very significant") included lack of time (72%), inadequate training (61%), lack of privacy (52%), and spiritual care better offered by others (50%). Nurses and physicians significantly differed as professional caregivers concerning how private space, professional roles, and power differences influenced their spiritual care provision. Many of the differences between nurses and physicians are likely created by the historical and cultural differences that developed in each profession and its resultant ethos of patient care.

Table 5.5 provides a multivariate analysis that examines the relationship of reported barriers to actual spiritual care practices by nurses and physicians for patients recently seen in clinic. In multivariate models predicting lack of spiritual care provision, significant barriers experienced by both nurses and physicians included inadequate training, a belief that spiritual care is not part of the medical professional's role, and worry that the power inequity between patient and clinician makes spiritual care inappropriate. This underscores a distinction between barriers perceived as obstacles to spiritual care but not associated with actual frequency and those barriers that do measurably limit spiritual care provision. Surprisingly, the barriers thought by most medical professionals to significantly limit spiritual care were not associated with actual provision of spiritual care. Though insufficient time and private space are widely thought to impede spiritual care, as described by RSCC participants and reported elsewhere in the literature,[7-9] these barriers were not associated with actual spiritual care frequency. This suggests that though these issues may be important to address as felt barriers for clinicians, they are not actual barriers to the provision of spiritual care.

The study also sought to measure the cumulative impact of the barriers. Thus, each nurse and physician was rated using an overall spiritual care barrier score (scores ranged from 11 to 44). Scores were based on the 11-item questionnaire and measured the cumulative effect of the 11 barriers (higher scores indicating greater perceived barriers to spiritual care). Multivariate linear regression assessed physician and nurse characteristics and their relationship to overall spiritual care barriers scores. Among nurses, only lower spirituality predicted higher ratings of spiritual care barriers. In analysis assessing physician barriers, predictors of increased perceptions of spiritual care barriers included female gender, years practiced greater than 11, non-Christian religious denomination, and lack of spiritual care training.[iv] This analysis reveals that, for some medical professionals, there is a cumulative effect by which the barriers operate in tandem, increasing their perceived impact. There are also certain professional characteristics that increase perception of those barriers. For female physicians, their increased recognition of the barriers likely means that they are more sensitive and willing to provide spiritual care, but that they encounter a number of barriers to provision of such care. Other characteristics, such as lower spirituality among nurses and longer years in practice among physicians, are indicators that personal and cultural perspectives are intertwined with perception.

Table 5.4 **Nurse (N = 112)* and physician (N=195)** perceptions of barriers in providing spiritual care to advanced cancer patients**

Rank Order[c]		Nurse Barriers[a] n (%)	Physician Barriers[a] n (%)	p[b]
#1	Not enough time	79 (71)	142 (73)	0.39
#2	Lack of private space to discuss these matters with my patients	83 (74)	76 (39)	<0.001
#3	I have not received adequate training	67 (60)	121 (62)	0.94
#4	I believe that spiritual care is better done by others on the health care team	35 (31)	120 (62)	<0.001
#5	I'm worried that patients will feel uncomfortable	50 (45)	86 (44)	0.12
#6	I feel uncomfortable engaging these issues with patients whose religious/spiritual beliefs may differ from my own	37 (33)	94 (48)	0.04
#7	I am personally uncomfortable discussing spiritual issues	37 (33)	91 (47)	0.03
#8	I do not believe it is my professional role to engage patient spirituality	26 (23)	87 (45)	<0.001
#9	I'm worried that the power inequity between patient and [nurse/doctor] makes spiritual care inappropriate	27 (24)	84 (43)	<0.001
#10	Religion/spirituality is not important to me personally	23 (21)	54 (28)	0.40
#11	I don't believe cancer patients want spiritual care from [nurses/doctors]	16 (14)	39 (20)	0.04

* Sample size reduced from 118 with six respondents with missing data.

** Sample size reduced from 204 with nine respondents with missing data.

[a] Responses dichotomized to not significant (not/slightly significant) versus significant (moderately/very significant).

[b] p values based on X^2 test.

[c] Rank order combines nurse and physician responses on most highly endorsed barriers to spiritual care.

Table 5.5 **Multivariable predictors of barriers hindering actual spiritual care provision by nurses and physicians to advanced cancer patients**[a]

	Nurses			Physicians		
	Odds Ratio[b]	95% CI	p	Odds Ratio[b]	95% CI	p
Not enough time	.73	.29 to 1.85	0.51	1.72	.82 to 3.62	0.15
Lack of private space to discuss these matters with my patients	.88	.34 to 2.25	0.79	.93	.46 to 1.91	0.85
I have not received adequate training	.25	.09 to .67	**0.006**	.49	.25 to .98	**0.04**
I believe that spiritual care is better done by others on the health care team	.31	.13 to .77	**0.01**	.68	.34 to 1.35	0.27
I'm worried that patients will feel uncomfortable	.65	.28 to 1.50	0.31	.35	.18 to .70	**0.003**
I feel uncomfortable engaging these issues with patients whose religious/spiritual beliefs may differ from my own	.20	.07 to .56	**0.002**	.51	.26 to 1.00	**0.049**
I am personally uncomfortable discussing spiritual issues.	.46	.18 to 1.12	0.09	.27	.14 to .54	**<0.001**
I do not believe it is my professional role to engage patient spirituality	.21	.07 to .61	**0.004**	.37	.18 to .75	**0.006**
I'm worried that the power inequity between patient and [nurse/physician] makes spiritual care inappropriate	.32	.12 to .85	**0.02**	.39	.20 to .76	**0.006**
Religion/spirituality is not important to me personally	.52	.17 to 1.596	0.25	1.10	.47 to 2.61	0.83
I don't believe cancer patients want spiritual care from [nurses/physicians]	.62	.20 to 1.97	0.42	.25	.11 to .61	**0.002**

[a] Provision of spiritual care defined as any versus no provision of spiritual care during the course of a nurse or physicians' relationship with the last three advanced cancer patients seen in clinic. Frequency of spiritual care provision has been previously published.[12]

[b] Multivariable analysis controlled for gender (MD only), race (white vs. non-white), years of medical practice (>11 years vs. 11+ years), religiousness ("not at all/slightly religious" vs. "moderately/very religious"), spirituality ("not at all/slightly spiritual" vs. "moderately/very spiritual"), religious tradition (Christian vs. non-Christian), and intrinsic religiosity (strong disagree-neutral vs. agree/strongly agree, and religious service attendance (>1–3× per month vs. 1–3× per month or more).

These analyses confirm our hypothesis that some perceived barriers impede spiritual care provision. As Table 5.5 reveals, there are four perceived barriers, held in common by both nurses and physicians, which were significantly correlated with reported lack of spiritual care provision. These barriers include (listed in order from most commonly endorsed): (1) inadequate training, (2) spiritual discordance in patient–clinician relationship, (3) conviction that spiritual care is not one's professional role, and (4) concern that power inequities render spiritual care inappropriate. Each of these barriers is tied to basic conceptual questions related to the relationship of medical practice and religion/spirituality.

Those who contend that medicine, religion, and spirituality should remain separate have appealed primarily to ethical arguments that religion and spirituality fall outside professional boundaries, risk patient autonomy, and require extensive training.[3,10-12] From this viewpoint, barriers limiting spiritual care are not to be overcome per se but serve as the very groundwork justifying a necessary separation. However, as evidence has accumulated to demonstrate the central relevance of patient religion and spirituality to the experience of serious illness (see Chapter 2), including being major determinants of patient quality of life and medical care at the end of life (Chapter 3), these ethical arguments for separation are being remolded as critical issues to be considered in providing patient-centered spiritual care at the end of life. This transformation is reflected in the presence of international and national spiritual care guidelines highlighting both the central relevance of spiritual care within palliative care and the necessity for a patient-centered approach to spiritual care.

What especially stands out in this list of four commonly held barriers is the professional perception of inadequate training. This was the only barrier that was endorsed by a majority of nurses and physicians (60% and 62%, respectively). It is also the clearest barrier that can be intervened upon and measured. Conceptually, it is through training that the other perceived barriers can be engaged and potentially transformed. This then raises our sixth hypothesis.

Hypothesis 6: Spiritual Care Is Infrequent Because of Inadequate Training

The RSCC study hypothesized that prior receipt of training in spiritual care would predict its actual provision. Clinicians answered "yes" or "no" to the following questions related to spiritual care training: (1) "Have you ever received training in providing any type of spiritual care?" and (2) "Would you desire further training in how to appropriately provide spiritual care to your patients?"[v]

Most nurses and physicians had never received spiritual care training (88% vs. 86%, $p = 0.83$). This finding is congruent with a national physician survey[13] but was surprisingly low for nurses given the profession's historical connection to religion[14] [p. 189-190] and the presence of spiritual care as part of nursing education guidelines. The availability of spiritual care training has increased recently for physicians,[15] but training remains largely voluntary and self-selecting.[16] In evaluating the correlation between receipt of training and actual provision of spiritual care, nurses were 72% more likely (risk ratio = 1.72, $p < 0.001$) to provide spiritual care and physicians 87%

more likely (risk ratio = 1.87, $p < 0.001$) if they had received prior training in spiritual care. This finding is a strong indication that spiritual care training plays a major role in influencing whether clinicians talk to their patients about religion and spirituality.

Is Spiritual Care Provision Driven by Training or Professional Preferences?

There are clearly other factors that might influence whether a clinician is likely to provide spiritual care. The most obvious predictors are the clinician's personal endorsement of religion and spirituality. Do nurses and physicians provide spiritual care if they have a predisposition to be sensitive to spiritual issues? And might this be a better predictor than insufficient training when it comes to the infrequency of spiritual care provision at the end of life? In order to test this possible rationale, we used univariate and multivariate linear and logistic regression analyses to identify predictors of actual spiritual care provision for nurses and physicians. Multivariable models included demographic characteristics, nurse and physician professional characteristics, religious/spiritual variables (religiousness, spirituality, affiliation, religious service attendance, and intrinsic religiosity), the barrier of lack of time (since it was the most widely endorsed reason hindering spiritual care), and receipt of spiritual care training.

Table 5.6 demonstrates that lack of spiritual care training does contribute to the lack of its provision at the end of life. In corroboration of this hypothesis, this analysis indicates that lack of spiritual care training is the strongest predictor of spiritual care provision, after accounting for other confounding variables, including the clinicians' own religion, spirituality, and other demographic characteristics. These findings suggest that training medical clinicians in spiritual care provision is a primary means of better incorporating spiritual care into end-of-life care, in keeping with national palliative care guidelines. If all versus none of the healthcare providers were given training, our results suggest that, of the spiritual care provided to patients, 34% of that provided by physicians and 36% of that provided by nurses would be attributable to spiritual care training.

Among physicians, this analysis highlights two other predictors related to spiritual care provision: gender and intrinsic religiosity. Female physicians were 66% more likely than males to have provided spiritual care to the last three terminally ill cancer patients seen in clinic. In the RSCC survey, male physicians were most likely to be Jewish (30%) and female physicians were most likely to be Catholic (50%). Males rated themselves as more religious than female physicians (45% vs. 40%), but female physicians reported much higher ratings of being spiritual (76% vs. 45%). These data point to one longer term implication of the medical profession transitioning to an equal distribution in gender. Others have shown how the feminization of medicine holds profound implications for communication within the patient–physician relationship and the increasing importance of psychosocial issues among female doctors.[17] In the RSCC study, female physicians were far more likely than males to indicate that they occasionally desire to provide spiritual care (65% vs. 46%), highlighting their proclivity to naturally shift patient care in this direction. Consequently, the spiritual predispositions of female physicians are shifting the profession toward an enhanced

Table 5.6 **Univariable and multivariable predictors of nurses and physicians providing spiritual care to advanced cancer patients[a]**

	Univariable Analyses			Multivariable Analyses[b]		
	Odds Ratio	95% CI	p	Odds Ratio	95% CI	p
Nurses						
Female			NE			NE
Non-Christian Affiliation	1.60	.44 to 5.78	0.48	2.70	.93 to 7.69	0.07
Moderately to Very Religious	1.34	.63 to 2.87	0.45	1.24	.42 to 3.69	0.69
Intrinsic Religiosity	1.47	.67 to 3.19	0.34	1.09	.43 to 2.79	0.85
Religious Service Attendance	.76	.33 to 1.73	0.51	.34	.011 to 1.10	0.07
Moderately to Very Spiritual	2.92	1.15 to 7.42	0.02	2.67	.90 to 7.95	0.08
Lack of Time	.91	.40 to 2.08	0.82	.79	.31 to 2.01	0.62
Received Spiritual Care Training	10.42	1.3 to 83.19	0.03	**11.20**	1.24 to 101	0.03
Physicians						
Female	2.86	1.59 to 5.13	0.004	**2.23**	1.09 to 4.55	0.03
Non-Christian Affiliation	.63	.36 to 1.10	0.11	.81	.39 to 1.69	0.57
Moderately to Very Religious	1.31	.73 to 2.33	0.37	.82	.32 to 2.10	0.68
Intrinsic Religiosity	4.05	2.22 to 6.98	<0.001	**3.32**	1.58 to 6.96	0.002
Religious Service Attendance	1.3	.68 to 2.49	0.43	.90	.35 to 2.35	0.83
Moderately to Very Spiritual	3.85	2.12 to 6.98	<0.001	2.25	.95 to 5.33	0.07
Lack of Time	1.62	.85 to 3.07	0.14	1.56	.74 to 3.29	0.25
Received Spiritual Care Training	5.89	2.14 to 16.22	<0.001	**7.22**	1.91 to 27.30	0.004

NE, Not Estimable.

[a] Provision of spiritual care defined as any versus no provision of spiritual care during the course of a nurse or physicians' relationship with the last three advanced cancer patients seen in clinic.

[b] Multivariable analysis performed with all variables entered simultaneously into the model.

spiritual sensitivity, and this suggests that physicians will become more aligned with patients' spiritual needs over the next generation.

Table 5.6 also accentuates that measures of intrinsic religiosity among physicians independently predict physician provision of spiritual care. Intrinsic religiosity is the extent to which religiousness permeates one's daily life, including one's vocation.[18] Intrinsic religiosity was assessed using a one-item measure tailored to the medical context based on a previous national survey of physicians[19]—"Please indicate the degree to which you agree with the following statement: My religious/spiritual beliefs influence my practice of medicine"—and was measured on a 5-point scale from "strongly agree" to "strongly disagree."

While a sizable minority of Boston physicians agreed with this statement (41%), it was endorsed by 58% of physicians nationally.[19] Physicians who self-reported agreement with the intrinsic religiosity measure were 94% more likely than those who disagreed to provide spiritual care to the last three terminally ill cancer patients seen in clinic. These findings suggest that physicians are influenced by their own spiritual worldviews. This moves in both directions, so that those who consciously foster religious faith as an influence on their medical practice provide more spiritual care, and those who do not allow such influence to take place are ostensibly less likely to provide spiritual care. Each side invites potential problems by either overemphasizing spirituality in patient care or missing it as a key factor in the patient's experience. The RSCC data (hypothesis four), however, suggest that the imposition of religion is an abnormal occurrence, whereas a neglect or an avoidance of spirituality is the norm. This then reinforces our finding that routine and mandatory spiritual care training may be required to overcome spiritual care infrequency and to achieve patient-centered religious and spiritual competence in life-threatening illness.

Predictors of Spiritual Care Training

We also sought to better understand who might desire future spiritual care training. Clinicians answered "yes/no" to this question: "Would you desire further training in how to appropriately provide spiritual care to your patients?" Most clinicians desired spiritual care training, though more nurses than physicians agreed (79% vs. 51%, $p < 0.0001$). A minority of nurses and physicians said they did not desire future training in spiritual care, with lower spirituality being the most notable predictor.[vi]

Notably, while a majority of nurses and physicians would like to receive spiritual care training, only 12% of nurses and 14% of physicians actually have prior training. In addition, these findings indicate that the desire to receive spiritual care training is influenced by personal characteristics. Nurses with lower self-reported spirituality had a fivefold reduced odds of desiring spiritual care training in comparison to more spiritual nurses. Likewise, several characteristics (lower spirituality, male gender, 11+ years in practice, and low intrinsic religiosity) predicted physician lack of desire for spiritual care training. Hence, the gap between national guidelines and current practices[20-22] will likely remain unaltered until spiritual care training becomes standardized within routine medical curricula[13,16,23] for all professional staff caring for patients in serious illness. Training in spiritual care provision would assist those nurses and physicians who desire to provide spiritual care more frequently than actual practice (Figure 5.2) by providing an educational foundation needed to overcome barriers to spiritual care.[24] Likewise, those clinicians who are predisposed to not seek spiritual care training because of personal characteristics would be better equipped to recognize patients' religious and spiritual needs as described in Chapter 2, draw upon other spiritual care providers within the medical team, and therefore employ a more patient-centered approach to care at the end of life.[25] While the Joint Commission already requires staff education concerning the unique needs, including those that relate to patient religion and spirituality, of patients at the end of life,[26] the RSCC study indicates that this training requirement is seldom fulfilled. If training were provided it would significantly increase frequency of spiritual care in life-threatening illness.

Conclusion

Based on evidence gathered from the RSCC study, this chapter has evaluated six potential hypotheses that may hinder the provision of spiritual care. After testing all six hypotheses, we concluded that a lack of spiritual care training is the strongest predictor of clinician's refusal to offer spiritual care provision after accounting for other confounding variables including religion, spirituality, and other clinician demographic characteristics. These findings suggest that training of medical clinicians in spiritual care provision is an important means of better incorporating spiritual care into serious illness, in keeping with national hospital and palliative care guidelines.[27-28]

These empirical data help clarify what medical professionals do in relation to spiritual care among seriously ill patients and help evaluate factors that explain the frequency of spiritual care by clinicians. Clearly, this is not a complete story, however. Consider, for example, that while the evidence links medical professional practice to the infrequent receipt of spiritual care training, it does not explain why there has been so little training among clinicians. Why have nurses and physicians been infrequently trained? In addition to this, even if every medical student received standardized training, there are still hidden cultural values within medicine that would likely undermine and at least partially negate the formal curriculum.[29-31] What factors and historical contingencies have created a culture that erects barriers to spiritual care?

In order to engage these questions on a deeper level, we now turn from direct empirical considerations, which provide helpful but limited perspectives, and in the next chapter explore historical and sociological evidence that further explains the separation between spirituality, religion, and medicine. This separation is now completely normalized, suggesting a deep socialization in cultural beliefs that shapes how we think about illness and its relationship to spirituality.

Notes

i. Nurse and physician responses were "never," 1%/3%; "rarely," 8%/9%"; "seldom," 4%/8%;"occasionally," 27%/37%; "frequently," 24%/23%; "almost always," 22%/15%; "always," 14%/5%. Nurses and physicians (87% and 80%, *p-value for difference* = 0.16). Nurses were more likely than physicians to indicate that spiritual care should be provided (*p* = 0.03).

ii. In multivariable patient models, increasing education (AOR, 1.26; 95% CI 1.06–1.49; *p* = 0.01), religious coping (AOR, 4.79; 95% CI 1.40–16.42; *p* = 0.01) and previous spiritual care (AOR, 14.65; 95% CI 1.51–142.23; *p* = 0.02) were significantly associated with positive perceptions of spiritual care. Other patient characteristics were unrelated to perceptions of spiritual care.

iii. In response to having a desire to provide spiritual care, nurse and physician responses included "never" (8%/11%), "rarely" (6%/11%), "seldom" (13%/16%), "occasionally" (34%/20%), "frequently" (18%/23%), "almost always" (11%/8%), and "always" (9%/3%). A majority of nurses and physicians desire to at least "occasionally" provide spiritual care when caring for patients with terminal illness (74% vs. 60%, respectively; *p* = 0.002).

iv. Among nurses, only lower spirituality predicted higher ratings of spiritual care barriers ($\hat{\beta}$ = 3.44,p = .038). In analysis assessing physician barriers, predictors of increased perceptions of spiritual care barriers included female gender ($\hat{\beta}$ = 5.56, p = .02), years practiced greater than 11 ($\hat{\beta}$ = 5.1,p = .001), non-Christian religious denomination ($\hat{\beta}$ = 3.51,p = .03), and lack of spiritual care training ($\hat{\beta}$ = 3.01,p = .04).

v. These questions are distinct from the perceived barrier of "inadequate training" (hypothesis five) because it measures perception of adequacy, whereas hypothesis six measures actual prior receipt of training.

vi. In multivariate models predicting nurse lack of desire for spiritual care training, only lower spirituality (OR = 5.00, 95% CI 1.82–12.50, *p* = 0.002) was significantly associated with lack of desire for spiritual care training. Physician predictors for lack of desire for spiritual care training include lower spirituality (OR = 3.33, 95% CI 1.82–5.88, *p* < 0.001), practicing greater than 11 years (OR = 2.00, 95% CI 1.09–3.57, *p* = 0.02), low intrinsic religiosity (OR = 1.92, 95% CI 1.09–3.45, *p* = 0.02], and male gender (OR = 3.03, 95% CI 1.67–5.56, *p* < 0.001).

References

1. C. D. MacLean, Susi B., Phifer N., Schultz L., Bynum D., Franco M., Klioze A., Monroe M., Garrett J., Cykert S. Patient preference for physician discussion and practice of spirituality. *J Gen Intern Med.* 2003;18(1):38–43.

2. NCP Clinical Practice Guidelines for Quality Palliative Care. National Consensus Project. 2009; 2nd Edition: http://ww.nationalconsensusproject.org/guideline.pdf. Accessed March 1, 2010.

3. S. G. Post, Puchalski C. M., Larson D. B. Physicians and patient spirituality: professional boundaries, competency, and ethics. *Ann Intern Med.* 2000;132(7):578–583.

4. B. Lo, Kates L. W., Ruston D., Arnold R. M., Cohen C. B., Puchalski C. M., Pantilat S. Z., Rabow M. W., Schreiber R. S., Tulsky J. A. Responding to requests regarding prayer and religious ceremonies by patients near the end of life and their families. *J Palliat Med.* 2003;6(3):409–415.

5. M. H. Monroe, Bynum D., Susi B., Phifer N., Schultz L., Franco M., MacLean C. D., Cykert S., Garrett J. Primary care physician preferences regarding spiritual behavior in medical practice. *Arch Intern Med.* 2003;163(22):2751–2756.

6. N. F. Pembroke. Appropriate spiritual care by physicians: a theological perspective. *J Relig Health.* 2008;47(4):549–559.

7. F. A. Curlin, Lawrence R. E., Odell S., Chin M. H., Lantos J. D., Koenig H. G., Meador K. G. Religion, spirituality, and medicine: psychiatrists' and other physicians' differing observations, interpretations, and clinical approaches. *Am J Psychiatry.* 2007;164(12):1825–1831.

8. S. Ronaldson, Hayes L., Aggar C., Green J., Carey M. Spirituality and spiritual caring: nurses' perspectives and practice in palliative and acute care environments. *J Clin Nurs.* 2012;21(15-16):2126–2135.

9. L. M. Ramondetta, Sun C., Surbone A., Olver I., Ripamonti C., Konishi T., Baider L., Johnson J. Surprising results regarding MASCC members' beliefs about spiritual care. *Support Care Cancer.* 2013;21(11):2991–2998.

10. R. J. Lawrence. The witches' brew of spirituality and medicine. *Ann Behav Med.* 2002;24(1):74–76.

11. R. P. Sloan, Bagiella E., Powell T. Religion, spirituality, and medicine. *Lancet.* 1999;353(9153):664–667.

12. R. P. Sloan, Bagiella E., VandeCreek L., Hover M., Casalone C., Jinpu Hirsch T., Hasan Y., Kreger R., Poulos P. Should physicians prescribe religious activities? *N Engl J Med.* 2000;342(25):1913–1916.

13. K. A. Rasinski, Kalad Y. G., Yoon J. D., Curlin F. A. An assessment of US physicians' training in religion, spirituality, and medicine. *Medical Teacher.* 2011;33(11):944–945.

14. Gary B. Ferngren. *Medicine and religion: a historical introduction.* Baltimore: Johns Hopkins University Press; 2014.

15. C. M. Puchalski, Blatt B., Kogan M., Butler A. Spirituality and health: the development of a field. *Acad Med.* 2014;89(1):10–16.

16. Marta Herschkopf Najmeh Jafari, Puchalski Christina. Religion and spirituality in medical education. In: John Peteet, Balboni Michael, eds. *Spirituality and religion within the culture of medicine.* New York: Oxford University Press; 2017:195–214.

17. Ann K. Boulis, Jacobs Jerry A. *The changing face of medicine: women doctors and the evolution of health care in America.* Ithaca, NY: ILR Press/Cornell University Press; 2008.

18. D. E. Hall, Meador K. G., Koenig H. G. Measuring religiousness in health research: review and critique. *J Relig Health.* 2008;47(2):134–163.

19. F. A. Curlin, Lantos J. D., Roach C. J., Sellergren S. A., Chin M. H. Religious characteristics of US physicians: a national survey. *J Gen Intern Med.* 2005;20(7):629–634.

20. A. B. Astrow, Wexler A., Texeira K., He M. K., Sulmasy D. P. Is failure to meet spiritual needs associated with cancer patients' perceptions of quality of care and their satisfaction with care? *J Clin Oncol.* 2007;25(36):5753–5757.

21. T. A. Balboni, Vanderwerker L. C., Block S. D., Paulk M. E., Lathan C. S., Peteet J. R., Prigerson H. G. Religiousness and spiritual support among advanced cancer patients and associations with end-of-life treatment preferences and quality of life. *J Clin Oncol.* 2007;25(5):555–560.

22. M. J. Balboni, Sullivan A., Amobi A., Phelps A. C., Gorman D. P., Zollfrank A., Peteet J. R., Prigerson H. G., Vanderweele T. J., Balboni T. A. Why is spiritual care infrequent at the end of life? Spiritual care perceptions among patients, nurses, and physicians and the role of training. *J Clin Oncol.* 2013;31(4):461–467.

23. H. G. Koenig, Hooten E. G., Lindsay-Calkins E., Meador K. G. Spirituality in medical school curricula: findings from a national survey. *Int J Psychiatry Med.* 2010;40(4):391–398.

24. A. C. Phelps, Lauderdale K. E., Alcorn S., Dillinger J., Balboni M. T., Van Wert M., Vanderweele T. J., Balboni T. A. Addressing spirituality within the care of patients at the end of life: perspectives of patients with advanced cancer, oncologists, and oncology nurses. *J Clin Oncol.* 2012;30(20):2538–2544.

25. C. Puchalski, Ferrell B., Virani R., Otis-Green S., Baird P., Bull J., Chochinov H., Handzo G., Nelson-Becker H., Prince-Paul M., Pugliese K., Sulmasy D. Improving the quality of spiritual care as a dimension of palliative care: the report of the Consensus Conference. *J Palliat Med.* 2009;12(10):885–904.

26. The Joint Commission. 3.7.0.0 ed: E-dition; 2013:PC.02.02.13.

27. World Health Organization. *Palliative care.* 2004.

28. National Consensus Project. *NCP clinical practice guidelines for quality palliative care.* 2013; Third Edition:http://ww.nationalconsensusproject.org/guideline.pdf. Accessed March 28, 2013.
29. M. J. Balboni, Bandini J., Mitchell C., Epstein-Peterson Z. D., Amobi A., Cahill J., Enzinger A. C., Peteet J., Balboni T. Religion, spirituality, and the hidden curriculum: medical student and faculty reflections. *J Pain Symptom Manage.* 2015;50(4):507–515.
30. J. Bandini, Mitchell C., Epstein-Peterson Z. D., Amobi A., Cahill J., Peteet J., Balboni T., Balboni M. J. Student and faculty reflections of the hidden curriculum. *Am J Hosp Palliat Care.* 2017;34(1):57–63.
31. F. W. Hafferty, Franks R. The hidden curriculum, ethics teaching, and the structure of medical education. *Acad Med.* 1994;69(11):861–871.

6

Social Structures Separating
Medicine and Religion

In the previous chapters, we explored empirical data (Chapters 2–5) that partially explain why spiritual care is infrequent in life-threatening illness. In this chapter, we shift to examining how the infrequency of spiritual care is caused by underlying cultural beliefs and structures. These cultural presuppositions encourage nurses and physicians to unconsciously neglect or avoid spiritual care despite their own recognition of its appropriateness and its benefits to patients as well as clinicians' own private religiosity and spirituality. This analysis is intended to clarify why separation has become the norm even though a large minority of physicians indicate that the practice of medicine is a "calling,"[1,2] that significant majorities consider spiritual care to be appropriate and beneficial, and that a majority indicate that their religion influences medical practice.[3]

When trying to understand the cultural complexities related to spirituality and religion in its relationship with medicine, it is critical to highlight how mostly unstated assumptions concerning this relationship are imposed from within a larger social construction influencing individual consciousness. Peter Berger described these unstated assumptions as "plausibility structures,"[4 [p. 45]] defined as particular social processes that legitimate socially held beliefs and practices, giving them a matter-of-fact quality. The assumption that medicine and religion should remain separate remains largely unquestioned throughout medicine, especially in academic medical schools and teaching hospitals. It is a perspective further legitimated by influential medical institutions— such as hospital structures, medical school training, and medical journals—where religion and spirituality are thought of as secondary concerns that need to be overcome as a problem by the medical team or utilized as a tool for medical goals of care. Because so many conceptualize separation as a matter of fact, the onus falls on those who challenge this model to make their case for integration.[i]

We outline three plausibility structures that help explain why the separation model dominates the practices of medicine within life-threatening illness. The basic legitimating ideas behind these structures are that (1) hospitals are domains of technology, (2) physicians are primarily scientists, and (3) thinking about our mortality can and should be avoided. We argue that these factors mutually reinforce one another and socialize patients, clinicians, and the general public toward accepting that religion and medicine are an "unholy alliance."[5]

Institutional Identity: From Care to Cure

As institutions, hospitals have undergone evolutionary changes, from focused on care to now fixated on technological cure.[ii] An examination of these changes uncovers a plausibility structure supporting the separation model. The following briefly provides a history of institutional change in hospitals in order to highlight unconscious beliefs concerning what we think hospitals are and should do.[iii]

Hospitals as Institutions of Recovery and Cure

During the Renaissance, as modern European states shifted their focus to protecting and restoring their productive members of society, the original religious shelters came under the jurisdiction of local municipalities and national governments.[iv] They now splintered into institutions with somewhat overlapping functions: hospitals, hospices, asylums, and prisons. In Catholic countries, large shelters or general hospitals warehoused a broad spectrum of individuals—the elderly, the chronically ill, lunatics, vagrants, and criminals. Many institutions were transformed into houses of rehabilitation aimed at specific populations. Members serving in the armed forces needed to be mended and returned to active duty or retired as invalids. To serve their needs, nations created networks of military and naval hospitals. Workers were herded into civilian establishments for both physical and moral recovery. Such secular goals led some institutions to hire more members of the medical profession to supplement the caregiving staff.[6] At the same time, the Protestant Reformation led to legislation that closed many monasteries and the hospital wards housed within them.[7] New hospitals emerged, but these had no direct ecclesiastical ties, relying instead on the financial support of local governments.[7,8]

By the eighteenth century, state power was even more focused on economics and science. Health became both an individual and social good and death an undesirable outcome, kept at bay through good health management and medical treatment. As part of the Enlightenment's utopian hope in the powers of science and reason to overcome the human condition,[9] hospitals came to focus on the physical recovery of diseased individuals, striving to become houses of cure that could overcome human mortality through advancing technologies.[10] While shelter, food, clothing, and moral rehabilitation still remained institutional goals, medical and surgical treatments became paramount.

As hospitals were transformed from caring facilities to primarily medicalized spaces, the cultural meaning of institutionalized death changed, prompting a redrawing of the hospital's boundaries and the displacement of the traditional hospice function. Indeed, dying patients quickly became institutional liabilities because mortality rates reflected adversely on hospital performance. High death rates threatened a hospital's reputation as a healing place and jeopardized public and private support for its upkeep. After 1750, for example, the Royal Infirmary of Edinburgh was proud to consistently boast a low 4% mortality rate among its patients. This statistical feat could be achieved by admitting only young people with acute, self-limited ailments who could recover spontaneously.[11]

Hospitals also participated in the education of medical, and later nursing, professionals and contributed decisively toward the creation of new knowledge about health and disease, especially medical theory and practice. Emphases on systematic clinical observations, treatment and experimentation with drugs, and bedside learning transformed hospitals into houses of teaching and research. Caregivers no longer acted as partners in death. People selected by academics for experimental management and teaching were segregated in teaching wards and subjected to postmortem dissections.[12] Very sick patients were often discharged well before a fatal outcome would mar the institutional record. Others left voluntarily to die at home surrounded by their family, friends, and possessions according to traditional customs.[13]

Hospitals as Institutions of Science and Technology

With advances in knowledge and technology, the early twentieth century witnessed the emergence of hospitals as houses of science and technology. During American medicine's so-called Golden Age of Medicine,[14] hospitals multiplied and expanded. They deliberately presented themselves as "houses of recovery," a status achieved by means of scientific insights and medical technology.[15] Equipped with clinical laboratories and x-ray facilities for diagnosis and treatment, hospital space was divided according to new medical specialties and equipment. Now affiliated with academic institutions, many hospitals were transformed into centers of biomedical research and training to bolster prestige.[15] In attempts to achieve social legitimacy and increase public demand, hospitals sought to drastically reduce mortality rates, shedding their remaining convalescent and dying functions by transferring chronic and terminal individuals to nursing homes and hospices. As acute, short-term facilities, hospitals even concealed death's presence through architectural designs that relegated the morgue and pathology department to the basement.[15] Management of near-death patients came to be focused almost exclusively on arresting or reversing their almost-fatal conditions with practices in harmony with the basic disease orientation of biomedicine. Despite their apparent futility, deathbed rituals in modern hospitals came to include specialized consultations and intensive care units with their aggressive employment of medications and technology, including sophisticated resuscitation techniques. By waging war on serious disease, hospitals sought doggedly to prolong life regardless of cost.[16,17]

As Risse (1986) observes, while "the early Christian shelters provided great spiritual solace but minimal physical comforts. . . . Modern hospitals, by contrast, have reversed this emphasis and now focus primarily on individual physical rehabilitation in more fragmented and depersonalized environments."[11 [p. 680]] Most hospitals in the United States no longer uphold an overtly religious mission and have decentralized the primacy of religion and spirituality within their central institutional characteristics. Most hospitals are not financed by religious groups or by philanthropists who require religious activities. Most hospitals are not overseen by clergy or religious groups who exert religious direction as administrators or trustees. Hospitals do not hire staff based on creed; in fact, many would conceptualize such a practice as discriminatory. Most hospitals no longer serve particular patient populations who adhere to particular cultural-religious perspectives. Finally, most hospitals no longer offer institution-wide spiritual rituals (e.g., morning prayer over the hospital audio system) but circumscribe religious rituals to selective spaces in order not to superimpose a religious practice on the entire institution. Thus, on an institutional level, religion and spirituality have been decentralized so that they hold no explicit role or formal purpose in the structures of "hospitals of high technology."

While there are several forces that have cemented the transformation of hospitals from places of care to places of cure, the single most dominant reason is deeply connected to economic shifts. Hospitals are part of a large, complex economic healthcare system that is one of the largest industries in the United States (employing one in ten Americans). Stevens has shown how American hospitals have been forced to be "adaptive institutions"[18 [p. xi]] in order to navigate shifting economic structures, market forces, and social healthcare policies. Their financial vulnerability has led to a large increase in the rates of outpatient services, pressure to decrease length of hospital stays, and emphasis on high-technological services in order to maximize income. Hospitals are in competition with one another for "customers," and, for those within a managed care system, they must navigate the reality that the locus of financial decision-making now resides primarily with the government and private insurers. With the establishment of Medicare and Medicaid in 1965, a profusion of government funding turned hospitals into gigantic financial and bureaucratic institutions, equipped with expensive diagnostic and therapeutic devices. The influences of government, health insurance, and pharmaceutical companies mutually reinforce one another, decisively consolidating the image of contemporary hospitals as houses of high technology.

Dimensions of medical care have been increasingly commodified in a way that influences how hospitals make institutional decisions and understand their own mission. For example, the ill are now increasingly called "customers," caregivers "health service providers," and hospitals "medical centers." This is a shift in terminology framed by business and commerce. Primary institutional decision-makers are now increasingly administrators and business executives rather than clinicians. These changes have altered the characteristics of hospitals as institutions and have decreased or eliminated once prominent spiritual institutional identities. Most hospitals are now secular, suggesting they have no overt association with a partnering religious denomination or community. Instead, hospitals increasingly "provide only what they do best: highly technical, intensive care, ranging from neonatal nurseries to near-terminal geriatric lifesaving."[19 [p. 677]]

In summary, institutional identity and hospital structures have played a critical role in making the separation of medicine and religion plausible. The current institutional ethos is one in which the presence of religion is surprising, not the norm. The emphasis on cure establishes expectations focused primarily on the physical dimensions of illness and an institution's technological prowess to heal the body. How our current institutions' primary identity and mission affect their offerings of spiritual care becomes more noticeable when put in the context of hospitals' historic approaches to religion and spirituality. A historical context also makes clear that many of these changes have occurred as unintended consequence of market and bureaucratic forces, reshaping their purpose and mission. The focus on cure now functions as an institutional plausibility structure[20] that makes cure of the body an obvious and unquestioned mission and care of the soul a questionable or disjointed activity in terms of the institutional ethos. In Chapter 7, we will return to matters of institution considered within a larger secular social structure and the effects of secularization.

Physicians as Scientists

Another plausibility structure that has socialized a separation of religion and medicine concerns the authority of physicians. According to sociologist Jonathan Imber, the initial ascendance of the medical profession during the nineteenth century was due in part to the fact that physicians were allied with and morally commissioned by Protestant clergy. Imber has argued that Protestant clergy endorsement directly led to public trust of physicians.[21 [pp. 3–21]] However, in the final years of the nineteenth century, the profession's relationship with the clergy changed. Clergy began to move away from describing a physician's calling as grounded directly in religion, replacing that with an emphasis on "humanitarianism."[21 [p. 75]] These changes occurred in a larger social context that emphasized trusting doctors mostly because of their professional competence, not their moral character.[21 [p. 78]]

The American public originally received physicians as a credible profession based on the authority of the clergy and the clergy's religious explanations, which framed the profession as one of high character and religious compatibility, but the profession gradually transitioned from a religious authorization to an internal authority based upon physicians' competencies, guild associations, and personal identities. As authority grounded in religious affiliation waned, doctors began to claim authority by presenting themselves to the American public as scientists.[22] By aligning with science, physicians in the mid-nineteenth century were able to differentiate themselves from "medical quacks" offering inferior, superstitious therapies. This association also enabled a professional monopoly over prescription privileges, eligibility for state-funded research, and reimbursements for patient care. In its contemporary form, the medical profession's scientific credentials remain its fundamental authority and justification for prestige.

The Conflict Thesis

The contemporary authority of physicians is embedded within scientific knowledge of the body and illness, along with technological expertise. Cultural authority is now constructed around a claim of technical competence to heal as well as standardization of training and evaluation that provides confident evidence to society that physicians are legitimate.[22 [pp. 17–21]] These internal claims of authority are credibly combined with externally validated and well-publicized scientific advancements that have dramatically improved health and led to the lessening of human suffering through the eradication of certain diseases.[23] Major medical advances over the past 150 years, which have been spread over a variety of subspecialties in healthcare (from anesthesia, to vaccines, to rheumatoid arthritis, to laparoscopic surgery) have demonstrated and reinforced our social confidence in physicians as authorities of diagnosis and therapy. But the tethering of the medical profession to scientific knowledge and technologically powerful therapies has led to a necessary avoidance of religious and spiritual associations.

While historians now largely reject the notion that conflict is the most appropriate lens through which to view a relationship between science and religion, warfare remains an enduring cultural metaphor.[5,v] Any large-scale association between the medical guild and religion is therefore perceived as a threat to the profession's cultural authority[24] because when the medical profession began to tether itself primarily to science, the profession took on the conflict thesis as part of its identity. Consequently, spirituality and religion are interpreted as a threat to the profession itself. It is this narrative that has become a plausibility structure in how our society conceptualizes physicians *qua* physicians.

Thus, describing medicine and religion as "the unholy alliance"[5] makes sense within a culture that believes these two domains are irreconcilable. Because the physician's guild historically staked its cultural authority on this dichotomization, notions of partnership or harmony are viewed as immediate threats to the guild's expert knowledge and its monopolistic hold over the social structures of healing. A practice of separation of medicine and religion is embedded within the fabric of a profession that transitioned from a religious to scientific narrative in grounding its cultural authority.

The Camouflaging of Death

A third contributing plausibility structure that justifies the separation of medicine and religion is the distancing of death and dying from our public awareness. Medicine has allied itself with the preservation of health and life in the United States and has both fostered and directly benefited from a cultural denial of death. Medicine creates a code of silence around death and dying based on a social upholding of philosophical immanence.[25] In contrast, many religions violate this code of silence by openly acknowledging death and orienting themselves around the goal of life after death. Religion's emphasis on life after death strikes against immanence, and thus it has been marginalized within medicine.

From Tame to Forbidden

The work of Philippe Ariés described how Western attitudes toward death dramatically shifted during the nineteenth and twentieth centuries.[2] Ariés suggested that for most of Western history, the dominant social attitude toward death was that it was "tamed" by religion, viewing death as inevitable and temporary. Such a view of death was that it was received with a sense of not only resignation, because nothing could be done about it, but a sense of trust: death was not the end, just a temporary "sleep" that led to a new beginning.[2 [pp. 101–102]] The social view of death was that it was an entity foreseen by those who were ill and prepared for through socially understood practices.[2 [p. 7]] The ill person was active in managing the personal and social impact of illness rather than being a passive agent. Death was a public event with socially prescribed rituals intended to instill acceptance and hope. Ariés also shows that death was "close"[2 [p. 14]] in that it took place at home and involved family directly caring for the dying. The body was handled by family members, and burial sites remained in proximity to family and religious communities.

In contrast, Ariés described death in the twentieth century as "shameful and forbidden."[2 (p. 85)] He claimed that current attitudes toward death are marked by a "total suppression of everything reminding us of death."[2 (p. 100)] Death avoidance as a constructed practice has its antecedents in the eighteenth century, but this attitude rapidly expanded in the twentieth century, accelerated by social structures that promoted and reinforced the camouflaging of dying and death and squelched communication about death even among the ill and elderly.[26] At the turn of the twentieth century, family members and caregivers often kept fatal conditions hidden from the patient. While such a practice is less tolerated in American medicine because of an emphasis on patient autonomy, patients themselves practice death avoidance: one study reported that 86% of chronically ill patients did not wish to talk with their physician about end-of-life issues; they said they would "rather concentrate on staying alive than talk about death."[27]

Lack of communication is therefore driven by a combination of patients, families, and clinicians, leading to a conspiracy of silence.[28] Patients and families may avoid discussion of death because of powerful emotions (e.g., anger and fear) related to a life-shortening diagnosis. Clinicians may also avoid discussions about dying because they identify primarily as healers, and discussing preparations for death admits defeat.[29] These underlying communication issues between patient and physician have socialized a widespread distancing of death that makes honest communication about it ever more difficult.

According to Ariés, several factors have led to the perception of death as taboo.[2 (pp. 85–107)] First, dying has been medicalized and institutionalized. The primary caregivers of the ill are no longer family members and local community members (including clergy) but medical professionals. This medicalization has distanced families and communities from their role in caring for the sick and has also distanced medical professionals from the role as caregivers of the sick, refocusing them on material and bodily concerns. The physical domain of illness has also dramatically shifted away from the home to institutional locations, including hospitals and nursing homes.[2] During the nineteenth century, almost all Americans died at home—only the indigent and those without relatives died in hospitals.[30 (p. 18)] The institutionalization of dying increased exponentially with the increased demand for healthcare in the 1930s and 1940s and a focus on cure rather than a peaceful death. By 1940, approximately a third of deaths took place in hospitals,[18] and institutionalized death appears to have reached its apex in the early 1990s (estimated at 78%),[13] catalyzed by both the creation of Medicare in 1965 and President Nixon's declaration of war on cancer in 1970.

Though many Americans continue to express a wish to die at home,[31] and the establishment of a Medicare hospice benefit in 1982[32] has affected the location of death away from hospitals,[33,34] the reality is that institutional death is still the norm: in 2007, 75% of all deaths took place in institutional contexts outside the home,[35 (p. 105)] including hospitals and nursing homes.[vi] The fact that most Americans still die outside the home has made dying distant and unfamiliar to the American experience. The location of death functions as a social structure that removes dying and death from our psychological awareness. We are less physically confronted with it unless we choose to go visit the dying in their isolated locations.

Second, Ariés emphasized that multiple social actions related to the deceased body have socialized the camouflaging of death. With most dying outside the home, the responsibility for handling the dead body has fallen to professionals, such as funeral directors, rather than to intimate family members. The deceased are either removed quickly from the home or never return home after dying in a hospital or nursing home. These practices make caring for the dead unfamiliar and impractical. This removal of the body into the hands of professionals has also allowed for the American practice of embalming and beautifying the dead through cosmetic enhancement, which curbs the devastating effect of death on the body and further pushes the reality of death outside our public consciousness. "She looked so good" is an odd but frequently heard statement at an American funeral.

Third, we have seen a dramatic shift in mourning practices. Historically, mourning was a lengthy and public ritual marked by the bereaved dressing in black for an extended period of time; this practice served as a public reminder of death's presence. Mourning has now become a private affair, where emotional outbursts or public displays of grief through dress are considered abnormal. Under recent definitions of mental disorders, extended grief (beyond two weeks) over the loss of a loved one could be diagnosed as depression rather than part of an understandable and socially accepted response to loss.[36] This confirms Ariés's observation that mourning is now considered a "morbid state" requiring treatment.[2 [p. 99]] This dramatic shift in mourning practices has made death nearly invisible—the emphasis seems to be on keeping death from impacting or confronting those outside the immediate circle of mourners.

This structural distancing of death, says Ariés, is finalized when the dead are cremated—a practice that gets "rid of the body" and "excludes pilgrimage"[2 [p. 91]] —or when burial grounds are moved outside cities and away from the path of everyday life. These structural changes reinforce cultural patterns that deny or maintain distance from the inconvenient truths concerning death.

The Forces Leading to Repression of Death

What explains these incredible changes in communication about death, the location of death, or the social practices of mourning, funerals, and burial location? We conjecture that there are at least three interconnected forces—psychological, epidemiological, and socio-political—that partially explain our cultural transition from tame to forbidden death.

First, a growing literature in the fields of anthropology and social psychology has provided evidence that there is a near universal human impulse that fears death and consequently represses that fear through a variety of social coping strategies.[16] In Becker's classic formulation of this perspective, he argued that modern societies produce cultural hero systems, which at their core function as psychological diversions and repressive practices that overcome human terror of "extinction without meaning."[16] [p.67] Religion can fulfill this function by providing transcendent meaning in response to death, therefore increasing social cohesion by managing fears that would create greater social chaos and increase death.[37] While Durkheim's claim that basic human fear produces religion goes well beyond the empirical evidence for causation,[38] there is strong suggestive evidence that cultures construct coping responses to death in order to create structural stability and daily normalcy.[4]

But with the rise of a secular age,[25] religion's influence on socially constructed meaning-making in response to our fear of death has waned. What takes the place of religion in managing death anxiety in our contemporary culture of immanence? Part of the new cultural strategy that arises in the absence of religion and transcendent meaning-making is partial death denial. According to Hayslip,[39 [p. 36]] death denial manifests itself in multiple intrapsychic and interpersonal forms, including "selective attention (purposeful ignorance or avoidance of death stimuli), selective responding (hiding one's feelings from others), compartmentalizing (allowing incongruences, such as understanding a terminal diagnosis and making long-term plans), purposeful deception (lying), and resistance (not giving up or giving in to death)."[39 [p. 36]] These individual and cultural strategies provide a psychological lens for explaining Ariés's observation of the cultural shift from a tame to forbidden death. This provides a rationale on why death has been removed from the home toward institutions, why public mourning is no longer acceptable, and why cemeteries are now out of sight.

Second, an epidemiological shift has occurred, with mortality rates falling dramatically in the United States since the end of the Civil War. Demographers generally believe that mortality rates began to fall in the latter part of the nineteenth century as a result of improved standards of living.[40 [p. 189]] The twentieth century then saw a dramatic decrease in death rates; in 1900, the crude death rate was estimated at 1,719 deaths per 100,000 people, and in 2000 it was 874 deaths per 100,000.[40 [p. 190]] During the same period, life expectancy increased from 47.3 years (in 1900) to 76.9 years (in 2000). These changes have buttressed a cultural shift away from recognizing death for the simple reason that it is less frequently encountered within our lifespan, and we have the impression that our own death is far off. As we encounter the fact of death less, a psychological confrontation with death becomes an exception rather than the rule. The result of these falling mortality rates may be a reduction in the felt importance of religion and its functional purpose in a society.[41] The palpable rise of our social health simultaneously reduces the need for religion in explaining death and justifies a collective repression of death.

Interconnected with these previous two points, a third factor that explains a cultural shift toward death is the rise of existential security grounded upon sociopolitical dynamics prevalent in modern societies. Modernization includes cultural processes of industrialization, rising levels of wealth and education, urbanization, and the proliferation of technology. Democratic societies provide imperfect but increased demographic equality (e.g., gender, race, etc.), stable governmental systems, greater systems of justice through the courts and policing, and cultural processes that peacefully adjudicate social differences without turning to civil war. Within this matrix of sociopolitical dynamics, rates of existential security within a culture rise dramatically.[42] An increased sense of existential security comes from having fewer perceived and objective threats to one's livelihood, decreased anxiety of external threats such as poverty or war, and an increased sense of hope in human development and the potential for success.

These sociopolitical factors also play a critical role in people's felt need for religion. As Norris and Inglehart (2011) have shown based on data from the World Values Survey, cultures under greater threats of poverty and war are far more likely to turn toward religion, whereas increasing existential security appears to diminish religious practices and religious coping. We hypothesize that levels of existential security from sociopolitical and cultural dynamics are similarly related to that culture's recognition of and engagement with dying and death. Social and political stability together with human flourishing provide cultures with an aura of invincibility and diminish the need to contemplate religion. Thus, existential security may cause a decline in religious coping, strengthen a culture's upholding of immanent structures and attitudes,[25] and further justify a cultural repression of public acknowledgment of our human frailty and mortality.

Medicine's Role in Repressing Death

Within these larger dynamics that have yielded a cultural denial of death,[16] the medical field has perhaps been exploited by society—but willingly so—in justifying and accelerating a cultural repression of death. This mutually beneficial relationship is grounded in two deeply held convictions embedded within medicine's own identity: (1) the obligation to restore health and resist death and (2) a well-grounded optimism regarding constant scientific advancement.

Restore Health and Prolong Life

The first conviction is that medicine is under a moral imperative to restore human health and utilize its therapeutic powers to counter death. Within the Hippocratic tradition, physicians historically held an uncompromising "respect for life," refusing to offer therapeutic abortion or euthanasia.[43 (p. 41)] However, a physician also was required to recognize the limits of medicine by not offering therapies for patients who were "overmastered by their diseases."[43 (p. 34)] Eminent historian Darrel Amundsen suggested that these attitudes began to shift in the late Middle Ages when religious ethicists began to emphasize the moral imperative that patients be given medical therapy against their will as a duty of love.[43 (p. 44)] This shift was cemented in the seventeenth century by Francis Bacon, who argued that medicine's explicit aim is to prolong life. Bacon argued that the aim of prolongation of life was "the most noble of all" medicine's purposes since it most fervently demonstrated the physician's act of nonabandonment of the patient in their suffering.[43 (p. 41)] Bacon chided physicians for failing to treat incurable diseases; he believed that the employment of medical powers in all cases would either advance medical knowledge, thus making an incurable disease curable, or, at a minimum, soften the harshness of dying through palliative strategies.[43 (pp. 41–42)]

Before the advancement of modern medicine, death was seen as a biological evil, but one outside of human control.[44 (p. 59)] But with the growth of medical powers, opposition to disease and death took on a moral obligation: "what can be done ought to be done."[44 (p. 61)] With the growth of modern technological medicine, physicians finally had the tools to push back death in many circumstances.

Scientific Optimism

Medicine's optimism in scientific advancement—a deeply held belief that the medical sciences are constantly improving and that they are always on the verge of a major advancement in the war against disease and dying—grew out of an Enlightenment esteem for science, and this optimism has powerfully motivated the medical community to consider "no illness incurable."[10] Medicine's self-confidence in overcoming illness is grounded on an unquestioning commitment to the scientific method, its incredible *vitae* of modern successes in following this method, and, perhaps more subtly, its social and financial esteem within our culture.

The medical field and the general public have strong reasons for this optimistic belief in medical advancement: Scientific medicine and public health have made dramatic advances that have greatly benefited mankind,[23] from the eradication of polio, to the cure of childhood leukemia, to the efficacy of vaccines and penicillin, to the development of technological advances in surgery and medicine such as anesthesia, chemotherapy, and radiologic imaging. Many of these advances took place between 1860 to 1960, "the Golden Age of Medicine."[45] With these advances, healthcare's social and economic power in the United States grew enormously. But as the medical field embraced its growing reputation to cure and bring health, it had to distance itself from dying and death institutionally[13] and professionally.[21] Because medicine has been rewarded socially and financially for its efforts to restore health and prolong life, it is highly motivated to maintain this reputation by lowering mortality rates in hospitalization[15] and utilizing its growing arsenal of technological abilities in treating life-threatening illness with a hope of prolonging life.

Coping Strategies Leading to Death Denial

These convictions—the moral imperative to restore health and the optimism that any disease can be overcome through the diligence of science—must be framed within the larger cultural dynamics of death anxiety. Surely Lavi is accurate in arguing that physicians are not self-conscious agents of a social repression of death[46 [pp. 55–56]]—physicians have always been motivated to provide patients hope since hope stimulates action whereas despondency creates inaction[46 [p. 57]]—but multiple prior[26,47] and recent studies[48] have suggested that medical professionals repress their own thoughts concerning death. As medical trainees encounter suffering and dying, they may be socialized early on in their training to protect themselves from difficult and powerful emotions using repression or compartmentalization as coping schemes.[48,49] Repression ignores and blocks internal emotions from arising as a response to the pain and suffering experienced by those who are dying. Compartmentalization is a coping strategy where self-states are kept separate, enabling medical caregivers to objectify a patient as a body and not engage the patient as a person. After the medical professional leaves the medical setting, he or she switches back to engaging others as persons. Clinicians hold a series of "masks" that act as shields between themselves and their dying patients.[49 [pp. 451–452]] As coping strategies, these approaches may enable individual clinicians to successfully navigate pain and suffering.

Beyond the individual, the medical profession's optimism that it can conquer illness and its commitment to restore health may also function as a collective coping strategy in which the reality of dying is subconsciously repressed. Patients who are dying serve as a powerful embodiment of medicine's limitations: "The dying represent a category of identity that is strongly at variance with the purposes of the institution and are therefore most likely to be confronted by both aversive reactions and negative moral meanings.[49 [p. 455]] As a hypothesis, medicine's collective repression of death is difficult to fully measure empirically,[vii] but it has been a popular view for more than a century; for example, it is a key theme in the novel *The Death of Ivan Ilyich*.[50]

When medicine does engage with death, the impulse is often to do so through active technological interventions. While this social activity has been credibly self-interpreted as motivated by compassion and a track record of overcoming illness, there remains a notable unwillingness to acknowledge the inherent limits of medicine.[51,52] One Harvard medical historian remarking on the implicit values of medicine said, "Most of us harbor a pervasive faith in the world of scientific medicine, a visceral and inarticulate hope of a temporal salvation: modern medicine will extend life, avoid pain, provide a gentle death."[53 [p. 191]] What is the source for this "visceral and inarticulate hope" that leads many to feel that medicine has or may soon gain a "power to banish mortality"?[44 [p. 59]] It is this unswerving hope in medicine, both structured in the cultural imagination and socialized among medical professionals, that substantiates the hypothesis that technological intervention is a cultural manifestation of a social psychological repression of dying. As long as medicine is acting against the dying process, it need not acknowledge the obvious reality of our shared mortality or of the unambiguous but unacknowledged dying process actively taking place before nurses and physicians.

The Implausibility of Medicine and Religion

What do these three plausibility structures have to do with medicine and religion? These three plausibility structures partially illuminate why contemporary medicine and spirituality have been separated and why change is exceptionally difficult. These social structures are unstated cultural assumptions that legitimate socially held beliefs and practices, socializing patients and medical professionals to keep medicine and spirituality discrete. Each plausibility structure interpenetrates and reinforces one another, giving the cultural sense that medicine and religion should be separated its matter-of-factness.[5] The first plausibility structure is the now-accepted belief that hospitals are spaces set apart for advanced technological interventions—places for cure, not care.[19] The second is that physicians, as the leaders of the healthcare team, are scientists whose social authority to act and intervene for our health is grounded primarily in the scientific method.[21] Finally, there is a cultural repression of dying that is in tension with religious sensibilities. The ethos within medicine striving to restore health and extend life is incongruent with the message of the world's religions, which fundamentally acknowledge human mortality. To the degree that medicine is collectively controlled by ambitions to forestall death, it is at best ambivalent toward social understandings that highlight either the limitations of medicine or the unavoidability of our own dying.

If we are correct in our argument that our culture at large and medicine in particular are largely controlled by and perpetuate psychological processes that camouflage and repress death, what does this have to do with social structures separating medicine and religion? All the major world religions *de facto* reject repression as a constructive coping strategy in the face of death.[54] While world religions obviously differ in many crucial particulars concerning issues of illness, dying, and death, they all uphold the importance of acknowledging our mortality. They all order spiritual realities over the material and encourage letting go of this life as our health wanes. A collective repression of dying, as expressed in contemporary American culture, grinds against the fundamental questions that each major traditional religious belief system attempts to answer. Human mortality serves as the fertile soil upon which religious engagement begins to take on greater meaning. Rather than repress death, traditional religions acknowledge this reality and build upon it as a crucial truth.

Repression of dying and death, woven into American culture, adopted as the *sine quo non* of modern medicine's twentieth-century project, is therefore in inevitable tension with religion. In our culture's imagination, it is only when the doctor's arsenal runs out, there is no hope for cure, and death seems imminent that medicine can create a socially acceptable space for religion.[55] In the cultural imagination, the medical profession represents life, whereas palliative care and, even more so, clergy represent death. From this vantage point, medicine's project of restoring health and prolonging life, especially to the degree that it serves as a collective system of repressing death anxiety, would be substantially undermined if religious voices were more extensively present in shaping medicine's cultural purpose. Thus, religion has been minimized within medicine's own social structures, further enabling the camouflaging of death. Hospitals and physicians are places of knowledge, hope, science, and greater human life. Religion brings a counternarrative that does not fit and is unwanted.

This is especially important as it pertains to explaining how spiritual care can be so infrequently provided by medical professionals despite their own individual beliefs to the contrary. While contemporary medicine asserts that it socializes its medical trainees to avoid spiritual care because they lack the necessary expertise to engage in religious dialogue,[56] we are suggesting that a more subtle or unconscious reason is because it would undermine our "visceral and inarticulate hope of a temporal salvation"[53 [p. 191]] represented by medicine's most visible healers—our doctors and nurses. If clinicians begin talking about traditional spirituality during illness, then our unquestioned faith in medicine's ability to extend life will be critically and permanently destabilized. The plausibility structure of medicine that denies death requires the absence of traditional religious logic, which is far too prone to start with an acknowledgment of our inherent insecurity, weakness, and undeniable mortality.

These plausibility structures help partly describe why medicine has been uneasy with traditional spirituality and religion. It clarifies why many prefer a typology of separation.[5] These plausibility structures therefore help explain why spiritual care remains infrequent even in life-threatening illness. Yet there is more to the story then we have described in the chapter because the plausibility structures that advocate for separation run deep down into the way we conceptualize human nature, knowledge, and society at large. Chapter 7 describes dualisms that further enable separation between medicine and religion.

Notes

i. The plausibility of separation is socially constructed and maintained by both what is stated as well as what remains unstated. Consider, for example, that the only article the *New England Journal of Medicine*, academic medicine's most influential and highest impact journal, has ever published on this issue is an opinion piece by RP Sloan et al. ("Should physicians prescribe religious activities?" N Engl J Med. 2000;342(25):1913–1916) that argues for strict separation. The fact that the *New England Journal* has never published an original research article investigating religion and spirituality may illustrate and legitimate a separation model. Is it that no studies have been of the necessary quality to be published by them? Or do the underlying plausibility structures provide an aura of obviousness and facticity to the separation of religion and medicine that influences editorial choices about publishing empirical research regarding the intersection of medicine and religion? The *NEJM* did publish several letters to the editor that argued against the separation model put forward by Sloan. However, there remains a significant advantage given to a perspective piece in the amount of space allotted to make an argument and the specific location of the article within the print version. Authors are also given the opportunity to reply to the letters written to the editor. It is hard to make a compelling argument that there was an attempt to be fair in weighing different opinions on these issues.

ii. As a historian, Risse warns that the generalizations that he offers in his concluding chapter easily overgeneralize the complexity of every individual hospital. Risse offers case studies that point to general shifts that may or may not specifically apply to any one case (see G. B. Risse.)[19]

iii. Portions of this section were published previously in G. B. Risse and M. J. Balboni.[13]

iv. Much of this story is told in G. B. Risse.[19] Our brief account of hospitals is indebted to his mageristerial volume, and we point readers to this book for a far more detailed acccount.

v. Historian Colin Russell argued that maintaining a metaphor of war between these domains is a socially constructed myth, an oversimplification, and at times "a deception."[24 [p.10]] He suggested that it has been aimed to "enhance the public appreciation of science" (p. 10) and simultaneously minimize religious influence from exerting itself within scientific endeavors.

vi. The hospice and palliative care movements in the United States, which slowly began in the 1970s, reflect both financial concerns from overutilization of medicine and technology and a frustration toward institutions that have provided poor-quality care to terminally ill patients (see KE Clemens, Jaspers B, and Klaschik E. The history of hospice. In: D. Walsh, ed. *Palliative medicine*. Philadelphia: Saunders; 2009:18–23). The establishment of a Medicare hospice benefit in 1982[32] appears to have begun a shift of location of death away from hospitals (see also S.Weitzen et al.[33]) and J. Flory et al.[34] While most Americans express a wish to die at home (see E. Bruera et al.[31]), it has been primarily since the establishment of the hospice benefit that the location of death has begun to shift away from hospitals. By 2009, 42% of all US deaths occurred at home or in nursing facilities while enrolled in hospice (see NHPCO Facts and Figures: Hospice Care in America. 2010. http://www.nhpco.org/files/public/Statistics_Research/Hospice_Facts_Figures_Oct-2010.pdf. Accessed January 5, 2012). The average days of hospice use among Medicare patients has increased from 12.4 days in 2003 to 18.3 days in 2007 (see D. Goodman, Esty A., Fisher E. S., CH C. Trends and variation in end-of-life care for Medicare beneficiaries with severe chronic illness. *A Report of the Dartmouth Atlas Project*. 2011. http://www.dartmouthatlas.org/downloads/reports/EOL_Trend_Report_0411.pdf. Accessed January 5, 2012).

This same report also shows a decline in the number of in-hospital deaths among Medicare beneficiaries from 32% of all Medicare deaths in 2003 to 28% in 2007.

Corresponding with these changes, palliative care programs have significantly increased within the past decade so much so that 63% of all US hospitals now have a palliative care program (including 85% of 300+ bed hospitals) (see S. Lutz[32]; D. E. Meier. Increased access to palliative care and hospice services: opportunities to improve value in health care. *Milbank Q*. 2011;89(3):343–380, 45; and R. S. Morrison, Augustin R., Souvanna P., DE M. America's care of serious illness: a state-by-state report card on access to palliative care in our nation's hospitals. *J Palliative Med*. 2011;14(10):1094–1096).

While palliative care grew out of hospice in the United States, palliative care proponents argue that they are not synonymous (Meier, 2011). Palliative care can be provided concurrently with a therapeutic aim of cure throughout the disease process, whereas the hospice benefit requires patients to forego curative treatments, limited to the last six months of life (Meier, 2011).[32] Consequently, the growth of palliative care, rather than functioning primarily as a separate, parallel system from traditional medical institutions—has blossomed as a new medical discipline within hospitals focused on the relief of suffering, management of symptoms, attention to patient communication and decision-making, and multidisciplinary psycho-social-spiritual support of patients and families at any stage of illness (see J. Hauser, Sileo M., Araneta N., et al. Navigation and palliative care. *Cancer*. 2011;117(15 Suppl):3585–3591, 47; and F. D. Ferris, Bruera E., Cherny N., et al. Palliative cancer care a decade later: accomplishments, the need, next steps—from the American Society of Clinical Oncology. *J Clin Oncol*. 2009;27(18):3052–3058). Palliative care includes general competencies for all professional caregivers as well as a growing medical specialty requiring certification. The underlying aim of palliative care is to systematically reintroduce the human dimensions of compassion and benevolence for the support of the sick and dying.

Most recent data may indicate that the rise of the hospice benefit has begun to reshape how the United States as a nation faces death—with location of death serving as an important marker. Future growth of hospice utilization may point to a critical epidemiological shift away from hospitals as the place where Americans die. What affect that this external change might have on hospitals remains to be seen. Simultaneously, the growth of palliative care within academic medical centers may point to internal change within hospital departments leading away from aggressive, technological care as the *modus operandi*. The impact of these trends is impossible to predict.

vii. There is good reason to imagine here testable hypotheses that could be roughly measured within large, public health cohort studies. A cultural fear of death could somewhat be accounted for if larger studies were conducted in a variety of human cultures, which would then allow for a more robust comparison.

References

1. J. D. Yoon, Shin J. H., Nian A. L., Curlin F. A. Religion, sense of calling, and the practice of medicine: findings from a national survey of primary care physicians and psychiatrists. *South Med J*. 2015;108(3):189–195.
2. P. Ariès. *Western attitudes toward death: from the Middle Ages to the present.* Baltimore: Johns Hopkins University Press; 1974.
3. F. A. Curlin, Lantos J. D., Roach C. J., Sellergren S. A., Chin M. H. Religious characteristics of US physicians: a national survey. *J Gen Intern Med*. 2005;20(7):629–634.
4. P. L. Berger. *The sacred canopy; elements of a sociological theory of religion.* 1st ed. Garden City, NY: Doubleday; 1967.
5. R. P. Sloan. *Blind faith: the unholy alliance of religion and medicine.* 1st ed. New York: St. Martin's Press; 2006.
6. O. P. Grell. The Protestant imperative of Christian care and neighborly love. In: O. P. Grell, Cunningham A., eds. *Health care and poor relief in Protestant Europe 1500–1700.* London: Routledge; 1997:43–65.
7. N. Orme, Webster M. E. G. *The English hospital 1070–1570.* New Haven: Yale University Press; 1995.
8. M. J. Balboni, T. A. Balboni. Medicine and spirituality in historical perspective. In: John Peteet, D'Ambra Michael, eds. *The soul of medicine: spirituality and world view in clinical practice.* Baltimore: John Hopkins University Press; 2011:3–22.

9. G. P. McKenny. *To relieve the human condition.* Albany: State University of New York Press; 1997.

10. G. P. McKenny. *To relieve the human condition: bioethics, technology, and the body.* Albany: State University of New York Press; 1997.

11. G. B. Risse. *Hospital life in enlightenment Scotland: care and teaching at the Royal Infirmary of Edinburgh.* Cambridge/New York: Cambridge University Press; 1986.

12. T. N. Bonner. *Becoming a physician: medical education in Britain, France, Germany, and the United States, 1750–1945.* New York: Oxford University Press; 1995.

13. G. B. Risse, Balboni M. J. Shifting hospital-hospice boundaries: historical perspectives on the institutional care of the dying. *Am J Hospice Palliat Med.* 2013;30(4):325–330.

14. J. C. Burnham. American medicine's golden age: what happened to it? *Science.* 1982;215(4539):1474–1479.

15. E. K. Abel. "In the last stages of irremediable disease": American hospitals and dying patients before World War II. *Bull Hist Med.* 2011;85(1):29–56.

16. E. Becker. *The denial of death.* New York: Free Press; 1973.

17. M. Fulop. The teaching hospital's modern deathbed ritual. *N Engl J Med.* 1985;312(2):125–126.

18. R. Stevens. *In sickness and in wealth: American hospitals in the twentieth century.* Johns Hopkins paperbacks ed. Baltimore: Johns Hopkins University Press; 1999.

19. G. B. Risse. *Mending bodies, saving souls: a history of hospitals.* New York: Oxford University Press; 1999.

20. P. L. Berger, Luckmann T. *The social construction of reality; a treatise in the sociology of knowledge.* 1st ed. Garden City, NY: Doubleday; 1966.

21. J. B. Imber. *Trusting doctors: the decline of moral authority in American medicine.* Princeton: Princeton University Press; 2008.

22. P. Starr. *The social transformation of American medicine.* New York: Basic Books; 1982.

23. R. Porter. *The greatest benefit to mankind: a medical history of humanity.* 1st American ed. New York: W. W. Norton; 1998.

24. C. A. Russell. The conflict of science and religion. In: Ferngren G. B., ed. *Science and religion: a historical introduction.* Baltimore: Johns Hopkins University Press; 2002:3–12.

25. C. Taylor. *A secular age.* Cambridge, MA: Belknap Press of Harvard University Press; 2007.

26. B. G. Glaser, Strauss AL. *Awareness of dying.* New Brunswick, NJ: Aldine Transaction; 2005.

27. E. Knauft, Nielsen E. L., Engelberg R. A., Patrick D. L., Curtis J. R. Barriers and facilitators to end-of-life care communication for patients with COPD. *Chest.* 2005;127(6):2188–2196.

28. K. Elbert-Avila, Tulsky A. J. Problems in communication. In: Walsh D., ed. *Palliative medicine.* Philadelphia: Saunders; 2009:625–630.

29. S. D. Goold, Williams B., Arnold R. M. Conflicts regarding decisions to limit treatment: a differential diagnosis. *JAMA.* 2000;283(7):909–914.

30. C. E. Rosenberg. *The care of strangers: the rise of America's hospital system.* New York: Basic Books; 1987.

31. E. Bruera, Russell N., Sweeney C., Fisch M., Palmer J. L. Place of death and its predictors for local patients registered at a comprehensive cancer center. *J Clin Oncol.* 2002;20(8):2127–2133.

32. S. Lutz. The history of hospice and palliative care. *Curr Probl Cancer.* 2011;35(6):304–309.

33. S. Weitzen, Teno J. M., Fennell M., Mor V. Factors associated with site of death: a national study of where people die. *Med Care.* 2003;41(2):323–335.

34. J. Flory, Yinong Y. X., Gurol I., Levinsky N., Ash A., Emanuel E. Place of death: US trends since 1980. *Health Affairs.* 2004;23(3):194–200.

35. Health, United States, 2010. U.S. Department of Health and Human Services: 2010; http://www.cdc.gov/nchs/data/hus/hus10.pdf. Accessed May 7, 2018.

36. Living with grief. *Lancet.* 2012;379(9816):589.

37. M. Weber. *The sociology of religion.* Boston: Beacon Press; 1963.

38. E. Durkheim, Fields K. E. *The elementary forms of religious life.* New York: Free Press; 1995.

39. B. Hayslip. Death denial: hiding and camouflaging death. In: C. D. Bryant, ed. *Handbook of death & dying.* Thousand Oaks, CA: SAGE; 2003: 34–42.

40. V. L. Lamb. Historical and epidemiological trends in mortality in the United States. In: C. D. Bryant, ed. *Handbook of death & dying.* Thousand Oaks, CA: SAGE; 2003:185–197.

41. E. Durkheim, Cosman C., Cladis M. S. *The elementary forms of religious life.* New York: Oxford University Press; 2001.

42. P. Norris, R. Inglehart. *Sacred and secular: religion and politics worldwide.* 2nd ed. Cambridge: Cambridge University Press; 2011.

43. D. W. Amundsen DW. *Medicine, society, and faith in the ancient and medieval worlds.* Baltimore: Johns Hopkins University Press; 1996.

44. D. Callahan. *The troubled dream of life: living with mortality.* New York: Simon & Schuster; 1993.

45. Brandt, AM, Gardner M. The golden age of medicine? In: Cooter and Pickston, eds. *Medicine in the Twentieth century.* Netherlands: Harwood Academic Publishing; 2000:21–37.

46. S. J. Lavi. *The modern art of dying: a history of euthanasia in the United States.* Princeton, NJ: Princeton University Press; 2005.

47. E. Kübler-Ross. *On death and dying.* New York: Macmillan; 1969.

48. M. J. Balboni, Bandini J., Mitchell C., et al. Religion, spirituality, and the hidden curriculum: medical student and faculty reflections. *J Pain Symptom Manage.* 2015;50(4):507–515.

49. C. Edgley. Dying as deviance: an update on the relationship between terminal patients and medical settings. In: C. D. Bryant, ed. *Handbook of death & dying.* Thousand Oaks, CA: SAGE; 2003:448–456.

50. L. Tolstoy. The Cossacks; The death of Ivan Ilyich; Happy ever after. In: *The death of Ivan Ilyach and other stories.* Baltimore: Penguin Books; 1960.

51. I. Illich. *Limits to medicine - medical nemesis: the expropriation of health.* Harmondsworth/ New York: Penguin; 1977.

52. H. S. Chapple. *No place for dying: hospitals and the ideology of rescue.* Walnut Creek, CA: Left Coast Press; 2010.

53. C. E. Rosenberg. *Our present complaint: American medicine, then and now.* Baltimore: Johns Hopkins University Press; 2007.

54. H. G. Coward, Stajduhar K. I. *Religious understandings of a good death in hospice palliative care.* Albany: State University of New York Press; 2012.

55. P. J. Choi, Curlin F. A., Cox C. E. "The patient is dying, please call the chaplain": the activities of chaplains in one medical center's intensive care units. *J Pain Symptom Manage.* 2015;50(4):501–506.

56. R. P. Sloan, Bagiella E. Spirituality and medical practice: a look at the evidence. *Am Fam Physician.* 2001;63(1):33–34.

7

The Secular–Sacred Divide in Medicine

In the previous chapter, we argued that important societal structures including depictions of hospitals as spaces of technology, physicians seen as primarily a guild of scientists, and understandings of human mortality that repress dying have each contributed to the plausibility of separation between medicine and religion. This separation is normal and matter of fact within contemporary society. In this chapter, we examine a final set of plausibility structures that function as a linchpin separating medicine and religion: the dichotomy of secular and sacred, often conceived in clearly demarcated modes of human reasoning and applied to our spatio-temporal experiences.

Definitions for Religion and Secular

A Western cultural view of social reality is based on the division of secular and sacred. This separation usually requires little defense or explanation as it functions as a social norm at the center of our cultural assumptions. In order to identify how the dichotomization operates, it is necessary to define religion. It is not possible to define what "secular" refers to without first defining or at least assuming some meaning for religion. Religion is "the West's most characteristic concept, around which it has established and developed its identity."[1] [p. 6]

Definitions for the secular tend to contrast or reverse meanings related to religion. "Secular" refers to what is temporal rather than ultimate, what is ordinary experience rather than what is beyond the ordinary, and what is immanent and within rather than beyond or transcendent. Precise meanings for "secular" are elusive to the degree that multiple meanings may be at play.[2] In Charles Taylor's view,[3] there are three meanings of secularity. The first sense of secular refers to an institutional separation between religious groups and the state—so that government is no longer connected to faith or God. This is what may be commonly conceived as the separation of church and state. A second sense of secularity refers to the norms and deliberations taking place within shared social spheres being emptied of religion. Secularity entails differentiation between institutions so that religious discourse no longer is an accepted public rationality within nonreligious social institutions such as economics, education, or medicine. Finally, he argues for a third sense that is more than social differentiation, referring to "a move from a society where belief in God is unchallenged and indeed, unproblematic, to one in which it is understood to be one option among others, and frequently not the easiest to embrace."[3] [pp. 1-3] Taylor suggests that it is especially this final sense of the secular which now depicts our time: "A secular age is one in which the eclipse of all goals beyond human flourishing becomes conceivable; or better it falls within the range of an imaginable life for masses of people."[3] [pp. 20-21]

Thus, both the religious and the secular are difficult to pin down conceptually. In the popular imagination, adopted by some of the most prominent scholars engaging religion, religion refers to what persons perceive to be ultimate, beyond ordinary experience, outside or transcending human experience, or superhuman.[4] Religious perceptions become systematized in a social order by including communal organization and spiritual practices that are aimed toward ultimate ends. The secular refers to all domains of human existence that are perceived to be temporal, ordinary, and immanent. These perceptions of what is secular have led to a social differentiation that circumscribes religion to particular social institutions, whereas institutions that are concerned with temporal and ordinary realities are deemed nonreligious. Within the context of healthcare, medicine comprises nonreligious institutions as it engages with temporal and material realities related to bodily health. How religion is defined in opposition to things of a temporal order inherently establishes separation, making any integrated approach between medicine and religion objectionable nearly *en toto*. By limiting religion to organized religion oriented around transcendent, supernatural realities and to what directly pertains to what is superhuman,[4] a separation has already been made plausible and unavoidable.

Bifurcation of Social Structures

Embedded within this popular understanding that separates religion from the secular is a multiplicity of related dichotomies or dualisms that underlie the structures of both Western society in general and, for our purposes, particular expressions as seen within contemporary medicine. Table 7.1 highlights how each level of human

Table 7.1 **Spiritual and nonspiritual plausibility structures governing socialization processes and institutions of medicine**

	Domain	*Separated Social Structures*		
		Immanence	*Transcendence*	*Significance*
1	Anthropology	Body	Soul	Human nature
2	Epistemology	Science	Revelation	Rationality
		Objective Fact	Subjective Value	Production of knowledge
3	Society	Public	Private	Social interactions
		State	Church	Political, legal
		Secular	Sacred	Space and time

experience follows a repeating pattern of bifurcation or division. The bifurcation is grounded upon the definitions for religion and secular previously suggested.

In Table 7.1, three domains of human existence are separated based on a division of religion or the transcendent on the one side and the secular or the immanent on the other. The first domain concerns perceptions of human anthropology. This broadly concerns how we conceptualize the nature of being human. The second domain concerns epistemology or the nature of knowledge and how that knowledge is discovered and identified as true. The third domain relates to the larger structures of society enabling how Western culture interprets spaces, time, various human institutions, and structures that orientate human power.

Body and Soul

In regards to anthropology, human nature is imagined as divided into a material and an immaterial self. The human body falls on the side of the immanent, whereas our immaterial selves—if they are believed in—come under the domain of the transcendent. By dividing our conception of the human person, different domains of society and specific professions may make particular claims of jurisdiction over one aspect or another of the human person. In this understanding, the State holds no jurisdiction over the human conscience or metaphysical beliefs, but the State will hold claims over material bodies, especially when the state itself is under threat.[5] Clergy may reasonably focus on the soul, but for them to espouse opinions concerning material realities comes dangerously close to crossing professional limits. Likewise, within medicine, modern disease theory has perpetuated the "dualism of the disease as object and the patient as subject."[6 [p. xii]] The body has been conceived of as an object that is separable from a subjective person.[6 [p. xiii]] Diseases of the body can be objectively evaluated, and, upon understanding the mechanisms of a disease by reducing the component parts of the body in a cause–effect relationship, medicine can intervene and treat the body. Medicine's jurisdiction pertains to the cause-and-effect aspects of the material body and is silent as it relates to human meaning or ultimate purpose.[7] Within this bifurcation of material and immaterial, physicians have little to say about the nonphysical, value-laden, subjective dimensions of illness because these fall outside their domain.[6,7] Thus, this separation in our understanding of human nature between material and immaterial works as a plausibility structure informing how the professions conceive their foci. As an underlying dualism, it is an important feature explaining why a separation between medicine and spirituality exists, and it informs why some find it a bewildering idea for medical professionals to engage patients' spiritual concerns.

Fact and Value

The bifurcation of immanence and transcendence impacts our epistemological conceptions in how we produce, authorize, and conceive the nature of knowledge (Table 7.1). The production of knowledge branches into two distinct and non-overlapping domains. There is knowledge produced through the scientific method and knowledge received through divine revelation and human wisdom.[8] The scientific method promises to produce knowledge that is objectively derived through processes that are open to all to falsify or reproduce. In the creation of knowledge, methodological naturalism approaches all causal relationships under purely immanent explanations without appeal to outside forces, whether God or other supernatural entities. This is not philosophical atheism, as Berger points out, simply the pursuit of human knowledge "as if God did not exist."[9 pp. 52–53] Knowledge from immanent processes is classified as objective fact, which implies its independence of human construction, and thus is universally applicable. The empirical method broadly defined across many fields including biology, epidemiology, and social policy are perceived to produce a "set of objective neutral principles, by which objective, universal judgments can be made.[10 pp. 152–153] Science produces facts that are believed to be true and universal. Though accepted knowledge ("facts") can be disputed through the same scientific procedures, they are widely received as true, irrespective of subjective feeling. As objective fact, there is a social expectation obligating reception and conformity to this knowledge. In contrast, knowledge derived from religion, whether by special revelation or based on theological assumptions, is nonuniversal, subjective, and value-based. People are free to submit to religiously based claims of knowledge privately, but there is no obligation since they are unverifiable claims. Separation of these two types of knowledge directly impacts acceptable forms of social discourse. Within the immanent realm, only knowledge produced by the physical and social sciences is considered valid. Thus, any religious claim within the process of science itself is a *non sequitur*. Religious discourse lacks rationality within any public domain because the underlying religious assumptions are not recognized as universally applicable.

Within the realm of healthcare, all claims to objective, universal truths must be grounded in scientifically testable processes. Medical knowledge is exclusively committed to a knowledge of the physical body and, in particular, a mechanistic conception of efficient causation.[7] As a public discipline medicine follows an evidence-based practice. Any association of medicine with religion, whether in its theories of disease, procedures of cure, or relational practices of patient care, serve as a threat to the objective and public basis of medicine's universally received discourse. The separation of religion and medicine is formed by a conception of knowledge leading to the conclusion that the two realms rightly remain disentangled.[i]

Public and Private

The bifurcation of immanence and transcendence also informs social structures governing human relationships maintaining separation of medicine and spirituality. Probably the most important form of institutional division is the separation between government and religious organizations. Reference to a division of church and state can hold several meanings, including the formal separation of government and religious organizations and a division on the level of rational discourse (e.g., the kinds of arguments appropriate to make), as well as a larger social differentiation between religion and those state-influenced institutions such as in education, social welfare, and healthcare, which are all concerned with the collective good.

Beyond the division of church and state, the idea of social differentiation refers to the division of labor within modern societies. Durkheim argued that religion functions within society by creating social cohesion, and he predicted that with the growth of the state in providing various social goods, there would be an overall decline in religion because it has lost its function in creating social cohesion.[11] As a theory of secularization, Durkheim's view has increasingly been contested as religion has remained a powerful phenomenon despite modernization around the globe.[12-14] While religious beliefs and practices have hardly disappeared in the United States or in most of the world,[14] many do affirm secularization if defined as social differentiation caused by a division of labor in modern societies where organized religion has less influence over society.[9,13] Among our shared social institutions—directly or indirectly related to state influence—religion is perceived and categorized as one of many institutionally discrete entities. As a domain unto itself, religion has not diminished, but it has been increasingly privatized to its own domain and is thus able to exercise less influence over "nonreligious" sectors of a culture, whether the market, public education, or the healthcare system.

As Table 7.1 illustrates, social differentiation is most popularly conceptualized in the categories of public and private, one of the "grand dichotomies" of Western thought.[15 [p. 1]] The boundaries between public and private are ambiguous and contested because imagery related to each varies considerably.[15,16] In general, social institutions (e.g., schools, justice system, corporations, hospitals, etc.) and their corresponding professions (e.g., teachers, lawyers, police, business professions, and medical professionals) are often conceived as public institutions to the degree that they serve our larger, collective society. On the other side of the division lies the realm of the private, which often is conceived to include the individual, family, and friends, as well as religion. Within this framework, medicine and religion are perceived to fall on opposing sides of the line. Scheurich argues for a "separation of church and medicine" model whereby medicine remains value-neutral toward patient religion, neither affirming or denying it.[17] Since religion is an extremely private affair, and because it is alleged that religion has little to do directly with the purposes of medicine,[18 [pp. 191-193]] it follows that medicine is for the collective public good of social health, whereas religion is a voluntary choice disconnected from health. Thus, as people consider the relationship of medicine and religion, the plausibility structure of public–private inevitably rises as a distinction that serves as critical objection to integration or partnership.[17,18]

Secular and Sacred

The bifurcation of reality divides on the lines of immanence and transcendence as it pertains to our conceptions of space and time. Constructed social structures, especially architecture and time, are informed by notions of secular and sacred. In Western Christianity, the idea of the secular has been used in previous times to distinguish professional roles, the import of space, and the telling of time.[3,9,19] The institutional church has in some eras utilized this distinction as a mode to make claims on persons or property or to protect itself from counterclaims from non–church leaders.[19] With the privatization of religion, space and time have undergone substantial reinterpretations as to their significance. Space and property are often seen as sacred or hallowed and may have especially strong connections to transcendent interpretations with the use of transcendent symbols or unique architectural designs that signal ultimacy or point to the divine. For example, hospitals in the Christian tradition were frequently constructed in the shape of a cross.[20] This architectural design imbued transcendent meaning into the literal walls of buildings where the sick received care. In modern societies, most healing spaces are typically viewed in terms of being *this worldly* and, consequently, part of ordinary and mundane meaning and experience. Indeed, postmodern hospital design has "entirely eschewed religious themes and iconography" in building structure and art,[21 [p. 2]] creating instead contemporary hotel-like space. The structure of contemporary healing spaces points to immanent comfort without confronting or reminding hospital visitors of transcendent themes. Secular space voids markers that signal a spiritual reality that stands "above," "beyond," and ultimately "greater than" our current moment.

Similarly, the social structure of time, in religiously oriented societies, was experienced through spiritual symbols and activities. Time itself was interpreted or marked by transcendent signals and social practices. In Christian societies, the church bells tolled, calling the neighborhood to service. Church bells rang on the hour, tethering the hour to a transcendent-pointing institution. In Islamic cultures, the *adhan* is publically called five times a day, which structures the experience of time according to a shared spiritual practice. In twentieth-century Catholic hospitals, the days began and ended with prayer over the intercom, routinizing the experience of time through social action oriented toward the transcendent.[22,ii] The etching of space and time with transcendent ideas marked the dominion of healing with an aura of the sacred and thus normalized spiritual care provision to patients in healing spaces as the expectation. In contrast, secular time lacks transcendent markers. The measurement of time through the clock "by its essential nature dissociated time from human events and helped create the belief in an independent world of mathematically measurable sequences."[23 [pp. 12–15]] Within contemporary medicine, the lack of transcendent markers in healing architecture and social structures related to time make attention to patients' spiritual needs seemingly out of context. These invisible social structures have increasingly been framed without reference to any transcendent realities. This division of space and time through processes of modernization reinforces a separation of medicine and religion as social structures embedded within medicine have shifted from sacred to secular frameworks. As the spatiotemporal dimensions of medicine have lost visible markers of transcendence, spiritual care of patients has also vanished, aided by the diminishment of a context that justifies and gives it meaning.

Medicine's Immanent Frame

As part of a larger cultural context, we are arguing that the separation of medicine and religion is justified and reinforced by plausibility structures that divide perceptions of reality into categories of immanence and transcendence (Table 7.1). Religion is perceived to be largely an institutionally circumscribed domain of life compartmentalized to the realm of the private. Religion is a subjective preference based on voluntary association and is separable from other domains of human existence, especially the realm of objective knowledge and spheres of social life that aim for the collective, public good. Healthcare and medicine are among these public goods that must avoid association with religion within its social structures, including the human imagining of space and time. Charles Taylor refers to this as the "immanent frame." He defines the immanent frame as a constructed social order that reconfigures space, time, rationality, and nature all in immanent terms—a full-blown human social system aimed toward human flourishing that contains no necessary contingency on the reality of transcendence undergirding human flourishing.[3,iii]

The immanent frame contextualizing medicine excludes religion in at least three critical ways. From an institutional perspective, the primary context of medicine remains the hospital. As public institutions, hospitals have been increasingly differentiated from transcendent associations in their stated missions, their philanthropic supporters, organizational character, identities of staff and patients, and their ritual care activities.[22 [p. 4]] With few exceptions, hospitals no longer orient themselves by a transcendent framework within their institutional organizations. Hospitals are institutions of technological immanence, organized by "this worldly" goals and foci.[iv]

From the professional perspective, nurses and physicians have frameworks that are guided by an immanent social formation and knowledge. Religion and spirituality have no bearing on the qualifications for being a medical professional. Knowledge of religion is deemed unnecessary and tertiary to the actual practice of medicine (although knowledge of religions may clearly assist a clinician when navigating medical issues with a highly religious patient). Formation in a spiritual tradition in preparation to care for patients may not only be viewed by some as unnecessary, but even as a threat to patient care. Knowledge required for professional guilds to competently care for patients are oriented primarily by facts, evidence, and mastery of technical skills. While many moral ideals for the profession remain intact for now,[24] formation within those morals is seldom directly attempted by the profession and can be awkwardly undermined by actual practices.[25] Nurses and physicians as professional guilds perceive spirituality and religion to be extrinsic to their professions. Thus, transcendence holds no role in the formation of medical professionals or in what is believed to be intrinsic to competent practice.

Likewise, based within a sociology of knowledge there is an underlying expectation that medical caregivers incorporate practices of compartmentalization as they pertain to the care of patients. Modern consciousness segregates reality into domains that can be conceived and lived as distinct realities. Sociological theorists have argued that modern consciousness adheres to multiple realities by which we employ distinct vocabularies, definitions, and actions depending on which reality is our primary reference.[9,v] With medicine as the reference point, nurses and physicians act upon their role as "medical professional," which includes knowledge, skills, and actions relevant to this role. The private life is not relevant when acting as a medical professional. Hence, physicians and nurses cross a professional boundary when they discuss their subjective viewpoints on serious matters, share personal information about where they live, provide details about family life, and, if religious, fail to circumscribe religious commitments from professional identity. Compartmentalization socializes medical professionals to adhere to a social consciousness framed by immanent concerns. Embedded within our own psychological identities is a compartmentalized sense of the self in which multiple sets of realities—which may in degrees conflict with one another—coexist within our own presuppositions and actions. Modern consciousness requires not only a division of labor across society but a division in the mind. "A general insight of sociology is that every institution, if it is to function in society, must be internalized in the minds of individuals."[9 [p. 60]] The compartmentalization of medicine and religion in the contemporary social imagination creates a situation in which religious claims are considered alien to healthcare and medicine. Within this context, accounts that seek to integrate medicine and religion seem implausible, strange, or simply coercive. Within the plausibility structures of modernity, medicine must be on the side of the immanent and should resist transcendent claims from religion that seek to inform the practice of medicine or its social structures.

Conclusion

As we have sought to explore the reasons for the infrequency of spiritual care within medicine, even in serious illness, our argument has identified several plausibility structures that keep medicine and religion separated. In the previous chapter, we suggested that the social forces of technology and scientific rationalism have come to dominate the hospital context and serve as the primary identity for clinicians. The previous chapter also argued that there has been a major shift in repressing social engagement of dying and death, that medicine has played a key role in this repression, and that religion inherently undermines this repression—explaining why medicine may be motived to remain at a clear distance from religion.

In this chapter, we have argued that, in addition to these dynamics, modern consciousness is comprised of a series of related bifurcations of life (Table 7.1) and that medicine is a social institution that is informed by understandings of human nature, human knowledge, and social structures that fall on the opposite side of the wall from religion. We are not suggesting that medicine and religion cannot be generally differentiated, but rather that modern Western societies advance this dualism to such an extent that there appears to be no unity or interconnection between both spheres. In other words, noting a proper distinction between the spheres of medicine and religion does not by itself create our modern consciousness. Rather, there has been a loss of a larger unitive vision tying together multiple spheres into a greater whole. If we get physically sick, we turn to the doctor not the priest. This is merely differentiation of roles and spheres. But it is quite another step entirely, not demanded by differentiation, to conclude that a priest has nothing to say about sickness or that a physician has nothing to say about spirituality.

Nevertheless, considered together, these plausibility structures create a framework of meaning that is dominated by immanence, which is in turn structured into our notions of time, architectural space, and consciousness itself. These social structures form the bricks that comprise the wall of separation between medicine and religion. Or, to use another metaphor, the separation of medicine and religion is invisibly interspersed within our cultural oxygen so that all the members of society inevitably, perhaps unwittingly, have taken it into their depths. Working together, these plausibility structures carry forward a powerful, omnipresent socialization that further explains why clinicians are able to neglect and avoid spiritual care despite their own positive opinions related to the appropriateness of providing spiritual care, recognition of its perceived positive benefits for patients, and the express desire among patients to receive it.

Though socialization concepts are essential in understanding medical professionals' lack of engagement of patients' spiritual needs, Part II builds on these points by examining the separation of medicine and religion from a theological perspective. As readers will discover, we will argue that the divisions that underlie religion, spirituality, and medicine are based on problematic definitions around the concept of religion. The dualistic sacred–secular structure discussed in this chapter is based on a popular, but we believe ultimately a troubled definition of religion. "Separation" hinges on our meaning of *religion*. From what is *it* that medicine is separating? As we turn to Part II in our argument (Chapters 8–12), we suggest that there is a theologically grounded explanation that sheds light on the separation of medicine and traditional religions. To make this case, however, we must first discuss the meaning of spirituality and religion. To this we turn next.

Notes

i. This account, however, fails to take into account how a growing body of empirical research challenges these very assumptions. As argued in Chapters 2 and 3, the evidence suggests that these divisions simply do not work within patient experience of illness or in how medical decisions are conceived by many religious persons. The abundance of research demonstrates that these bifurcations of our reality are based more on ideology than evidence.

ii. To our knowledge, some Roman Catholic hospitals continue public prayers over the intercom as part of their opening morning routine. We are unaware of any systematic research documenting the proportion of hospitals that have retained this public practice in the United States.

iii. An immanent frame, according to Taylor, can be applied as either open or closed to transcendent ideas. An "open" immanent frame refers to a basic immanent system that can be punctured by moments of transcendence. There is mystery that is real and greater than the horizontal world around us, and it is characterized by a disposition "open to something beyond."[3 (p. 544)] A closed immanent frame may be defined as a disposition closed to the possibility that a greater reality exists beyond the natural, material world. Whether open or closed, an immanent frame structures human experience of social reality—space, time, rationality, and a metaphysical view of nature—nudging everyone toward a basic disposition of immanence.[3 (p. 555)]

iv. What we will begin to show in Part II of our argument is that immanent-only conceptions of human flourishing function in religious-like ways because they are not based on empirical evidence. Part of the self-contradictory nature of an immanent-only framework of meaning is that human flourishing has not the necessary contingency upon transcendent aims. This is a values claim that is not based on objective, fact-based evidence. The contradiction lies in claiming a structural system of human flourishing that is areligious and yet, embedded within its own presuppositions, there are particular values of meaning that cannot be grounded beyond their mere claim.

v. Individual modern consciousness is characterized by one set of assumptions and discourses shared with most other people in everyday life and a second set of assumptions and discourses relevant to a smaller group of people (see A. Schutz and T. Luckmann. *The structures of the life-world*. Evanston, IL: Northwestern University Press; 1973). Shared cultural consciousness is shaped by the larger social forces of technology, bureaucracy, and pluralization of our social worlds, and these institutional forces shape individual ways of seeing the larger world (see P. L. Berger, Berger B., Kellner H. *The homeless mind; modernization and consciousness*, 1st ed.

New York: Random House; 1973). The use of the term "consciousness" does not mean that an individual is aware of how these social forces influence his or her own thinking. In fact, consciousness refers to the unquestioned presuppositions that most individuals are not aware that they absorb and use within their engagement of everyday life (Schutz and Luckmann, 1973). The carriers of modernization (especially technology, bureaucracy, and pluralization) have embedded within a rational discourse a structure that exerts force upon individuals to internalize patterns of thought requiring reductionism and compartmentalization. For example, in a modern division of industrial labor, individual workers see only pieces of the whole, operate by reductionist principles, and perform work without any intrinsic appeal to transcendent ideas. Berger, Berger, and Kellner argue that this form of compartmentalized thinking spills over into every form of modern consciousness: "Elements of consciousness that are intrinsic to technological production are transposed to areas of social life that are not directly connected with such production. . . . In so-called developed or advanced industrial societies . . . these carry-over effects are massive. . . . It is not necessary to be engaged in technological work in order to think technologically (Berger, Berger, and Kellner, 1973).

References

1. Daniel Dubuisson. *The western construction of religion: myths, knowledge, and ideology.* Baltimore: Johns Hopkins University Press; 2003.
2. Karel Dobbelaere. *Secularization: an analysis at three levels.* Vol no. 1. Bruxelles/New York: P. I. E.-Peter Lang; 2002.
3. Charles Taylor. *A secular age.* Cambridge, MA: Belknap Press of Harvard University Press; 2007.
4. Christian Smith. *Religion: what it is, how it works, and why it is still important.* Princeton, NJ: Princeton University Press; 2017.
5. William T. Cavanaugh. *Torture and Eucharist: theology, politics, and the body of Christ.* Oxford, UK/Malden, MA: Blackwell Publishers; 1998.
6. Eric J. Cassell. *The nature of suffering and the goals of medicine.* 2nd ed. New York: Oxford University Press; 2004.
7. Jeffrey Paul Bishop. *The anticipatory corpse: medicine, power, and the care of the dying.* Notre Dame, IN: University of Notre Dame Press; 2011.
8. Stephen Jay Gould. *Rocks of ages: science and religion in the fullness of life.* 1st ed. New York: Ballantine Publishing Group; 1999.
9. Peter Berger. *The many alters of modernity.* Boston: De Gruyter; 2014.
10. Kenneth R. Craycraft. *The American myth of religious freedom.* Dallas, TX: Spence Publishing; 1999.
11. Emile Durkheim, Fields Karen E. *The elementary forms of religious life.* New York: Free Press; 1995.
12. Peter L. Berger. *The desecularization of the world: resurgent religion and world politics.* Washington, DC/Grand Rapids, MI: Ethics and Public Policy Center/W. B. Eerdmans Publishing; 1999.
13. José Casanova. *Public religions in the modern world.* Chicago: University of Chicago Press; 1994.
14. Pippa Norris, Inglehart Ronald. *Sacred and secular: religion and politics worldwide.* 2nd ed. Cambridge: Cambridge University Press; 2011.
15. Jeff Alan Weintraub, Kumar Krishan. *Public and private in thought and practice: perspectives on a grand dichotomy.* Chicago: University of Chicago Press; 1997.
16. Paul Starr. The meaning of privatization. In: S. B. Kamerman, Kahn A. J., eds. *Privatization and the Welfare State.* Princeton, NJ: Princeton University Press; 1989:15–48.
17. N. Scheurich. Reconsidering spirituality and medicine. *Acad Med.* 2003;78(4):356–360.
18. Richard P. Sloan. *Blind faith: the unholy alliance of religion and medicine.* 1st ed. New York: St. Martin's Press; 2006.
19. John Milbank. *Theology and social theory: beyond secular reason.* Cambridge, MA: Blackwell; 1990.
20. Nicholas Orme, Webster Margaret. *The English hospital 1070–1570.* New Haven, CT: Yale University Press; 1995.

21. Stephen Verderber. *Innovations in hospital architecture.* New York: Routledge; 2010.
22. Guenter B. Risse. *Mending bodies, saving souls: a history of hospitals.* New York: Oxford University Press; 1999.
23. Lewis Mumford. *Technics and civilization.* New York: Harcourt; 1963.
24. Project Medical Professionalism. Medical professionalism in the new millennium: a physicians' charter. *Lancet.* 2002;359(9305):520–522.
25. W. A. Kinghorn, McEvoy M. D., Michel A., Balboni M. Professionalism in modern medicine: does the emperor have any clothes? *Acad Med.* 2007;82(1):40–45.

PART II

THEOLOGICAL PERSPECTIVES ON THE SEPARATION OF MEDICINE AND SPIRITUALITY

8

Defining Religion and Spirituality

Evaluating the operating definitions of religion and spirituality underlying this book's argument is central to understanding the relationship between spirituality and religion on the one side and medicine on the other. Those who argue against the role of religion or spirituality in medicine operate on certain assumptions about the nature of religion and spirituality that we believe fail to acknowledge the complexity of these concepts. Additionally, within the field of health, the concept of religion is sometimes perceived as settled, whereas definitions for spirituality remain contested. These critical misunderstandings must be addressed in order to reveal a more accurate picture of the potential role for spirituality and religion in medicine.

In this chapter, we begin with our definitions for religion and spirituality, highlight key features of these definitions, expand on their origins within a larger conversation, discuss whether it is possible to treat religion and spirituality as conceptually distinct concepts, and then, based on these definitions, describe the meaning of "theology." This chapter is needed to lay a scholarly foundation for how to conceptualize the relationship of religion as it pertains to medicine. The impact of this discussion will become clearer especially in Chapters 11 and 12.

Formal Definitions of Religion and Spirituality

Though there are many different proposals defining spirituality and religion, we begin by proposing the following definitions:[i]

- *Spirituality*: Life centered in the person(s) and/or object(s) of one's chief love—however individually understood and pursued.
- *Religion*: The individual and social structures that flow from and facilitate a chief love, including beliefs, practices, relationships, and organizations.

There are five features of these definitions that we want to highlight. First, the idea of "chief love" within our concept of spirituality highlights that spirituality is not only cognitive but also part of a person's will and affect. (Affect refers here not only to its psychological association with emotion but especially to the idea of inner drive and desire.) Although spirituality does concern ideas and beliefs, its central mark is what is most deeply desired and loved. Of course, most human beings follow many desires and loves. This definition assumes that human nature follows a hierarchy of loves—primary (chief), secondary, and tertiary. But because individuals may have multiple primary desires around which their life is centered, they may have more than one chief love.

The second feature concerns the concept of "centering." Spirituality is organized by how a person's life is centered. Though an individual's attestation of a chief love is obviously an important factor, this does not necessarily correspond to how he or she lives. There are times, perhaps quite often, when theory and practice diverge in our lives—when we assert belief in one thing but live in a contrary fashion.[1,2] Therefore, we refer to spirituality as focused on how one actually lives life in relation to objects or persons that function as chief desires and loves.

Third, our definition of spirituality is not limited to certain objects or persons that are independently identified as worthy of being one's chief love. Instead, spirituality is inherently self-referential. The object of chief love is dependent on individual choices and pursuits. Thus, any object or person, including those that are considered by others to be truly worthy of human love and those that are deemed trivial and ephemeral, can be the chief object around which an individual centers his or her life. In this definition, what makes something "spiritual" is not the object's or person's independent qualities or content but the level of affection placed upon them. Some have concluded that a definition of spirituality that depends on a person's perception in this way makes the concept of spirituality so diffuse that it becomes meaningless as a construct[3] This is a misunderstanding, however, since our definition contains a clear object that identifies spirituality; namely, the elevation of an object to what is deemed ultimate. Again, the object chiefly loved is not itself constitutive of spirituality. Rather, spirituality is identified as the activation of a chief love combined with the object of that love. Thus, spirituality may conceivably encompass a diverse set of potential objects including God (a transcendent object), marriage (a human good), baseball (an ephemeral good), or heroin (a destructive human addiction).[ii] Each of these has the potential to become a spirituality when it operates as a chief love within a person's life and becomes what that person centers life around.

Fourth, within our definition, there is a constructive and necessary relationship between spirituality and religion. This will be discussed in more detail later in the chapter, but, in short, we define spirituality and religion as intrinsically interconnected so that every religion is grounded within a spirituality, and every spirituality inevitably produces a functional religion.[4] There is no sound conceptual option either of depicting spirituality versus religion, as Pargament has rightly argued,[6] or of understanding them as potentially non-overlapping constructs.[7] The difference between spirituality and religion is that the former is the underlying affection of the heart, whereas the latter is the individual and collective outworking and experience of that ultimate love. Spirituality is the invisible connectedness of one's desire toward the object of one's chief love, and religion is the visible human manifestations of that love aimed at serving and enabling a chief love. Spirituality refers to the real, albeit invisible, chief love that produces a corresponding religion. In turn, religion serves a spirituality.[iii]

The relationship between spirituality and religion can be compared to a marital relationship. The love and commitment shared between a couple is akin to spirituality, as it serves as the guiding aim and desire constituting the relationship. The necessary social structures of marriage—such as living in the same house together, shared practices in sexual relations, raising children, financial cooperation, taking care of one another's physical and emotional needs, and regularly eating meals together— are akin to religion. The daily business of marriage should flow from love and commitment, but these practices and structures are also necessary to giving expression to and sustaining love. Without social practices and structures, sustaining human love is impossible, suggesting that the structures are constitutive for marital love. Yet most also recognize that the social structures and shared practices are not themselves the *sine qua non* of marital love but expressions of an immaterial but real human phenomenon. Just as marital love and its social structures are distinct yet interdependent concepts, spirituality and religion function with a similar dynamic interdependence.

A fifth feature, closely related to the fourth, is that it is important to resist false dichotomies between religion and spirituality. For example, our definitions resist depicting spirituality as primarily individual and religion as primarily collective.[8] Such a view does not hold up under scrutiny because all religions have clear individual dimensions, and all spiritualities have collective expressions.[9] Nor does adhering to the concept of an "inner" core for spirituality and an "outer" shell for religion adequately capture the relationship.[10] [pp. 8–11] Spirituality cannot function without religion's embodiment and human structures, which provide it shape but also shape it in turn.[4] Religion should also not be considered a subsphere of spirituality, so that spirituality is the larger domain that religion falls within.[11] [p. 14] This view conceives of some human experiences as being spiritual but lacking religious dimensions. But this is conceptually problematic because it is based within a sociopolitical position rather than sound conceptual reasoning.[12]

In our view, spirituality and religion are not independent concepts but are so closely related that one always leads to and requires the other. Spirituality refers to the immaterial but real love directed toward the object or person chiefly desired. Religion refers to the material dimensions of that love expressed in human forms of practices, relationships, organizations, and supporting beliefs. Since these two concepts are inherently related, mutually producing one another, we adopt the nomenclature of "religion/spirituality" or use the terms interchangeably in some instances throughout this book.

Origins of Our Understanding of Spirituality and Religion

Our concept of "chief love" has roots in two understandings of religion that we believe adequately merge substantive (emphasizing belief in something superhuman or beyond material reality)[13–15,iv] and functional (emphasizing the relationship that a system has toward a human need or end)[v] definitions. Both the substantive and functional approaches to defining religion have clear strengths and limitations. The major strength of substantive definitions, especially those that focus on what is supernatural or superhuman, is that they carry a high level of clarity in classifying human phenomena. They make identifying religion relatively easy. However, substantive definitions are plagued by their inability to identify any one object that can be applied to all phenomena typically perceived as religious. Applying the idea of God, divinity, the supernatural, or the superhuman works among monotheistic phenomena such as Christianity, but it does not fit certain Eastern belief systems, which have normally been recognized as world religions but do not entail such objects as part of their systems.[vi]

In contrast, functional understandings, rather than being too restrictive in defining religious phenomena, are intentionally vague in order to apply to a wider variety of phenomenon. Functional definitions for religion can therefore open the concept up to a broader array of phenomena popularly not perceived as religious, such as political ideologies like Marxism or secular society itself.[16] This can lead to the description of certain groups as religious even if adherents within that group or ideology self-consciously reject any religious identity. Marxism serves as a striking example of this conflict—though its adherents believe that religion ("the opium of the people") must be eradicated, its overall function could lead the ideology of Marxism to be described as religious.[13] [pp. 110-111] While some scholars of religion are comfortable in describing religious phenomena in this way, most lay people feel puzzled by functional understandings of religion that allow for these contradictions.

In our view, the best manner forward is to follow religious historian Martin Marty and health psychologist Ken Pargament, who both suggest a bridge between the substantive and functional definitions.[17] [pp. 29-33] Martin Marty identified five characteristics related to the phenomena of religion: a focus on an ultimate concern, important roles for myth and symbol, reliance on rite and ceremony, behavioral or ethical obligations, and the presence and role of community.[18] [p. 10-12] The most critical building block of Marty's definition is the meaning of "ultimate concern." He indicated that this refers to an "overarching purpose," that is, what we care about most and would be willing to die for.[18] [p. 12] This perception of ultimacy, in Marty's view, becomes systematized in a social ordering that we typically recognize as a religion. Marty's identification of "ultimate concern" has blended substantive and functional elements into a single identifying principle.[vii]

Pargament, a leading psychologist in the field of spirituality and health, defined religion as "a search for significance in ways related to the sacred.[6] [p. 33] viii This definition ties religion to spirituality and recognizes functional dimensions. The concept of *search* depicts religion as an ongoing journey and relationship rather than as a static and stale entity. The concept of *significance* acknowledges the functional dimension of religion, that is, its role in creating psychological meaning, social cohesion, and physical health within a person's life. The concept of the *sacred* acknowledges the substantive dimension of religion; that is, the proper object in which one can identify religion's presence or absence. Pargament's use of the *sacred* is inclusive of both theistic conceptions of God or a higher power and nontheistic conceptions, including "other aspects of life that are perceived to be manifestations of the divine or imbued with divine-like qualities, such as transcendence, immanence, boundlessness and ultimacy. . . . [V]irtually any part of life, positive or negative, can be endowed with sacred status."[6] [p. 33] An object held as sacred is one that is "set apart" from all others and upheld for its unique, central importance to an individual's life.[ix]

We believe that there is a general equivalence between Marty's and Pargament's use of "ultimate concern" and "the sacred" and our own accent on "chief love." Each provides a clear way to identify functional religion as opposed to nonreligion. Our preference for the phrase "chief love" is that it is a more readily understandable phrase that does not carry philosophical or traditionally religious overtones. Marty's "ulti-mate concern" emphasizes a mental concentration and conscious focus on the thing held most important. However, "concern" can hold negative meanings including worry, anxiety, and consternation, which are inherently too negative to aptly describe the construct's meaning. Pargament's "sacred" is too closely associated with objects of religious worship, failing to capture the breadth of potential meaning. Although Pargament clearly used "sacred" with the intent of going beyond religious theism, the term "sacred" may be too closely connected to substantive definitions associated with Judaism and Christianity and thus fail to increase clarity.

In comparison, our suggestion of "chief love" is relatively clear in its reference to "what is loved the most," avoiding any necessarily theistic connotations. Most recognize that "love" involves emotion, commitment, and the giving of oneself over to the object of love in both mind and body. The term "chief" signals that this is not a secondary love but the central energy and will that drives a person throughout his or her daily routines. Our concept of "chief love" is thus dynamically equivalent to ultimate concern and the sacred, but it emphasizes a slightly different perspective.

Implications of Broadening the Understanding of Religion

The typical catalog of world religions, which is largely based on substantive definitions, is no longer adequate if applying our broader understanding of religion based on the concept of chief love. When theistic or superhuman definitions of religion are replaced with self-referential functional understandings, then the concept of religion refers to any object deemed worthy of chief love. These objects, including objects that others perceive as unworthy of esteem, are set apart from all others because of the central role that they hold in an individual's life, irrespective of content.

By naming a diverse set of sacred objects under the single category of functional religion, we do not suggest that there is a common human experience[19 (p. 43-44)] irrespective of the object of ultimate concern. It is necessary to move beyond a generic or context-free conception of religion toward greater levels of specificity.[20] If religion can include radically distinct objects deemed sacred, it can also create sometimes radically distinct human experiences, beliefs, practices, and relationships.[x]

By way of analogy, the category of "sports" refers to a wide range of physical activity, play, and competition that include a diversity of experiences such as golf, football, cycling, and fly-fishing. While each of these shares some characteristics, they dramatically differ in aim, physical activity, required skills, tools employed, mental strategies, and whether and in which ways they involve teamwork. Describing all as "sports" has utility since they have levels of resemblance,[21] but it is important to understand that no one plays "sports-in-general."[20] Describing them all as sports does not make them interchangeable phenomenon.

Religion, like sports, refers to a constructed category of convenience that identifies a broad range of human activities that are loosely affiliated with one another but not interchangeable.[xi] While certainly some claim that all roads lead to the same mountain peak,[22] it should equally be stressed how distinct objects of ultimate concern produce distinct beliefs and practices that are organic to or flow from their central object of affection. Even traditionally recognized world religions such as Christianity, Buddhism, and Islam hold radically distinct objects as sacred.[23] And these distinct objects lead to, for example, practices of prayer that are only vaguely similar. Some religions pray to the Divine-Creator, some pray to ancestors, some use prayer as a means of self-reflection without intent of communicating to another, and some do not pray at all. The meaning and experience of prayer is sufficiently different between many religions that describing all manifestations under the single term "prayer" risks masking the differences that exist to those not familiar with each intent. Care must be taken in using the term "religion" at all since it is a broad term that categorizes a variety of phenomena that have similarities but should not be equated with one another.

Returning to the sports analogy, many sports use balls, but the balls are distinct from one another and cannot be interchanged (e.g., compare the qualities of a golf ball, basketball, or tennis ball). The nature of the ball itself is organically connected to the rules, strategies, and skills necessary to the game. American football would dramatically change on every level if a tennis ball were substituted. Sport fishing would be nearly impossible if a golf ball were attached to the fishing line. Similarly, among the world religions, while it remains broadly helpful to recognize family resemblances, including the practice of prayer,[24] each holds distinct beliefs, practices, and aims, making it necessary to recognize not only the general fact of whether they employ a specific activity but also the composition and intent of the activity and how it shapes the person and is shaped by the sacred object.

Though those on each side of the religion–secular divide will lose something if the definition of religion is properly broadened beyond substantive definitions, we also might anticipate important gains. First, rather than needing to decipher if something is religious or secular, which we believe is intractably arbitrary and based within motives of power, there will be a wider acknowledgment that groups have claims grounded in their own most deeply held loves and ultimate concerns.[xii] Social issues of power and control could be settled on the principle of equity and fairness irrespective of the group's central guiding love (this concept is explained in Chapter 15 in our discussion of structural pluralism). While this may appear like a radical proposal, we will argue in Chapters 11 and 12 that this is already fully taking place but has been disguised by the sacred–secular framework. Second, a broader understanding organized around functional religion removes confusing and unnecessary rhetoric around the relationship between spirituality and religion. As we will argue next, synthetic divisions separating spirituality and religion are partly motivated by power dynamics and have been based on theistic and superhuman conceptions of religion rather than a broad conception of religion.

The Problem with Separating Religion and Spirituality

As noted earlier, our approach to religion and spirituality precludes a conceptual separation of the two terms. However, it is helpful to understand the history behind why the two have been separated and how this has impacted the provision of spiritual care within medicine. Spirituality has been a historically Christian term,[3,7] but, since the 1960s, it has also been favored—and in some cases co-opted—by those in the New Age movement.[3,25]

Spirituality has been increasingly employed as a construct that consciously seeks to be differentiated from traditional religion.[9]

As a specific example related to our focus on medicine, there has been a growing consensus that, within the patient–clinician relationship, employing the language of spirituality is preferable to the language of religion because it is inclusive of both patients of prototypical religions (e.g., Christianity) and those who do not identify with a traditional religion.[26] This assertion that spiritual care should be underpinned not by a historically rooted religion per se but by generic spirituality has developed in correspondence with a widening recognition of the diverse cultural and religious practices and beliefs operating in American society. This approach understands spirituality to be rooted in the human person prior to religious or theological formulation.[7] Spirituality scholar Sandra Schneiders suggests that spirituality "has become a generic term for the actualization in life of the human capacity for self-transcendence, regardless of whether that experience is religious or not."[7 [p. 168]] Proponents of this approach have suggested that understanding spirituality in this way enables dialogue between different religious groups by emphasizing the common starting point of a shared humanity. Some, such as Peter Van Ness, argue that spirituality is viewed as a shared human experience that precedes theological and religious attempts to describe that experience.[27,xiii] This approach understands spirituality to be rooted in the human person prior to religious or theological formulation.[7,11,27] Such inclusion enables spiritual care to be provided in pluralistic contexts to those who either do not identify with religion or are for some reason alienated from their religious community.[xiv] This approach appears to serve as theoretical background for the 2009 Consensus Conference definition of spirituality.[28,xv]

However, attempts to separate spirituality from religion on a conceptual level have been critiqued from within a variety of disciplines, including the sociology of religion,[1,9] the psychology of religion and health,[6] medicine,[29,30] philosophy,[31] and theology[3,32–37] Additionally, Ammerman showed through in-depth interviews of participants in Atlanta and Boston that, as recently as 2013, most Americans conceptualized spirituality and religion as mutually dependent concepts.[1] This finding is consistent with our own interviews of seriously ill patients discussed in Chapters 2 and 3.

Even when individuals attempt to separate the two by describing themselves as "spiritual, not religious," the eminent sociologist of religion Robert Wuthnow has shown that they are still depending on underlying beliefs that function as a theology, institutional social structures that operate as a community, particular moral codes marked by autonomy, and spiritual practices that function as rituals.[9,xvi] Religious scholar Candy Brown has further argued that even ostensibly nonreligious spiritual practices such as yoga are "theory-laden" and cannot be completely detached from the religious systems that produced those practices.[33]

Therefore, while it may be common, especially in the medical literature, to divide spirituality and religion, this separation is difficult to maintain upon closer analysis.[xvii] All spiritual practices have underlying presuppositions regarding the nature of humanity and of the universe that can be considered theologies, even if they are latent or unacknowledged. This has led Cadge to astutely conclude that the rhetoric that differentiates spirituality from religion is a "strategically vague frame,"[38 [p. 14]] which is employed to navigate the sacred–secular sociopolitical divide rather than being a conceptually comprehensive position. Those who are motivated to divide spirituality from religion may do so because they have strongly formed negative feelings toward a particular religion like Christianity or Judaism.[9] It may be that they grew up in a particular religious tradition and have rejected those doctrines and/or organizational forms but still maintain some vaguer sense that there is something beyond the material realm.[25] Some with these negative feelings may turn toward forms of spirituality that have arisen precisely in response to the forms of religion that have been consciously rejected. Those who describe themselves as "spiritual, not religious" are often responding to particular theological beliefs, moral codes, or organizational structures that have been found oppressive, objectionable, or hypocritical. The irony, however, is that despite their rhetorical claims, in function they often hold to beliefs that are effectively doctrines and submit on some level to a social organization and hierarchy. For example, if someone believes in the authority of the individual, engages in yoga, and ardently reads Oprah or Deepak Chopra, they may be functionally engaging in religious activity: their belief in their own authority is a socially shared doctrine. Their practice of yoga contains an embedded theology aimed at an internally defined transformation toward salvation.[33] And spiritual gurus hold as much functional authority as clergy do in the lives of traditionally religious people. While people in this group may not acknowledge that their spirituality generates religious structures, it is not difficult to see that these social structures are operative.

In conclusion, there are serious conceptual problems in agreeing to separate spirituality from religion.[xviii] We concur with many who identify conceptual differences between these two constructs but deny that they are separable.[27] Under our approach to spirituality, based on life centered around a chief love, this separation is neither necessary nor possible. While it has become popular to think of spirituality as being an experience that can be isolated and independent from religion, it is precisely at this point that we believe the argument has transitioned to an ideological grind against certain religions. Every spirituality, no matter how seemingly individualistic, depends on external social structures in the form of beliefs, practices, and relationships. Spirituality thus produces functional religion, and religion in turn serves as an embodied infrastructure that every human affection requires in its action. While we recognize that this conclusion contradicts the self-understanding of those who understand themselves as "spiritual, not religious," it is our view that the recent construction of this self-identity is a specific reaction to Western religions. Those who embrace the nonreligious spiritual identity are affirming a nonmaterialist belief system and simultaneously rejecting Western forms of monotheistic spirituality. This experience and perspective is still developing and should be respected. However, the claim that it lacks religious structures or should not be categorized as a religion is, on its face, untenable. Serious conversation about the relationship of religion, spirituality, and medicine will not proceed far if advocates within medicine continue to champion this deeply problematic and flawed construct.

We believe that broadening the understanding of religion and acknowledging the intrinsic link between religion and spirituality will open the door to a more productive discussion regarding the place of spirituality and religion in medicine.

Defining the Scope of Theology

Our approach to spirituality and religion also carries implications for the meaning of theology as an academic discipline, which we will rely upon beginning in the next chapter. Relying on "theology"[xix] may strike readers as a strange turn in argument, especially if we are trying to persuade skeptics. However, the concept of theology is a reflection on what one fundamentally believes to be the truth about reality. That reality shapes how we live, what we consider important, that which deserves our time, and, ultimately, where our affection is centered. If spirituality refers to what is chiefly loved, and religion is in reference to the structures supporting that chief love, then *theology is reflection and reasoning that springs out of a relationship and experience of that chief love*. The goal of theology is simply to enable lovers of that object to more fully and consistently understand, relate to, and show affection for the object of their chief love. As a scholarly discipline, theology concerns itself with a systematic and rigorous form of thinking on understanding what is loved and how to love that object more fully. Correspondingly, practical theology is a reflective practice that especially focuses on obstacles of a chief love and how those obstacles may be overcome.[xx]

Keeping Theology Out of Medicine

We must begin by reconsidering how theology and secular medicine relate to one another. However the secular is specifically defined—and its exact meaning and intent remains debated—it generally refers to a human domain where appeals to nonmaterial realities are denied. In the popular imagination, there is a separation of that which is characterized by its *this worldly* character and that which is set apart unto that which is other worldly. Upon entering the secular, there is a certain type of rationality that is condoned and other kinds of knowledge that are classified as inimical, such as theological reasoning. In a popular account, theology by definition cannot function within secular medicine. The secular is often identified with certain spaces or locations. It also includes certain human relationships and institutions. When applied to the concept of secular medicine, its knowledge, professions, and institutions become fully implicated.

From the viewpoint of secular medicine, spirituality and religion are not denied, despised, or denigrated. Rather, they are separate domains that, within their space and time, have full freedom to exercise whatever pursuits are deemed good and desirable. Certainly, some appear to advance a form of secularism that appears to be motivated by an ideology that seeks to undermine and destroy traditional religious belief. Setting aside strident ideologies, most who adopt a secular medicine do not appear to have an agenda against religion itself[39] but believe that these two domains best function unto themselves, maintaining division to the benefit of both. This more discreet view of the secular is to a degree extremely attractive because of some obvious benefits. One benefit that is rooted in early Hippocratic experience of healing is that the secular lens enabled healers to see more clearly the material cause of some diseases and eventual identification of powerful cures.[40,41] When medicine and spirituality were blurred, spiritual theories became obstacles in properly understanding certain cause-and-effect relationships. Most religious traditions have had a tendency to provide interpretations of disease and healing that created conditions preventing physical healing from taking place. Another obvious benefit is that it creates structures keeping the different religions from fighting or competing with one another.[42] There should be no tolerance for religious wars or acts of power against one another in the realm of illness, where the sick are in desperate need of physical care and compassion. Theology sometimes causes conflict. There are enough of these historical and contemporary examples demonstrating the import of keeping these domains separate.

Medicine Cannot Function Without Certain Theological Presuppositions

On the other hand, advocates of a closer relationship between medicine and spirituality have highlighted how religious rationales have been essential both to medical care and scientific thought. For example, Christian theology was the driving force that created and developed hospitals because this theology sanctified illness as a state where God was especially present rather than, as previously believed, absent.[43-45] With this new theology of illness, the care of the sick became a high privilege and responsibility, rather than deeming the ill as being rightly punished for their sins. With the rise of the scientific method as applied to medicine, a theological belief in a rational God who has created a rational universe has shown itself to be a contingent presupposition for cause-and-effect reasoning.[46] Human recognition of a coherent, cause-and-effect relationship in the material universe developed, not despite of theology, but precisely because of the theological belief in a Rational Creator who inculcated within the universe a reflection of God's rational and orderly nature.[47] While theology has hampered the practice of medicine at certain times and in certain cultures,[44] it has more decisively provided the necessary conditions for societies to embrace their obligation to care for the sick and to employ scientific reasoning in the practice of diagnosis and therapy.[xxi]

Despite these important historical examples illustrating a constructive and beneficial relationship of medicine and theology, it is also the case that historical examples do not prove that there is a necessary or contingent relationship. Secular medicine and its partnership with science could have developed apart from theological presuppositions. There is no counterfactual to prove that one set of beliefs in a culture (theological in nature) spawned another set of beliefs and practices (science and secular medicine). Even so, the relationship should give pause, and it provides the opportunity to more deeply entertain that secular medicine not only needs theology but in fact holds to a theology that undermines its very claim to be secular.

To the degree that our previous chapters have accurately described why spiritual care is infrequent (Chapters 5–7), particularly our understanding of compartmentalization of medicine and religion (Chapter 7), the failure to raise theological perspectives merely supports the de facto position of compartmentalization. Thus, we would ask readers who have journeyed with us thus far to extend patience as we unpack a theology in understanding the separation of medicine, spirituality, and religion. While we understand that many readers will not share with us key theological assumptions, this will not ultimately undermine the direction we encourage readers to deliberate. Whatever your theological presuppositions, we will have been successful merely if readers are willing to consider the underlying grounds for their values and motives as they inform the practice and institutions of medicine.

With these operating understandings of spirituality, religion, and theology in hand, we now turn in the next chapter toward the values of Western religion as they have informed the practice of medicine. Some of these theological values remain latent within contemporary medicine. Nevertheless, there are also other theological ideas functionally operative in medicine that are alien to Western religions, and so the importance of this approach will become clearer in Chapters 11 and 12.

Notes

i. One senior scholar of the study of the sociology of religion remarked in a private meeting, "The definition of religion is wholly uninteresting." What this scholar meant by this statement is that definitions cannot be solved and are therefore not worth serious attention. Although we agree that it is unlikely that there will be academic consensus on conceptualizing religion and spirituality, scholarly attention must continue to adequately attend to and describe underlying definitions when considering spirituality, religion, and related concepts such as the secular. Unfortunately, many scholars within the field of spirituality and health provide definitions but do not justify their views beyond a bare claim. This pattern of not justifying one's definitions harms debate and hinders a constructive move forward. A scholar may not be able to persuade readers to his or her understanding of religion or spirituality, yet it is still incumbent to explain how a particular definition came into view. Being more forthcoming allows fellow thinkers to better understand where a scholar's argument is coming from, what underlying issues are being responded to, see potentially blind spots that may exist, and, finally, locate places of synergy that scholars can build upon to grow consensus. We uphold Ken Pargament as the preeminent example in this regard as he carefully offers ongoing engagement and explanation on how he understands these critical definitions.[6,17] Others have provided an important service to the field by reflecting on a diverse set of definitions and offering strengths and weaknesses.[21]

ii. Some have argued that drug addiction cannot be spirituality because of its destructive nature,[7] but this conclusion seems presumptuous because it assumes certain norms of flourishing based within a particular spirituality.

iii. Though certainly religion does not always serve the spirituality that it claims to serve. One of the many frustrations with certain embodiments of religious structures is that they might fail to serve the heart and soul of a particular spirituality. For example, in the Christian tradition, Jesus railed against outward religious expressions as "whited sepulchers with dead man's bones" (Matthew 23:27). He was naming the problem of when religious structures do not serve the spiritual structures that they claim to serve, but rather an alien spirituality. The important distinction to note here is that though religion may not always serve the spirituality that it claims to serve, this does not mean that it lacks an underlying spirituality.

iv. Substantive definitions demarcate religion from other social constructs based on "beliefs about the nature of reality."[13[p. 102]] One illustration of a primarily substantive definition comes from sociologist Peter Berger, who defines religion as "a belief that there is a reality beyond the reality of ordinary experience, and that this reality is of great significance for human life,"[14 [p. 17]] Built within Berger's definition is the idea that there are two realities, one the mundane and the other a reality beyond the normal that carries "great significance" for humanity. Berger's definition is grounded in a bifurcation of reality in the forms of lower and upper realms, where religion occupies belief in the latter. Another illustration of a primarily substantive definition comes from philosopher Charles Taylor. Though he avoids a formal definition of religion in his book *A Secular Age* (Harvard University Press, 2007), he suggests that religion is primarily concerning the transcendent in contrast to the immanent (Taylor, p. 15). Taylor conceives religion as that activity aimed for human flourishing conceived in terms of dependence upon that which is outside or beyond humanity itself. Berger and Taylor illustrate substantive perspectives on the meaning of religion, which in turn also produces clarity on what is secular or nonreligious. Berger and Taylor each identify religion using slightly different but still substantive criteria of beliefs. Berger identifies religion as a belief in an extraordinary reality with great significance. Taylor's conception of religion is organized by the idea of "transcendence," which refers to a greater good "higher than, beyond human flourishing" and extending beyond the natural cycle of birth and death (Taylor, p. 20). While slightly distinct objects of interest are being identified in these definitions, they are substantive definitions because they identify a specific object that must be necessarily present for it to be "religion."

v. In contrast, functional definitions of religion do not focus on particular object but on the role that a system holds toward a human need or end. The classic functional definition of religion was suggested by sociologist Emile Durkheim who identified religion as beliefs and practices that serve social unity (see E. Durkheim, Cosman C., Cladis M. S. *The elementary forms of religious life*. Oxford/New York: Oxford University Press; 2001). Since Durkheim, multiple proposals have been identified as the critical function of religion including that religion is an instrument for psychological coping and survival (see Malinowski, *A scientific theory of culture*, 1944), creation of stability through value and meaning (see T. Parsons. *The social system*. Glencoe, IL: Free Press; 1951), unifying society via a civil religion (R. N. Bellah, Hammond P. E. *Varieties of civil religion*. 1st ed. San Francisco: Harper & Row; 1980), that which provides a general order of culture (C. Geertz. Religion as a cultural system. In: M. Banton, ed. *Anthropological approaches to the study of religion*. New York: Praeger; 1966:1–46), and what enables the overcoming of struggle with suffering and death (J. M. Yinger. *The scientific study of religion*. New York: Macmillan; 1970). What makes religion is that "it concerns types of needs and satisfactions which can be said to be ultimate and transcendent because they concern those basic features of life and the world which threaten the human condition."[24] In contrast to a substantive perspective, functional definitions assume that religion is a universal phenomenon in every society because its meaning is tied to ultimate human needs and desires.

vi. For example, Zen and Theravada Buddhism are nontheistic but include temples, rituals, priests, monks, pilgrimages, and sacred texts (see W. Herbrechtsmeier. Buddhism and the definition of religion: one more time. *Journal for the Scientific Study of Religion*. 1993;32(1):1–18). Concepts including theism or the superhuman do not apply to these versions of Buddhism, but then to describe these as a philosophy rather than a religion strikes many as a miscategorization (see M. E. Spiro. Religion: problems of definition and explanation. In: M. Bantion, ed. *Anthropological approaches to the study of religion*. London: Tavistock; 1966: 85–126).

vii. The phrase comes from theologian Paul Tillich who taught that religion was about what was of ultimate concern, the object of whom would bring ultimate fulfillment (Paul Tillich, *Theology of culture*. Robert C. Kimball, ed. New York: Oxford University Press, 1964). Tillich asserted, "Religion, in the largest and most basic sense of the word, is ultimate concern" (p. 8). In Marty's estimation, this may include not only self-described religious systems such as Christianity but also ideologies such as Nazism or New Age astrology. For Tillich, as for Marty, the object of ultimate concern varies according to religion, but its distinguishing mark is that which is "ultimate" in contrast to secondary concerns, and from which we find total fulfillment. This perception of ultimacy, in Marty's view, becomes systematized in a social ordering that we typically recognize as a religion. Religion is life centered on what is ultimate and brings total fulfillment. Marty's identification of "ultimate concern" has blended substantive and functional elements into a single identifying principle. Its substantive dimension is the object perceived to be ultimate, and its functional aspect relates to the human fulfillment experienced as one enters the state of being ultimately concerned. The other four characteristics in Marty's definition flow out of this first characteristic.

It may also be clarifying to note that Marty has typically not employed the term "spirituality." His characteristics of religion include the spiritual dimension and the structures of religion. This is common in how most scholars used the term "religion" throughout the twentieth century, in that it was used to apply to a wide range of phenomena that has more recently been associated with spirituality. Thus, there is an equivalency in how Marty uses the term "religion" and our suggested definition that interconnects religion and spirituality.

viii. Pargament offered an updated definition for religion as "the search for significance that occurs within the context of established institutions that are designed to facilitate spirituality."[6]

ix. Also critical to this understanding of religion is its focus on "sacred" rather on than superhuman or supernatural ideas. Pargament's use of "sacred" is near if not identical with Marty's (and Tillich's) meaning of "ultimate concern." The object of religion can vary from traditionally recognized religious concerns such as God or enlightenment, to nontraditional, seemingly ephemeral concerns that are either positive (e.g., family), neutral (e.g., baseball), or negative (e.g., drug addiction). Any object can operate within a person's life as an ultimate concern, taking the status of a sacred object. Life may center on transient objects so that, for a person or groups of people, that object operates for them as the most important thing in life. This is religious in nature, and it functions with the same level of significance that theistic conceptions have within Judaism or Islam. It is also conceivable that social systems operate within a hierarchy of concerns without a single one being ultimate. Multiple objects may thus take on a sacred quality and should be considered simultaneously religious.

x. This is true not only when comparing across religions (e.g., comparing Buddhism to Islam) but also within major world religions such as Christianity. While "Christianity" shares core texts and stories, branches within Christianity relate to their ultimate concern in such diverse ways that it is not always clear to many Christians whether they substantively share the same faith in the same ultimate object.

xi. Oman has shown how religion and spirituality are difficult concepts to technically define because they are generally recognized through prototypical examples rather than core characteristics.[21] By way of analogy, although the concept of "vehicle" is an uncontested concept in human experience, phenomenological studies have shown that certain objects serve as prototypes for recognizing a category with high levels of consensus (e.g., automobile as a type of vehicle), whereas other examples are contested and unclear (e.g., surfboards and blimps as types of vehicles). In a similar fashion, religion and spirituality are general categories that describe a broad array of human phenomenon that have a "family resemblance." While the concept of religion is identified by prototypical examples including Christianity, Hinduism, Judaism, and Islam, other phenomena have been more highly contested including Buddhism, Confucianism, and Marxism. Thus, lack of conceptual clarity is due to ambiguity of the phenomena itself.

xii. Another important issue concerning definitions of religion and spirituality relates to who has authority to name a certain phenomenon as "religious" or "spiritual"? The issue at stake in this question concerns the acceptability of describing a group or a group's practices as religious when participants of that group do not consider themselves or their practices religious. Most would presumably agree that it would be ideal for adherents of a group to be the one's who determine if their group and related practices qualify as religious or spiritual (social scientists have called this the *emic* perspective, because it is an interpretation derived from within the people group). However, issues of motive and underlying power dynamics are at play concerning who names something religious or spiritual and on what grounds. Within Western societies, the Christian Church attempted to control social values and protect herself from outsiders using religious classification as a rationale for certain privileges. Milbank suggests that the Church created the categories of sacred and secular in order to expand its land holdings during the Middle Ages.[16] Religious groups continue to be motivated to self-define themselves as religious in order, for example, to gain tax benefits and be exempt from certain discrimination laws. Those committed to nontheistic worldviews have also been motivated by certain power dynamics attempting to control particular religious groups from exerting social influence over certain legal or political processes.[13] Naming certain groups and activities as religious and others as nonreligious can be motivated to keep religion outside of certain social domains and to exert control based on rationales perceived as "nonreligious." Within this matrix, proponents and antagonists of religion have mutually relied on substantively theistic definitions. Within Western societies, this consensus about what religion consists has generally worked because theistic groups (especially Protestants, Catholics, and Jews) and nontheistic groups have been relatively satisfied with the distribution of power.

There is increasing awareness of religious-like phenomenon through interactions with other cultures, clarifying that theistic definitions are not comprehensive. For example, many Buddhists deny that they are a religion (Herbrechtsmeier. Buddhism and the definition of religion). However, the consensus of religious scholars has been to see Buddhism as a religion, though it does not inherently affirm theism. This is also true of Shintoism and Confucianism, both nontheistic traditions originating in Japan and China, which are nevertheless religion-like when using a functional definition. Most scholars consider these religions even though adherents of them deny this category.

Or consider scholars who have begun analyzing nontheistic movements such as Nationalism, Nazism, or even the New Atheism in terms of describing these as religions. For example, Stephen Prothero claims that dogma espoused by the New Atheism, despite their ardent arguments against the dangers of religion, is itself a de facto religion.[23]

Within American evangelicalism, some, like Billy Graham, claimed that "Christianity is not a religion but a relationship." Others like Dietrich Bonhoeffer advocated for a "religion-less Christianity." For many, this is not merely the rhetoric of zealots but a serious claim on how a relationship with Jesus is *sui generis* and cannot be cataloged with other religions. Some Evangelicals say they are not religious based on notable conceptual reasons and to differentiate themselves from other religious groups. Despite this claim, few people outside of evangelicalism perceive it as a nonreligious phenomenon.

Finally, consider practices of yoga and mindfulness, which have gained wider acceptance even in publically shared arenas such as hospitals and public schools because they are perceived to be secular practices. Religious scholar Candy Brown suggests that proponents of yoga and mindfulness have consciously described their practices as nonreligious in order to gain social acceptance and its related benefits. Brown argues that while practitioners of yoga and mindfulness have been widely successful in describing themselves as nonreligious, on a conceptual level they are clearly based on implicitly religious theories and generated within religious communities.[33]

Each of these examples is a sign that substantive definitions of religion oriented by theism and the supernatural are less convincing than in past times. Many religion-like groups do not perceive themselves to receive the necessary social benefits of being categorized as a religion or religious and have thus been reconceiving categories. There does not appear to be any definition of religion, including ours as "chief love," that can completely sidestep issues of social power and control.

One advantage of a broader definition for religion such as "chief love" is that it does not remove but instead mitigates issues of power around religion by expanding its boundaries. An expanded definition means that everyone has a religion since everyone lives within a hierarchy of loves. Such a perspective changes the jockeying of power between those who conceive themselves as religious and those who do not. We are all religious to the degree that we all seek, serve, and center our lives on what we love most. More narrowly conceived religious definitions amplify social motivations to declare one's group as religious or to purposively avoid this designation. Both create unnecessary categorical distortions and obfuscate phenomenon that are functional similarly. Groups who come under theistically derived conceptions of religion, especially Christians in the United States, will lose a level of power to the degree that they acknowledge nontheistic worldviews as being on par with their own religious beliefs. Room will need to be made in sharing social power with groups currently conceived as nonreligious. Likewise, groups who are currently considered nonreligions will lose a level of social control to the degree that they acknowledge their chief love as being essentially religious in nature.

Those on each side of the religion–secular divide will lose something, but we also might anticipate important gains. First, rather than needing to decipher if something is religious or secular, which we are arguing is intractably arbitrary and based within motives of power, there will be a wider acknowledgment that groups have claims grounded in their own most deeply held loves and concerns self-defined as ultimate or sacred. Social issues of power and control are to be settled on the principle of equity and fairness irrespective of the group's central guiding love. While this may appear like a radical proposal, we will argue in Chapter 12 that a particular spirituality is already operative in medicine but has been disguised by the sacred–secular framework. There will be greater potential fairness and equity for all if we begin to recognize that religion is a far broader construct than what nineteenth-century definitions imagined (see Jonathan Z. "Religion, Religions, Religious." In M. Taylor, *Critical Terms for Religious* Studies. Chicago: University of Chicago Press; 1998:269-284). Second, a broader definition of religion will remove the confusing and unnecessary rhetoric around the relationship between spirituality and religion. Synthetic divisions separating spirituality and religion are partly motivated by power dynamics and have been based on theistic and superhuman conceptions of religion rather than a broad conception of religion.

xiii. Three strategies are theoretically possible when relating spirituality and religion: (1) Spirituality is autonomous and independent from religious tradition. (2) Spirituality is primary, subordinating religion as ontologically second. (3) Spirituality and religion are in an equal, dialectical, and mutually informing relationship. Those who define spirituality and religion based on either the first two options employ what we would describe as an "anthropological approach," which presupposes spirituality to be either independent or primary to religious tradition. Peter Van Ness serves as an example of a scholar who has approached spirituality as fundamentally independent and without necessary engagement with a religious tradition.[27] He argues that spirituality itself is (1) derived phenomenologically rather than metaphysically or institutionally, and (2) it moves toward a psychological telos of human immanence. A preference for anthropological disciplines, sources, and methods results in a practice of spiritual care that subordinates historically rooted, theologically derived religious beliefs, symbols, and expressions.

In contrast, when definitions of or methodological approaches to understanding spirituality and spiritual care are conceptualized as equal to (or less than) other conventional sources, methods, and categories for religion, then we consider this a dialectical model—where spirituality and religion depend on and reinforce one another. Sandra Schneiders serves as an example of a scholar who, while arguing for a significant anthropological component to the study of spirituality, recognizes the important role for the discipline of religiously grounded theology as an interdisciplinary partner with the social sciences. In her view, spirituality and religion form a hermeneutical process in which spirituality and religion mutually work together in describing spiritual experiences, giving them meaning and form, and reevaluating religious theories to ensure that they conform to spiritual experiences (see Sandra Schneiders, "The Study of Christian Spirituality: Contours and Dynamics of a Discipline." In: Elizabeth A. Dreyer and Mark S. Burrows, ed. *Minding the Spirit: The Study of Christian Spirituality*. Baltimore: The Johns Hopkins University Press; 2005: 1-24.).

xiv. This view of spirituality has developed in correspondence with a widening recognition of the diverse cultural and religious practices and beliefs operating in American society. Proponents of this approach suggest that understanding spirituality in this way enables dialogue between different religious groups by emphasizing the common starting point of a shared humanity. The approach has an ability to soften stark differences and avoid unnecessary conflict. Its emphasis can inform and challenge static aspects of a religious tradition's beliefs and practices that fail to adequately account for human experience or new challenges that arise from new contexts. Likewise, this approach leverages its ability to have a more nuanced perspective on human nature and human problems through an interdisciplinary partnership with the social sciences. Finally, an anthropological spirituality aims to include those who do not indisputably fit within religious categories or definitions. Such inclusion, consequently, beneficially enables spiritual care to be provided in pluralistic contexts to those who either do not identify with religion or are for some reason alienated from their religious community.

xv. A consensus conference on spirituality for palliative care thus produced a broad definition of spirituality as the aspect of humanity that refers to the way individuals seek and express meaning and purpose and the way they experience their connectedness to the moment, to self, to others, to nature, and to the significant or sacred.[28] Spirituality may include religion and other worldviews but encompasses far more general ways in which these experiences are expressed, including through the arts, relationships with nature and others, and, for some, through the concept of secular humanism, the latter of which emphasizes reason, scientific inquiry, individual freedom and responsibility, human values, compassion, and the needs for tolerance and cooperation. Our definition of "chief love" or "ultimate love" differs from this definition in that the adjectives of "chief" and "ultimate" are absent from the 2009 Consensus Conference. In their absence, spirituality is impossible to consistently identify .

xvi. Robert Wuthnow in *After Heaven*[9] has helpfully argued that those who are classified in the group that he calls a "spirituality of seeking" have falsely understood themselves to be anti-institutional. He shows that no spirituality, no matter how individualistic it first appears, can exist without strong and deep institutional supports coming from, for example, publishing houses and generic spirituality authors, academic and spirituality centers, and small groups of people who gather to support themselves in their spiritual quest. Wuthnow's analysis supports how spirituality and religion are ultimately inseparable.

xvii. Some have critiqued an anthropological approach to spirituality and spiritual care because it can dehistoricize spirituality[20] (see also B. J. Zinnbauer, Pargament K. I., Kadar J. L. Religion and spirituality: unfuzzying the fuzzy. *Journal for the Scientific Study of Religion*. 1997;36(4):549–564), incorrectly envision spirituality as being noninstitutional and atheological[9] (see also J. J. Kotva. Hospital chaplaincy as agapeic intervention. *Christian Bioethics*. 1998;4(3):257–275), soften the identity and religious integrity of patients and practitioners (see Kotva. Hospital chaplaincy as agapeic intervention; S. Pattison. Dumbing down the spirit. In: Orchard H, ed. *Spirituality in health care contexts*. Philadelphia: Jessica Kingsley Publishers; 2001:33–46, 37; T. N. Fawcett, Noble A. The challenge of spiritual care in a multi-faith society experienced as a Christian nurse. *J Clin Nurs*. 2004;13(2):136–142), and can diminish spirituality into a functional tool subservient to bodily health.[37]

Moreover, those who resist the autonomy and/or primacy of anthropological definitions of spirituality are concerned that without complementary approaches to understanding spirituality, such as the historical-contextual and theological, the anthropological approach to understanding spirituality risks an unhealthy reductionism of knowledge (see C. Wolfteich. Devotion and the struggle for justice in the farm worker movement: a practical theological approach to research and teaching in spirituality. *Spiritus*. 2005;5(2):158–175) and may degenerate into "enthusiastic chaos, dangerous aberrations, or anemia" (S. Schneiders. Theology and spirituality: strangers, rivals, or partners? *Horizons*. 1986;12(2):253–274).

Thus, other spirituality scholars have argued for a dialectical and interdependent relationship between religion and spirituality[3,4,7] (see also S. Schneiders. A hermeneutical approach to Christian spirituality. In: E. A. Burrows, ed. *Minding the spirit: the study of Christian spirituality*. Baltimore: Johns Hopkins University Press; 2005:49–60; C. Wolfteich. Graceful work: practical theological study of spirituality. *Horizons*. 2000;27(1):7–21; and C. Wolfteich. Spirituality and social sciences. In: P. Sheldrake, ed. *The new Westminster dictionary of Christian spirituality*. 1st American ed. Louisville, KY: Westminster John Knox Press; 2005:68–73).

Likewise, building on the viewpoint that human spirituality is independent of religion and theology, some have argued that spiritual care can be given autonomously from theology and religious tradition (see G. Schmidt Kwa. A Christian for the Christians, a Muslim for the Muslims? Reflections on a Protestant view of pastoral care for all religions. *Christian Bioethics*. 1998;4(3):239–256; L. VandeCreek, Burton L. Professional chaplaincy: its role and importance in healthcare. *Journal of Pastoral Care*. 2001;55(1):81–97).

However, against an independent or an anthropologically primary practice of spiritual care, others have claimed that the nature of spiritual care must be informed by religious traditions and theological language and methods (see Pattison. Dumbing down the spirit; B. Miller-McLemore. Revisiting the living human web: theological education and the role of clinical pastoral education. *The Journal of Pastoral Care and Counseling*. 2008;62(1-2):3–17; C. Tollefsen. Meta ain't always betta': conceptualizing the generic chaplaincy issue. *Christian Bioethics*. 1998;4(3):305–315; B. Holifield. *A history of pastoral care in America: from salvation to self-realization*. Nashville: Abingdon Press; 1983; W. B. Oglesby. Theological education and the pastoral care movement, Protestant. In: J. Rodney, Hunter N. J. R., ed. *Dictionary of pastoral care and counseling*. Nashville: Abingdon Press; 2005:1261).

xviii. It is important to emphasize a distinction between popular or folk usage of a term (the *emic* interpretation) and an informed, scholarly understanding of a topic (an *etic* interpretation based on an outside observer). Within popular usage in Western cultures, the idea of religion has remained closely tied to nineteenth-century Christian views of religion, often conceiving of Judaism and Christianity as the prototype religions and comparing all others to them.[13] As a remnant of this heritage, most continue to conceive of the term in some reference to God and other superhuman beings (argued recently by Christian Smith).[15]

    Nevertheless, there are signs that this consensus of definition is fraying. Many scholars of religion have long-recognized that limiting religion to either God or the superhuman is based on an arbitrary consensus that leaves out swaths of human phenomena. A proliferation of functional definitions of religion beginning with Durkheim have been signs of correction toward the arbitrariness of Enlightenment conceptions of religion. While functional definitions such as the one employed by Geertz have not become widely accepted on a popular level, they are more widely embraced in academic religious circles because they are, on their face, conceptually sounder than supernaturally based substantive definitions.

xix. Practical theology refers to a meta-theological discipline involving four processes: (1) understanding the problem or question relying on nontheological disciplines (especially the empirical sciences) to describe the problem; (2) discerning the problem or question by turning to a theological tradition, including its fundamental beliefs and practices, in order to clarify truth in response to the problem or question; (3) imagining with practical proposals a correlation that yields human flourishing that transforms the situation in faithfulness and truthfulness; and (4) testing critically those proposals in their ability to bring about human fulfillment. Our approach has been informed by others[10] (including J. Swinton, Mowatt H. *Practical theology and qualitative research*. London: SCM: 2006; J. N. Poling, Miller DE. *Foundations for a practical theology of ministry*. Nashville: Abingdon Press; 1985).

xx. Clearly, it is the case that the term "theology" has primarily been a Western concept that literally means "the study of God" and harkens back to Greek philosophy preceding the rise of Christianity. For spiritual traditions that identify God or gods as their chief love, "theology" continues to be a fitting term that describes this activity of systematic reflection. For those with a chief love that excludes the divine, the term is somewhat anachronistic if taken literally. Irrespective of the term or its background, it is the activities represented by the term, which continue to hold an important position to the degree that it reflects systematic thinking about a chief love. If reconceptualized in this manner, metaphysical philosophy becomes a field of study that is difficult to differentiate from theology.

xxi. This theology in the West created the conditions necessary for science to operate and flourish. Since God's character is governed by order and reason, then the creation which reflects God's character will also operate with order and reason. The scientific method requires a presupposition that there is a cause-and-effect relationship between objects, even if there is no clear or obvious connection. For science to successfully proceed, it assumes there must be a connection, and so science continues in pursuit of identification of a causative relationship even after many frustrating attempts of understanding fail, believing that discovery will take place with enough time and systematic effort. Such a disposition to underlying reasons and connections in the natural order were formed through theological reflection on God's nature.

References

1. Nancy T. Ammerman. Spiritual but not religious? Beyond binary choices in the study of religion. *J Sci Study Relig.* 2013;52(2):258–278.

2. Meredith B. McGuire. *Lived religion: faith and practice in everyday life.* Oxford/New York: Oxford University Press; 2008.

3. Bernard McGinn. The letter and the Spirit: spirituality as an academic discipline. In: E. Dreyer, Burrows M. S., eds. *Minding the Spirit: the study of Christian spirituality.* Baltimore: Johns Hopkins University Press; 2005:25–41.

4. Philip Sheldrake. *Spirituality and theology: Christian living and the doctrine of God.* London: Darton, Longman & Todd; 1998.

5. National Consensus Project. *NCP Clinical Practice Guidelines for Quality Palliative Care.* 3rd:http://ww.nationalconsusproject.org/guideline.pdf. Accessed March 28, 2013.

6. Kenneth I. Pargament. *APA handbook of psychology, religion, and spirituality.* Washington, DC: American Psychological Association; 2013.

7. Sandra M. Schneiders. Religion vs. spirituality: a contemporary conundrum. *Spiritus.* 2003;3:163–185.

8. Harold G. Koenig, King Dana E., Carson Verna Benner. *Handbook of religion and health.* 2nd ed. Oxford/New York: Oxford University Press; 2012.

9. Robert Wuthnow. *After heaven: spirituality in America since the 1950s.* Berkeley: University of California Press; 1998.

10. Don S. Browning. *A fundamental practical theology: descriptive and strategic proposals.* Minneapolis, MN: Fortress Press; 1991.

11. Daniel P. Sulmasy. *The rebirth of the clinic: an introduction to spirituality in health care.* Washington, DC: Georgetown University Press; 2006.

12. Wendy Cadge. *Paging God: religion in the halls of medicine.* Chicago/London: University of Chicago Press; 2012.

13. William T. Cavanaugh. *The myth of religious violence: secular ideology and the roots of modern conflict.* Oxford/New York: Oxford University Press; 2009.

14. Peter Berger. *The many altars of modernity.* Boston: De Gruyter; 2014.

15. Christian Smith. *Religion: what it is, how it works, and why it is still important.* Princeton, NJ: Princeton University Press; 2017.

16. John Milbank. *Theology and social theory: beyond secular reason.* Cambridge, MA: Blackwell; 1990.

17. Kenneth I. Pargament. *The psychology of religion and coping: theory, research, practice.* New York: Guilford Press; 1997.

18. Martin E. Marty, Moore Jonathan. *Politics, religion, and the common good: advancing a distinctly American conversation about religion's role in our shared life.* 1st ed. San Francisco: Jossey-Bass Publishers; 2000.

19. David Tracy. *Blessed rage for order, the new pluralism in theology.* New York: Seabury Press; 1975.

20. D. E. Hall, Koenig H. G., Meador K. G. Conceptualizing "religion": How language shapes and constrains knowledge in the study of religion and health. *Perspect Biol Med.* 2004;47(3):386–401.

21. Doug Oman. Defining religion and spirituality. In: R. F. Paloutzian, Park C. L., eds. *Handbook of the psychology of religion and spirituality.* New York: Guilford Press; 2013:23–47.

22. Huston Smith. *The world's religions: our great wisdom traditions.* San Francisco: Harper Collins; 1991.

23. Stephen R. Prothero. *God is not one: the eight rival religions that run the world--and why their differences matter.* 1st ed. New York: HarperOne; 2010.

24. Peter B. Clarke, Byrne Peter. *Religion defined and explained.* New York: St. Martin's Press; 1993.

25. Elizabeth Spencer-Smith. Eclectic spirituality. In: John Peteet, D'Ambra Michael, eds. *The soul of medicine: spiritual perspectives in clinical practice.* Baltimore: Johns Hopkins University Press; 2011:133–151.

26. Harold G. Koenig. *Medicine, religion, and health: where science and spirituality meet.* West Conshohocken, PA: Templeton Foundation Press; 2008.

27. Peter H. Van Ness. *Spirituality and the secular quest*. New York: Crossroad; 1996.

28. C. Puchalski, Ferrell B., Virani R., Otis-Green S., Baird P., Bull J., Chochinov H., Handzo G., Nelson-Becker H., Prince-Paul M., Pugliese K., Sulmasy D. Improving the quality of spiritual care as a dimension of palliative care: the report of the Consensus Conference. *J Palliat Med.* 2009;12(10):885–904.

29. D. E. Hall, Meador K. G., Koenig H. G. Measuring religiousness in health research: review and critique. *J Relig Health.* 2008;47(2):134–163.

30. J. R. Peteet, Balboni M. J. Spirituality and religion in oncology. *CA Cancer J Clin.* 2013;63(4):280–289.

31. Jeffrey Paul Bishop. *The anticipatory corpse: medicine, power, and the care of the dying*. Notre Dame, IN: University of Notre Dame Press; 2011.

32. Claire Wolfteich. Spirituality and social sciences. In: P. Sheldrake, ed. *The new Westminster dictionary of Christian spirituality*. 1st American ed. Louisville, KY: Westminster John Knox Press; 2005:68–73.

33. Candy Gunther Brown. *The healing gods: complementary and alternative medicine in Christian America*. New York: Oxford University Press; 2013.

34. Jeffrey P. Bishop. Biopsychosociospiritual medicine and other political schemes. *Christ Bioeth.* 2009;15(3):254–276.

35. Jeffrey P. Bishop. Of idolatries and ersatz liturgies: the false gods of spiritual assessment. *Christ Bioeth.* 2013;19(3):332–347.

36. M. Therese Lysaught. Beguiling religion: the bifurcations and biopolitics. In: J. Levin, Meador K., eds. *Healing to all their flesh*. West Conshocken, PA: Templeton Press; 2012:150–187.

37. Joel James Shuman, Meador Keith G. *Heal thyself: spirituality, medicine, and the distortion of Christianity*. New York: Oxford University Press; 2003.

38. Wendy Cadge. *Paging God: religion in the halls of medicine*. Chicago/London: The University of Chicago Press; 2012.

39. Richard P. Sloan. *Blind faith: the unholy alliance of religion and medicine*. 1st ed. New York: St. Martin's Press; 2006.

40. Roy Porter. Religion and medicine. In: W. F. Bynum, Porter R., eds. *Companion encyclopedia of the history of medicine*. Vol 2. New York: Routledge; 1994:1449–1468.

41. Roy Porter. *The greatest benefit to mankind: a medical history of humanity*. 1st American ed. New York: W. W. Norton; 1998.

42. Wolfhart Pannenberg. How to think about secularism. *First Things*. 1996; June: https://www.firstthings.com/article/1996/1906/1002-how-to-think-about-secularism.

43. Gary B. Ferngren. *Medicine & health care in early Christianity*. Baltimore: Johns Hopkins University Press; 2009.

44. Gary B. Ferngren. *Medicine and religion: a historical introduction*. Baltimore: Johns Hopkins University Press; 2014.

45. Jean-Claude Larchet. *The theology of illness*. Crestwood, NY: St. Vladimir's Seminary Press; 2002.

46. Gary B. Ferngren. *Science and religion: a historical introduction*. 2nd ed. Baltimore: Johns Hopkins University Press; 2017.

47. Lesslie Newbigin. *Foolishness to the Greeks: the Gospel and western culture*. Grand Rapids, MI: W. B. Eerdmans Pub.; 1986.

|| 9 ||

Toward a Theology of Medicine

Introduction

In this chapter, we transition from a general discussion of definitions of religion to the particular religious traditions that have deeply influenced Western medicine. How have these traditions shaped medicine and the care of the sick? In this chapter, we examine the Abrahamic or monotheistic traditions, especially Judaism and Christianity, but also Islam, since these are the primary spiritual traditions that have historically most influenced Western medicine.[1] This relationship has tangible and ongoing effects in American medicine including many of the hospital institutions that currently exist, but, even more importantly, certain assumed values that have somewhat continued into contemporary practice.

These religious values have served as the foundation for care in Europe and the United States, but these values are also fraying because the effects of the partnership, which were once omnipresent and mostly assumed, have been diminished by rival considerations showcased by market forces, the bureaucratic role of government, and the rise of medical technology. What is too often not adequately recognized is that lying behind these social forces is a powerful spirituality that rejects and has replaced the Abrahamic traditions.[i] The values embedded in secular social forces will only become clearer, however, when they are situated in comparison to these traditional spiritual values that have carried Western medicine for two millennia.

In this chapter, we suggest that within medicine's partnership with the Abrahamic traditions there were three foundational values informing why and how medicine should be practiced in caring for the sick. These capture the original and most widely regarded motives driving medical practice. These include that (1) the human body and soul must be treated together, (2) that hospitality is the foundational motive driving clinicians and hospitals, and (3) that medicine is a divine gift. The Abrahamic traditions imbued into medicine these understandings, justifying medicine's proper use based on theological grounds. This theology is most clearly embedded in early encounters with Hippocratic medicine, which pushed Jewish and Christian thinkers to articulate perspectives that have penetrated these traditions from that time onward. The purpose of this chapter in our larger argument is to highlight how the Abrahamic traditions approached illness and medicine in order to better contextualize subsequent chapters that compare these traditional Western religious values to secular medicine.

The Synthesis Between Medicine and Monotheism

Why have the Abrahamic religions not only accepted the physician's art but equally incorporated it as part of their own traditions of care of the sick? It is because these religious groups have perceived physicians and medicine as a God-given gift to humanity, embedded within the creation,[ii] in addressing our suffering bodies. God's wisdom is the singular source of medicine, and thus physicians as its ministers should be received as a sign of God's loving mercy in response to our broken condition. Credit belongs to God, not physicians, who are mere servants of God's healing mercies. Such conclusions can be seen early on in both Jewish and Christian writings, and later in Islam. We discuss how each of these traditions interacted with medicine and have continued to exert influence.

Judaism and Ben Sira

In light of Israel's difference from other nations,[iii] Judaism resisted physicians and the medical arts because they were associated with idolatrous magic and because turning to medicine has the appearance of rejecting the belief that God alone heals (Exodus 15:26). In the Ancient Near Eastern understanding surrounding Mesopotamia, knowledge of medicines were originally associated with celestial beings, who revealed the mystery of the cutting of roots to heal to capture man's worship.[iv] Thus, Judaism was resistant to shamanistic (2 Chronicles 16:12) and Greek medicine[v] because it was strongly allied with spiritual mediums and magical remedies.

Responding to these religious worries in approximately in 180 B.C., Ben Sira, a Jewish scribe, provided a theological perspective on why the faith community should receive the physician's art.[2 [p. 8],3 [p. xxii]] The Hellenization of Judaism and its initial exposure to Greek medicine led Ben Sira to instruct his Jewish readers to: *"Make friends with the physician for. . . him also God has established in his profession"* (Ben Sira 38:1).[2 [pp. 438–439]] This affirmation of Hippocratic physicians by Ben Sira specifically addresses several key Jewish concerns about the embrace of medicine.

First, Ben Sira affirms the axiomatic belief that God alone is healer: "My son, when you are ill, delay not, but pray to God, for *it is he who heals*" (38:9). Ben Sira makes it clear that by recognizing the medical profession, he continues to affirm the Torah's teaching that Yahweh alone is their Redemptive-Healer.[vi] Ben Sira also affirms a traditional spiritual piety among the ill as part of their religious response to God.[vii]

Second, this foundational affirmation results in an embrace rather than a rejection of the profession of Hippocratic medicine. The affirmation is based upon several points that position medicine within a theological framework that perceives God as the fount, means, and ends of medicine:

1. The wisdom exercised by physicians comes from God who is its source. "From God the doctor has his wisdom" (38:2).
2. The medicinal agents discovered and used in the medical arts are part of God's continuing "creative work" (38:8) in which God "makes the earth yield healing herbs" (38.4). God is the source of medicinal agents, not humanity. The Torah itself

recognizes nonmiraculous *means* in which God provides healing. Again, Ben Sira appeals to Exodus 15:25, the verse immediately preceding the aforementioned foundational text, in which the bitter waters were made drinkable when Moses cast a tree into the water by God's command. Ben Sira is clearly identifying the use of a tree—given its organic and potential medicinal powers—as a divine endorsement of pharmacological agents. God's command to Moses to use a tree for "healing" in Exodus consequently does not undermine the theological claim that Yahweh is Redemptive-Healer, but, according to Ben Sira, it establishes its wise use as complementary to the Lord, Israel's Healer.

4. The glory does not go to the physician but to God who manifests his "mighty works" through medicine (38:6). It is to God's glory that medicine points, since healing through medical means is a testimony of God's providential display of power and mercy.

Last, a spiritual piety is not reserved for patients alone in Ben Sira's view, but will also be realized in the practice of spiritually minded physicians. The kind of physicians defended by Ben Sira are those who plead in prayer before God that (1) their diagnosis is accurate and (2) that their therapy is curative (38:14). In this way, the physician's art is infused with the practitioner's reliance upon divine wisdom and therapeutic potency. The physician does not claim special authority or power implicitly in self through either special knowledge or office or in appeal to foreign gods, but relies upon Israel's God for special attendance within medical practice. Especially through prayer, the physician's practice becomes permeated with God's revelation: "I am the LORD, who heals you" (Exodus 15:26). Similarly, when the patient is cured, the physician gives "glory in [God's] mighty works" (38:6). From Ben Sira's perspective, prayer to Yahweh who heals is the most decisive mark of a faithful and pious practice of medicine. Ben Sira's argument implies that, without the physician's heartfelt prayer as part of medical practice, a rational medicine stands at odds with Torah.

The theological perspective of Ben Sira has been generally affirmed throughout the Jewish tradition with emphasis on "a reverence for life, a belief in the sacredness of health, and a life-defining conviction that illness is an evil to be banished." There is a moral obligation to provide healing, for example, taken from Leviticus 19:16, where we are "not to stand idly by the blood of one's kinsman."[4] [p. 30] Jewish understanding of the doctrine of the image of God (*imago Dei*) was interpreted to mean that human life, in a psychosomatic unity, "possessed intrinsic value" in reflecting God's nature.[5] [p. 98] Within this tradition embodied in Maimonides' prayer,[6] bodily sickness and health were both secondary goods ordered on behalf of the spiritual life. The physician's vocation of restoring physical health was not a good unto itself, but was pursued, according to the tradition of Maimonides, "in order that his soul be upright to know the Lord."[7],viii This sentiment has led Jewish physicians to be carried by a deep charity to the poor.[8] [p. 18] "Personal concern for the poor and needy was an important theme in the Hebrew scriptures," Ferngren notes, which instilled in later Judaism the conviction "that almsgiving is a duty and even the highest virtue."[5] [p. 98] Physician services should be paid for, but it was such a human good that should never be withheld from the poor. In certain contexts during the Middle Ages, Jewish physicians even risked their own lives caring for Christians because of local church prohibitions against Christians seeking medical care from Jews.[8] [p. 17] This trend has continued in more recent times; speaking before the American Medical Association in 1964, Rabbi Heschel described physicians as partners with God and medical healing as the "highest form of *imitation Dei*."[4] [p. 33]

Jesus and Early Christian Interpreters

Reflecting on the teachings of Jesus, many Christians concluded that love for the sick was an act reflecting divine love (*agape*), first among the persons in the Trinitarian Godhead (John 15:9-10; 17:26), and then extending from God in Christ given to humanity (Romans 5:9; 8:39; 1 John 3:1) in the form of a Spirit-generated act (1 Corinthians 13) of a self-emptying love (Philippians 2:1-8) in the incarnation, crucifixion, and resurrection of Jesus (John 3:16; Ephesians 5:10). From the love of God in Christ, Christians were commanded to share in this love between Christians (Colossians 1:4; Hebrews 6:10; 1 John 4:8) and extending outwardly to include neighbors (Luke 11:42; Romans 13:10), enemies (Matthew 5:43-44), and the physically needy (1 Corinthians 13:3; 1 John 3:17). Caring for the sick, including the stranger, with agape love was part of the central logic that was a response to Christ's sacrificial love. To love was Jesus' new command (John 13:34).

Jesus' parable of the Good Samaritan, recorded by Luke, who was a physician himself (Colossians 4:14), provided moral clarity that one's neighbor includes anyone who had need (Luke 19:29–37). In this well-known parable, the Samaritan traveler had "compassion" on the Jewish man who was left half-dead by robbers. He then bandaged the man's wounds, applying medicinal agents of "oil and wine." At his own expense the Samaritan provided ongoing care in order for the man to get better. The parable ends with Jesus exhorting, "Go and do likewise." Jesus' teaching was seen by many as an implicit endorsement to care for the sick and authorization to employ medicinal agents in binding the wounds of others. Similarly, Jesus emphasis on corporeal acts of mercy, including the visitation of the sick, served as a powerful motivation for Christians to commit themselves to radical acts of mercy and compassion to the sick (Matthew 25:34–40).[ix] In the second and third centuries, this would lead to Christians earning a reputation for radical acts of love to those facing plague and "an active program of palliative care through hundreds of churches in cities throughout the Roman Empire."[5] [p. 145]

From the beginning of Jesus' message, Christians responded to the call to have compassion on the sick. These responses varied from healing miracles reported by Jesus' followers after Christ's resurrection, to the establishment of the diaconal office and its efforts to care for the needy and sick (Acts 7), to early hospice efforts among plague victims. A Christian integration of Hippocratic medicine followed a different course from the integration represented in the Ben Sira text because Hippocratic medicine was more firmly aligned with the Asclepian healing cult in the second and third centuries A.D.[x] It was not until the fourth century A.D. and thereafter,[xi] with a cessation of state persecution after 313 A.D.,[xii] that the Christian church clearly began to systematically employ[xiii] Hippocratic medicine as a partner in its *agape* mission of compassion for the sick.

One of the most influential early Christian engagements with Hippocratic medicine came from the instructions and practice of Basil, Bishop of Caesarea (d. 379). Two important aspects of Basil's legacy include his instruction to monastic communities concerning the use of medicine in his *Long Rules*[xiv] and the establishment of the first hospital in approximately 371 A.D. Basil's merger of health care and Christian mission has had a long-term effect on both Eastern and Western monasticism[xv]—including a substantial impact on Benedict's monastic vision—having a ripple effect in subsequent centuries in Christian thinking and practice.

Basil was trained in and practiced Hippocratic medicine but apparently refused its oath because of the Hippocratic Oath's pledge to Greek gods.[9] Toward the end of his life, after becoming archbishop, he started what most consider the first hospital[xvi] on the outskirts of Caesarea (in modern day Turkey)—described triumphantly by his eulogist as the "new city" since it was a relatively massive complex which modeled the highest Christian ideals of an archetypical city grounded in a church-governed institution guided by Christian love.[10,11] [xvii] Basil's personal familiarity and comfort with Hippocratic medicine[xviii] combined with the social conditions of rising poverty,[xix] changes within local government and citizenship laws,[xx] implications associated with theological debates,[xxi] and the elevated status of church bishops to engender a new alliance between Christian discipleship and the use of medicine.

Governing Basil's understanding of physicians and the medical arts are three theological concerns, highlighted as critical in order for Christianity to partner with medicine. These are an understanding of medicine as a gift of God; an interpretation of medicine as mirroring the salvation of the soul; and ordering medicine, not as an end in itself, but in relation to God as the true *telos*.

First, medicine is described as a gift of God aimed at addressing bodily infirmities that are ultimately due to human brokenness as a result of the Fall. The practice of medicine is comparable to other arts such as agriculture and clothes-making, both directly mentioned as part of the curse in Genesis 3, given partly "to relieve the ills which came of the curse." God made medicinal herbs out of his benevolent will for our help, for they did not according to Basil "sprout from the ground of their own accord."

Second, Basil stresses that medicine is a "pattern for the healing of the soul." This idea is mentioned six times in *Long Rules* 55 and permeates his entire argument. As a pattern, medicine's primary purpose in God's economy is to illustrate spiritual realities and truths to the sick. Basil gives several examples in order to be clear. Hippocratic medicine, grounded in the theory of humor excess and deficiency, illustrates the spiritual reality in which the soul is "advised to remove what is in excess or to make up what is lacking." This statement captures the alliance between Hippocratic theory and theology—the reference to "excess" and "lack" allude to the humor-based understanding of health and disease. Another medical example according to Basil includes painful medical procedures and "bitter drugs," which show how we must "accept the cutting effects of the word that exposes and the bitter drugs of penalties for the cure of the soul." Likewise, chronic diseases teach us that spiritual healing may take a long time and require "sustained prayer and prolonged repentance and a more laborious struggle than reason would suggest to us is sufficient for our healing." Basil spiritualizes medicine and disease, not in order to merely justify the use of medicine, but as an axiomatic principle ordering its God-given intention. This means that when medicine for the body is not directly teaching and forming the soul, then it is by definition not in accord "with the goal of piety" and, consequently, should not be relied upon. In Basil's view, physical health and healing were secondary goods serving and subject to the primary good of eternal salvation. Temporary disease and healing provide a hermeneutic for comprehending and experiencing spiritual truths.[12] Consequently, the entire medical profession became "one of Basil's most enduring analogies" for the care of the soul.[13 [p. 264]] It functioned similarly to a sacrament,[xxii] and, when a spiritual *telos* was not present, then medicine was useless and had no spiritual value. So, while Basil acknowledged that medicine was originally established in God's creative order, medicine's true, hidden purpose culminates in the way that it follows the pattern of Christian salvation and its applications for the advancement of the spiritual life. In Basil's view, Hippocratic medicine could only be rightly understood as a divinely created art that ultimately pointed to the story of the Bible culminating in Jesus Christ.

Third, Basil argues that medicine is finite so that health is not an end in itself but is ordered by our true and final *telos* or end in God. He calls those who completely "avoid the benefit of medicine" as having a "contentious spirit." God may use "means" in order to "accomplish the grace of healing," as in the case of King Hezekiah (whose healing came through the application of figs—2 Kings 20:7) or healing may come "invisibly." For Basil, the key is emphasizing the source of healing instead of focusing on its medium. The benefit of healing through means such as medicine is that, when rightly interpreted, it "often leads us to a keener perception of the Lord's grace." However, there are also important limits to the right use of medicine stressed by Basil. Physical health and healing should not be pursued to the extent that it "turns our whole life into one long provision for the flesh." In other words, the pursuit of bodily health and healing should not be an end in itself. Signs of misuse of the art include considering physicians as "saviors," placing all of one's hope in the power of medicine, "expecting medical remedies for every disease" by operating under a "craze for bodily health," and considering medicine as the only means for healing. In contrast, the right use of medicine must always give credit to God when healing takes place, should not exclude other forms of healing practices,[xxiii] must always serve the formation of the soul, and is an important moment within illness to discern why God has permitted it.[xxiv] Each are important factors when considering the proper ordering of medicine.

Deep Motives Behind Medical Care

Within the classical world that birthed Hippocratic medicine, according to medical historian Gary Ferngren, few felt any obligation to care for the poor or particular persons in need of care.[5] The obligation fell on family to care for their own during illness. Those without family protectors had little recourse or expectation to be protected or cared for during time of need. Kindness toward strangers was not the norm. Moreover, the Greek sense of philanthropy was focused not on an individual, but on gifts given to the entire community.[5 [pp. 89–90]] Motivations for philanthropy, including among physicians, was normed by personal honor and glory (*philodoxia*).[5 [p. 90]] Plato argued that even if physicians practice medicine out of self-interest and financial gain, this was irrelevant so long as the physician's technical competence resulted in the good of the patient.[5 [p. 91]] Moreover, human worth was not inherent to being human, but a dignity that was earned by being virtuous.[5 [p. 95]] Thus, in classical thought, many who lacked status or were not formed in the virtues could not claim human dignity. This included the unborn, orphans, slaves, and the physically handicapped.[5] [p. 96]

Building upon a Hebrew understanding of *imago Dei*, Christian philanthropy rejected *quid pro quo* motivations of self-interest, advancing instead a radical vision of *agape* or divinely motived love offered to all including "the least of these." This new ethic understood every person, irrespective of class, race, or gender (Galatians 3:28), as holding intrinsic value in the new humanity accomplished through the eschatological work of Christ. Christ's teaching about one's neighbor, explained in the parable of the Good Samaritan, demonstrated that love of the sick must cross ethnic and religious barriers. The lives of the most vulnerable were to be protected and loved because God's love goes beyond one's own family and community, extending even to those we are most prone to depersonalize or objectify. The ethic of *agape* was equally imperative since Christians, influenced by the ascetic and Nicene tradition, viewed hoarding temporary material goods to be inconsistent with a God who united the divine nature with human nature in the doctrine of Christ's incarnation. God's fusion with humanity was not with mankind in a state of human power and royalty, but with the lowliest and despised, as exemplified by those whom Christ identified as his representatives.[14]

> Then the righteous will answer him, saying, "Lord, when did we see you hungry and feed you, or thirsty and give you drink? And when did we see you a stranger and welcome you, or naked and clothe you? And when did we see you sick or in prison and visit you?" And the King will answer them, "Truly, I say to you, as you did it to one of the least of these my brothers, you did it to me." (Matthew 25:31–46)

For those in the monastic tradition, Christ's teaching meant that caring for the sick, housing them, and employing the medical arts for their benefit were pious acts of devotion and worship of God. This was a radical departure from Greek models of caregiving, altering how medicine would be used and who it was intended for. For example, in the Benedictine tradition of the sixth century, which spread throughout Western Europe and held influence for a millennia, the *Rule of St. Benedict* upheld the care of the sick as "before" and "above" all things, so that the sick were treated as if the sick person were Christ himself.[15] [ch. 36] Embedded within this care was an emphasis on self-effacement before strangers, including the sick visiting the monastery. Humility in the presence of the sick was considered a top priority. Beginning with the Superior or Abbot, the entire community would receive strangers with bowed heads or with "the whole body prostrated on the ground in adoration of Christ, who indeed is received in their persons."[15] [ch. 53] The ethic of the hospital resided in this groundswell of humble agape and honor given to strangers, many of whom were the rejected of society. The care of strangers, especially the sick, fueled an ethos of hospitality, a virtue applied to these new spaces which came to be called hospitals.[16] In Eastern expressions of Christianity, championed by Chrysostom, Gregory of Nazianzus, and Basil, during the fourth century, this same ethic was applied to lepers, from whom social stigma was removed and who were ironically seen within the religious-medical sphere as persons who "bring holiness and healing from spiritual diseases to those who touched them in order to assist them."5 [p. 103] This perspective clearly elevated the sick role, with the result that the ill were no longer viewed primarily in terms of being the just recipients of God's retribution, but rather as a fount of God's presence, able to bestow holiness upon the caregivers who serve them.

Islamic Medicine

Many of the ideas found in Jewish and Christian dispositions toward the sick are similarly embedded within the later rise of Islamic medicine after the seventh century A.D. There is dignity and unity among humans, so that wrongly killing one is to kill all: "And whoever saves one—it is as if he had saved mankind entirely" (Qur'an 5,32). Thus, the sick are counted among those who are to be cared for and helped, not discarded or abandoned. While illness was seen as part of God's will, the sick are not to be blamed for their illness: "If God touches you with affliction, no one can remove it except Him" (Qur'an 6,17–18). Muslims are obligated to care for the body as a divine gift, and this led to a natural alliance with Hippocratic medicine. Medicine itself was seen as part of God's will, as expressed by one Hadith: "There is a medicine for every ailment such that if a right medicine hits a corresponding ailment, health is restored by God's permission."17 [p. 34] Within medieval Islam, hospitals were well-endowed institutions supported by the wealthy, especially as acts of charity. This led to philanthropic endowments of hospital institutions (*waqf*) in order to ensure their perpetuity.1 [p. 128] As acts of philanthropy, the wealthy were especially motivated by the promise of divine merit, based within the purifying, religious act of *zakat*, one of the five pillars of Islam.

Islam has produced prominent physicians throughout its history, and many historians point out that medieval Islam played a critical role in maintaining Western (Galenic) medicine during a decline in Christian knowledge during this period. The physician or the *hakim*, which literally means "wise one," has always been a highly esteemed social position within Islam. To this day, Muslim physicians hold some of the highest positions within Islamic cultures, regarded as a service second only to faith in God itself (Rahman, 38).17 [p. 38] Patients should consider physicians "better than their best friends."17 [p. 93] The term *hakim* is one of God's names,17 [p. 94] and even so reflects some of God's attributes within his interactions with patients such as kindness, patience, and concern.17 [p. 96] In fact, many have believed that physicians must themselves be morally and religiously upright in order for their medical therapies to be effective.17 [p. 96] Islam also does not always make a distinction between medical and spiritual therapies; for example, a *hakim* might privately recite the Qur'an over his or her patient in order to effect physical healing.17 [p. 95]

For Islamic physicians, a primary motive behind care of the sick is that it earns the physician meritorious righteousness, necessary for hope in salvation, by caring for community members.1 [p. 127] One physician writing in the tenth century stated, "Visiting and healing the poor and needy patients is your special duty because a more meritorious work you cannot perform."17 [p. 93] One Hadith reports Muhammad making comments that identify the sick to be in close connection with God:

"God shall say on the Day of Judgment: 'O son of Adam! I was sick but you did not visit me.' 'My Lord! How could I visit you when you are the Lord of the whole world,' man will reply. God will say, 'Did you not know that so and so from among my servants [that is, human beings] was sick but you never visited him or her? Did you not know that if you had visited, you would have found me there?"[17 [p. 59]

Thus, similar to the teaching of Jesus recorded in Matthew 25, written in the first century, the sick hold a special place in God's economy. Whereas Christianity has tended to emphasize care of the sick as an act of grace, Islam has emphasized this as an especially unique opportunity of gaining righteous merit. Both have proved to be powerful motivations for care of the sick.

An Alliance Perpetuated

Deep in the psyche of monotheism is recognition that God alone heals. God is medicine's genius, and so, when healing occurs, all credit and thanks are returned to God. Medicinal agents, whether discovered in their natural form in the earth or manufactured by combining elements derived from what predates our existence, are gifts from God. The Gift Giver either placed them in the creation for us to discover or provided humanity with minds made in God's image, able to produce new healing agents. Similarly, the physician guild, though comprised of art, knowledge, and skill—discovered, learned, and passed down through years of laborious learning and practice—knows that it only assists in the healing process. After all, if physicians were to take credit for healing through surgical or medical practice, then they would also be responsible for all failed healing attempts. However, medical reflection has generally recognized that whatever the ultimate reason that one person recovers and another dies from illness, physicians are mere handmaidens to bodily processes that cannot ultimately be manipulated or controlled. Either the body's energy heals itself, or, as Judaism and Christianity have claimed, God operates providentially through the means of bodily processes, ultimately yielding healing or death. In the well-known words of French Protestant surgeon, Ambroise Pare (d. 1590 A.D.), "I bandaged him and God healed him."[18 [p. 42] Even so, physicians, caregivers, and health institutions are merely extensions of God's mercy and wisdom and subject to the many limitations of our finite lives.

Similarly, a religious ethic in the care of patients has cultivated a spirit of compassion based in Jewish responsibility to care for the *imago Dei* and its Christian extension to serve God in the holy presence of the patient. This humility and agape has largely governed the medical profession and its related institutions for two millennia in the Western tradition. This theological framework was embodied among caregivers both in practice and in a disposition toward patients. As we argued in Chapter 8, this disposition reflects an underlying spirituality, where the chief love is devotion to God *through* service to the sick and care of their bodies. Medicine practiced in this way was ordered by *religious* ideals as these were incorporated into the structures of medicine, not merely in private interactions or unspoken motives of individuals, but publicly.

While we can easily marshal many modern examples throughout the United States, here we offer two symbolic ones that illustrate how this alliance has remained embedded within American medicine, at least through the beginning of the twentieth century. These examples come from two of the most prominent academic medical institutions in the United States.

Near Harvard in Boston, a public emblem of the nineteenth-century perspective on partnership between medical science and religion is exemplified in the ether monument erected in 1868 in the Boston Public Garden.[19] The monument has served as a tribute to the discovery and first use of ether in surgery in 1846 by the renowned Harvard surgeon, John Collins Warren, one of the principal founders and the first surgeon of the Massachusetts General Hospital where the public ether experiment took place. With the benefits of anesthesia, the medical and surgical sciences advanced rapidly, and ether had numerous applications on the battlefield, in childbirth, and in the surgical theater. Ironically, an early controversy ensued on who should receive credit for discovering ether. This resulted in a public argument between William Morton, Horace Wells, and Morton's advisor, the Harvard professor Charles Jackson, MD. The monument itself, fitting within the theology previously described, gives credit only to God, failing to note any of the human actors involved.

In its north and south facing directions, the ether monument pays tribute to the benefits of ether on the battlefield and in the surgical ward. In its eastward facing direction, the monument depicts the angel of mercy descending over Adam in the "first" ether surgery (Genesis 2:21), in which God causes a sleep to fall over Adam before removing one of his ribs to create Eve. Inscribed with the angel are the words from Revelation 21:4: "neither shall there be any more pain." This depicts the analogical dimension of medicine suggested in Chapter 10 regarding how medicine points beyond itself to an eschatological future hope. In the monument's westward facing direction is a depiction of Lady Wisdom operating an ether machine. Inscribed is a verse from Isaiah 28:29, "This also cometh forth from the Lord of hosts, which is wonderful in counsel, and excellent in working." Bowing down to Lady Wisdom is a monk-like, religious pilgrim. Looking at Lady Wisdom with gratitude is the Madonna and child, suggesting the blessings of ether for childbirth. Finally, at the monument's crown is a statue of the Good Samaritan holding a half-dead man as he wipes the man's wounds. Like the oil and wine administered by the Good Samaritan, ether is a medicinal agent given to all mankind in God's wisdom and kindness, a gift bestowed upon all regardless of race or creed. It is to be given and received with thanksgiving in relief of suffering.

A second example of the historical alliance between medicine and religion can be found at John Hopkins University. There had been some public discontent with a lack of institutional expressions of religious piety from its beginning in 1876, and, in response, the university commissioned a white marble replica of the statue *Christus Consolator* in Copenhagen by Bertel Thorvaldsen. At its unveiling in 1896, the ten-and-half foot statue of the resurrected Jesus with outstretched arms and pierced hands was placed at what was then the center of the hospital complex. Some suggest that part of the reason for the commissioning of the statue was to assuage the deeply religious Baltimore public that John Hopkins was not entirely materialistic in its outlook.[20] The cost of the statue was paid directly by a religious philanthropist and supporter of the hospital. At its unveiling, Hopkins President Gilman said that the statue was created "with the outstretched hands of mercy to remind each passer-by—the physician and the nurse as they pursue their ministry of relief; the student as he begins his daily task; and the sufferer from injury or disease, that over all this institution rests the perpetual benediction of Christian charity, the constant spirit of 'good will to man.'"[20] [p. 14] Jesus' words at the base of the statue have been the source of comfort to many: "COME unto ME all ye that are weary and heavy laden and I will give you REST" (Matthew 11:28).

Many have claimed that the presence of *Christus Consolator* has been a source of hope and comfort, pointing people to look beyond themselves to a transcendent God who has not abandoned them. Accounts include collected stories[21] and journalistic accounts advocating the statue's symbolic power in providing comfort for those who gaze on it.[22,23] The statue is a reminder that there is much more than our present suffering—we can look beyond it to hope of life and rest. The original centrality of the statue located at the hub of the original hospital entrance is one of its notable features, as this suggests that religion is not at the margins of the illness experience but front and center. The iconographic predominance of the Christian religion, a not unreasonable assumption during the nineteenth century in a US city, is more challenging for non-Christians, whose encounter with *Christus* requires the person to either ignore the symbolism or perform a private "translation" of what it may mean for them from within their own alternative spiritual worldview.[22] Even with this challenge, *Christus Consolator* is at the very minimum a gesture that medicine and human material existence is not all there is or even the penultimate concern. While some hospital administrators are known to be embarrassed by the statue, patients' stories continue to abound of its symbolic power of encouragement and consolation.[24] [p. 82] It functions as an ongoing herald that medicine and religion can operate quite seamlessly together on an institutional level, even within elite academic medical hospitals.

Neither Harvard nor Hopkins have been bastions of religious fervor. One can make the case that the ether monument and *Christus Consolator* are not merely icons from days past but continue to serve an important purpose by offering signs of transcendence among the suffering ill and those who care for them. How such signs of transcendence might manifest in contemporary situations is an issue we will discuss in Chapter 15. At this point in our argument, however, we are identifying ways that Western medicine and religion have been in partnership and the specific value that religion has offered medicine.

Characteristics of a Religious Vision for Medicine

Within the Western tradition of medicine, a theological alliance between religion and medicine created an aura of sanctity around care for the sick and dying. As briefly mentioned in our introductory thoughts on Judaism, Christianity, and Islam, there have been three larger themes that have framed a theology of medicine and informed its practice which were drawn especially from the Abrahamic traditions.

Body and Soul

First, a prominent characteristic within the monotheistic traditions is that attention on *the material body is framed within and balanced by its order to the soul*, for both the patient and the clinician.

For patients, this means that physical illness is a spiritual experience, calling patients to not only deal with the material aspects of their disease but to include issues pertaining to the soul. For example, Ben Sira insists that the sick person should offer spiritual sacrifices and *"then give the doctor his place"* (emphasis ours). The sequential order suggests a difference of importance between the visible and invisible. This ordering of illness toward the spiritual life has been a common view throughout the Jewish tradition.[6] Likewise, Christians structured a proper use of medicine oriented by an understanding that the physical corresponds to the spiritual. Medicine is only properly received when it is done, as Basil described, "as a pattern for the care of souls."[13 [pp. 264-269]] A sacramental theology of medicine results in an essential tenet that whenever medicine is not ordered for instruction to the soul, then medicine's *telos* or purpose is misused. Or, positively, medicine for the body is intended to instruct the soul.

In practical terms, ill patients uphold an orderly balance between body and soul through spiritual practices such as prayer. Jewish and Christian thinkers regularly admonish patients to pray throughout the experience of illness. Ben Sira, for example, encourages the sick to pray to God because God is the source of healing: "My son, when you are ill, delay not, but pray to God, for it is he who heals" (Ben Sira 38.9). Similarly, Basil writes: "when we receive blows from God who so kindly and wisely orders our life, we first ask of him that we may understand the reason why he imposes the stripes, then we ask either release from the pain or endurance, such that with the trial he may also give us a way out, that we may be able to bear it" (55.3).[13] In Basil's theology, the sick ought to turn to God in prayer to discern God's spiritual purposes in illness—a purpose that is always geared to the patient's salvation or spiritual growth. It is upon understanding the spiritual rationale that God is teaching within illness that the patient may then petition God for physical healing or endurance. Patient prayer holds a key place in the way that a patient interfaces with illness. Physical illness becomes the material portal through which the patient grows into greater spiritual communion with God.

For clinicians, following this ordering of body and soul begins with rejection of a physical-only worldview, which limits the practice of medicine to disease processes, physical symptoms, and bodily cure or comfort. A clinician's domain is not confined *only* to the bodily needs of the sick but extends positively into spiritual and religious relationships. Speaking to the sick, Ben Sira admonishes them to make the appropriate ritual sacrifices ("offer your sweet-smelling oblation and memorial"), an action that would presumably require the services of clergy or the priesthood. While Ben Sira stresses the importance of the physician's prayers to God that medical therapy be accurate and effective, it is left unclear to what degree (if any) a physician engages directly in soul care. Ben Sira does make an important link between medicine and spiritual growth in that the use of medicine leads to "people learn[ing] his power" and "glory[ing] in his mighty works." In a rudimentary way, Ben Sira advocates for a sacramental understanding of medicine.

A sacramental theology becomes more fully developed in the thinking of Basil of Caesarea. Medicine and pastoral care are corollaries in that medicine is a "pattern for the care of the soul." Both the diagnosis and treatment of illness, per Basil, teach the sick about the realities and truths of the spiritual world. Spiritual realities are discerned through personal introspection, as well as through the diagnostic work of a spiritual superior and one's spiritual community.[13] Basil does not comment in either the Long Rules 55 or Short Rules 314 about whether a physician should also carry the responsibility for discerning the spiritual meaning and purpose of physical illness. However, in Basil's Letter (No. 189) To Eustathius the physician, he clearly extols the physician who does not confine the art of medicine to the body but also attends to the cure of the human soul.[xxv] Whereas Basil does not demand that physicians expand their responsibilities to include the spiritual, he applauds physicians who practice medicine as if they operated with "two right hands"—which is to say, soul care is as much as a domain of the medical art as bodily care.[xxvi]

While the Abrahamic traditions hardly demand or expect physicians to be intensely or regularly involved in the spiritual care of patients, they appear to imagine a deep partnership that upholds the patient's body and soul. Clinicians may hold a passive role in spiritual care of patients since within a deeply religious culture it would have been expected that patients' spiritual care would be provided by the patient's clergy and religious communities, as well as by a hospital context informed by an ethos of care for the soul and whole person. When the larger context was largely concerned with care of the soul, physicians were enabled to focus on physical care, being passive spiritual supporters. For example, in the Islamic tradition, medicine developed in a culture that viewed all of society to be in submission to Allah. Within a larger religious society, medicine itself could serve the sick while being indirect or more silent concerning theological motivations and rationales.[25 (p. 346)] Similarly, in the later English and American Christian context up until the nineteenth century,[26] a physician was not obligated by professional duty but by a more general obligation of love to gently address spiritual needs within illness.[xxvii] In the words of clergyman Richard Baxter, the physician's role was to speak "a few serious words" about faith. "Think not to excuse yourselves by saying, 'It is the pastor's duty.' For though it be theirs ex officio, it is yours also ex charitate. Charity bindeth every man, as he hath opportunity, to do good to all, and especially the greatest good."[27] In Baxter's context, shaped by English Puritanism, the greatest good cannot exclude care of the soul, especially regarding relationship with God. In Baxter's depiction, it was the physician's lay duty, not professional responsibility, that urged spiritual engagement. Baxter's view of the physician's role in spiritual care was characteristic of how most Protestant clergy in the United States expected physicians to engage the sick.[26]

There is then an important relationship between the physician's role in spiritual care and the larger system of care of the patient. Within institutions and in contexts where patients are spiritually well-tended by others, such as in countries dominated by one religious viewpoint, the physician's spiritual role may be circumscribed or unspoken. This may partly be the case in some contemporary Muslim societies.[25] However, in such contexts where spiritual care is neglected, the importance of upholding body and soul places additional responsibilities on clinicians to ensure that the nonmaterial needs of the patient are met. This may require that clinicians petition clergy and religious communities to be directly involved in the care of the patient. It may necessitate physicians to ensure that the medical or hospital environment is conducive to whole-person care. Or it may oblige physicians to be directly involved in spiritual care if no other qualified person is willing or able. Within the rationale of the Abrahamic traditions that upholds both body and soul within the care of the ill, it is incumbent on physicians as leaders of the care team to ensure that the patient's spiritual needs are adequately engaged. In medical contexts that are already deeply informed by religious perspectives, the physician's role may be largely passive. Thus, in a contemporary secular medical context, it becomes increasingly incumbent on clinicians who recognize the importance of the soul in serious illness to be active advocates and participants in spiritual care. If the larger system of healthcare functionally neglects or avoids patients' spiritual and religious needs, a duty falls on clinicians *ex charitate*.

Hospitality: In the Presence of the Divine

A second way in which the Abrahamic traditions have shaped the ethos of medicine has been in their central emphasis on hospitality since the patient is a bearer of God's image and, especially within Christianity, an identification of God within the suffering patient. The Christian perspective, which has arguably been the most pervasive throughout Western medicine in cultural influence, goes beyond "humanizing medicine" because it interprets the sacred presence of God within the patient–clinician encounter.[xxviii] To be clear, this does not mean that the patient is divine, since there is a radical demarcation between Creator and creature. Yet, within the human enactment, the sick signal transcendence because they function as human signposts that point beyond the purely human dimension, pointing toward God's attributes and presence mediated in and through the human encounter. Christians have historically emphasized these sacramental elements within the patient–clinician relationship.

Caregivers are employed to see and receive the suffering Christ, in, with, and through the presence of the patient. Jesus taught his disciples that they visit Him even as they visit or care for the sick (Matthew 25:31–46). As quoted earlier, this teaching has made an indelible mark on Jesus' followers, transforming Christian viewpoints on the previously stigmatized role of the sick. Against prevailing cultural values of Hellenistic culture, the sick person was to be visited as if he or she were the actual presence of God himself. This revolutionary interpretation of the patient catalyzed by Jesus' teaching creates new perspectives on the meaning of hospitality. Within this view, patients are not primarily vulnerable and weak human persons in need of human pity. Based on Christ's overturning of the social order, "the last will be first, and the first will be last" (Matthew 20:16), rather than being stigmatized, abandoned, or pitied, the sick (among several other marginalized groups) are held in highest honor.

The basis for esteem given to the sick is established within a theological viewpoint that perceives a deep analogy between the sick person and Christ's divine work of incarnation and crucifixion. The sick embody and represent Christ to the extent that they are signs and symbols of Christ's condensation in taking human nature, as well as his humiliation in his crucifixion. As one sees and visits an ill person, the human form of the sick is a witness of the self-emptying of God (Philippians 2) in his incarnation, even as many ill people travel the difficult journey from physical health into disease and dying. Just as Christ left heaven to take on mortal flesh, even so, in a less but still important way, the healthy leave the state of health and enter into illness. Of course, a key difference is that while Christ voluntarily gave up his perfect state of "health" and power out of love for humanity, sickness is a state that humans do not voluntarily enter.[xxix] In Christ's agape, he voluntarily took on human flesh, and it was his passion to die for the sins of humanity (Hebrews 10:5–10).

In Christian theology, intrinsically connected to the incarnation is Christ's crucifixion. The New Testament views Jesus as the fulfillment of the Suffering Servant of Isaiah 53, whereby the sins of the world are placed upon the Messiah. Christ's physical degradation is not because of his own sinfulness, but his imputation of the sin of others in order to remove sin according to the justice of God (1 Peter 2:21–24). In a similar fashion, while physical illness is connected to spiritual sickness and God's judgment,[28] the sin in view is not the patient's in particular, as Job (Job 1:1) or the man born blind (John 9:1–7) illustrate. Rather, illness is a symbolic or sacramental embodiment of an immaterial reality. Physical illness represents a spiritual sickness in the human relationship with God, diffuse among the whole race. Collapsed within this reality, the sick and dying patient also points to Jesus' crucifixion, in which he bore the sins of the world. Christ's close identification with sinners and human weakness comprises the internal logic in why caring for the sick is to receive Christ himself. Christ's dereliction is visibly signaled within the degradation of illness. Thus, what takes place in the material, human realm sacramentally mirrors this greater spiritual reality.

The implications of Jesus' teaching in care for the sick have been widespread, but perhaps no contribution has been more important than the resulting emphasis on the importance of hospitality. Within a sacramental imagination, hospitality goes in two directions between caregivers and patients.

First, caregivers, especially clinicians, are to receive and care for their patient as if they were caring directly for the Suffering Christ. Rather than objectifying or depersonalizing the patient,[29,30] an approach akin to those who participated in or stood by during Christ's crucifixion, medical caregivers address and enter into human suffering. Similar to the Benedictine communal practice of receiving visitors[15 [ch. 53]] and the care of the sick,[15 [ch. 36]] caregivers are humble before their patients, guided by heartfelt concern and attentiveness for the sick, understanding that their practice "rank[s] above and before all else,"[15 [ch 36]] including spiritual prayers and other spiritual practices. A humble disposition completely undermines a god complex,[31 [p. 348],32] which physicians may be prone to as an outcome of the power they gain through medical knowledge, technical competence, or swelling pride from grateful patients. It can often be only in the context of medical errors that this complex reveals its unfortunate character.[32] Contrary to a god complex that elevates the clinician, Jesus' teaching reflects a radical vision of religious hospitality that not only denies that the physician is godlike, but, more importantly, reveals the patient as reflecting the presence of God to the clinician! Failure by clinicians to embrace such a spirit of humility and hospitality before the patient merely symbolizes the medical professional's hubris, not just before the patient, but before the face of God. If such a radical vision of hospitality is taken seriously in the patient–clinician relationship, then it calls for nurses and physicians to enter into a profound state of humility before the patients they serve.

The act of medical care creates sacred spaces of highest hospitality where the clinician realizes that he or she is visiting Christ in the sacrament of the suffering patient.

The analogy also implies by inference an irony in that patients, as God's symbolic representatives of suffering, exhibit hospitality to others including their medical caregivers.[xxx] Whereas clinicians may show material hospitality to the sick, patients demonstrate spiritual hospitality because they sacramentally reflect Christ's divine passion. The language of Matthew 25 is that clinicians visit the sick. This suggests that *it is the sick who hold the role as hosts* since the patient is the one being visited. Caregivers are guests in the presence of the patient. Patients are not merely passive objects who hold the sick role[33] but are active agents offering hospitality, receiving guests, including their caregivers, into their presence under difficult circumstances. The analogical relationship expressed by Jesus in Matthew 25 suggests that patients represent and symbolize the Suffering Christ to their caregivers.

Within this surprising responsibility, the sick hold a unique obligation to prophetically speak truth to the physically healthy, who are often blinded to invisible realities because of good health. Acting in a priest-like role, patients lament sin, suffering, and death, and use their own suffering as a witness to God's promises of resurrection and eternal life. Verhey and Dugdale have recently described this active obligation of patients toward the healthy through the *ars moriendi* (art of dying well) tradition.[34,35] As a medieval Christian perspective developed in response to the Black Death,[35 [p. 6]] the *ars moriendi* highlights virtues and practices upholding the patient, in the same pattern of Christ, to actively fight against evil within suffering. But it is also the sick that instruct and give guidance to the healthy on how to live well. In other words, those who are ill ought to be understood to hold a role as a teacher, a prophet, and a guide. Sometimes these roles are directly expressed in words, but it may be just as often that those facing serious illness point others to transcendent realities and give a witness to life's deepest purpose and meaning.[xxxi] As they struggle with the evil of human mortality, dying, and death, the sick are confronted with life and its core meanings more urgently and with greater clarity than those who rest in the façade of temporal good health. Caregivers stand to receive from their hosts fresh reminders of the purpose of life. This by no means suggests that illness is good. It is an evil to be deeply resisted and lamented. Yet, given that illness as an inevitable experience, the Christian tradition interprets it as a spiritual state in which the patient metaphorically represents and potentially transmutes aspects of Christ's nature to anyone willing to receive it.

God's Gift of Medicine

Finally, *the source of medicine is received as a gift from God*. The powers of medicine reside not in man's genius or ability, but in divine mercy and benevolence, from the one who sees our frailty and provides means to alleviate suffering. If medicine is framed primarily as a gift, instead of a human right or an outflow of man's technological genius, it changes the basic framework and meaning in what takes place in the medical encounter.

For example, if medicine is a gift, then expectations and claims of healing do not rest on human powers. Patients cannot expect or demand healing from their doctors since clinicians do not ultimately have power or control over healing. Physical healing is a gift that is mediated through but ultimately located outside of human knowledge, scientific expertise, or technological capacities. When medicine is received as a divine gift, patients will not hold misplaced expectations on scientific medicine but will look beyond to seek the real source of healing. One does not put hope in the doctor's skills or medicine's technological ingenuity but in the final source of ultimate hope. Similarly, in this framework, physicians and scientists refuse to receive credit if healing takes place. Nor should they accept or place blame on themselves, as they are often tempted to do (apart from obvious cases of malpractice) when therapy fails to heal. Clinicians should strive for cure and provide the best care, but, ultimately, life and death are in God's not human hands.

Additionally, if medicine is a divine gift, then how can it be hoarded, bought, sold as a commodity, or demanded as a right? As a divine gift, it should be liberally given to others without compulsion and gratefully received by patients without demand or expectation. Though a gift, medicine remains a costly and extremely valuable service in terms of the enormous amount of time, energy, and devotion involved from bench research to the bedside of patients. Human participation in God's gift should clearly include expectations of fair reimbursement of medical professionals, scientists, and institutions that offer care. Recipients of the gift of medicine should not expect it to be free of charge but should generously support all those who give their lives in service of the sick. While there is no single agreed-upon religious financial model for healthcare, the concept of medicine as a divine gift seems most consistent with an economic rationality that resists both pure market forces that commodify medicine and legal-bureaucratic forces that frame medicine as a human right distributed based on some account of justice.[36] Both political perspectives from either the political right (that tends to depict medicine as a commodity) or the left (that tends to highlight medicine in terms of social justice) fail to depict medicine as a gift. Older healthcare frameworks, however imperfectly, reflected and understood medicine to be a philanthropic activity[xxxii] based in the voluntary calling and loving response of individuals and organizations who aim to care for the least of these.[37] While costs incurred need to be foreseen and engaged by sound business practices, any underlying motivations toward wealth generation, corporate greed, stock portfolios, and so on are corrupting influences within the service of the sick. If medicine is a divine gift, then humanity should not in turn treat it as a commodity for purchase or sale. Likewise, the sick should receive excellent care even if they cannot adequately pay the actual costs of care. Yet the religious rationale that frames medicine as a divine gift will not require or force human generosity through legal or financial compulsion.[36] The legal and bureaucratic forces unleashed upon American medicine are equally corrosive to practicing and receiving medicine in a sacred manner. Medicine should be freely given, motived by human love, upheld as a gift for all to hold in generosity and compassion. The Abrahamic vision of medicine grounded in agape stands in rivalry with some contemporary views of medicine.

Conclusion

In moving toward a Western theology of medicine, we have argued that medicine has been especially shaped by the theological presuppositions of the Abrahamic traditions. Threads of this synthesis remain with us to this day, especially the desire among many to provide patient-centered care. Some clinicians and patients may continue to interpret medicine within an explicitly theological framework, but these have also largely become private interpretations. There are now rival views expanding across medicine, replacing this older framework. There has been increasing rejection of medical concern for the soul since it does not fall within the purview of the material realm. This has resulted in a perception of the patient not as an agent of God's presence honored as sacred, but as a depersonalized object. As an object, these rival views transform the patient as primarily a sufferer into a "body" to be worked on, or a "customer" to be placated, or as a "number" within a bureaucratic machine. As these impersonal social forces have encroached on the meaning of medicine, its practice is no longer publically acknowledged as a divine gift but tends to be interpreted as a human achievement subject to whatever ends we so choose. Such rival views are incompatible with the synthesis that we have described in this chapter between medicine and Abrahamic perspectives.

These social forces are less "disenchanted" as Weber thought,[38] [p. 357] however, because Weber failed to see that increasing rationality not only overcame magical thinking but has embedded within it implicit goals that are religious-like. These impersonal social forces carry within them a new type of enchantment, one that has expelled the Abrahamic faiths and brought medicine under the spell of a new magic. Secular medicine has advanced itself under a claim that it is atheological, instrumental, and nonreligious. But, as we begin to unpack this claim in Chapters 10–12, we argue that secular perspectives carry veiled theologies that are not in themselves invalid within a pluralistic society but are functionally religious nevertheless. As we try to make this case, the next three chapters will show how secular medicine rivals the Abrahamic traditions in the ways outlined in this chapter. In Chapter 10, we examine medicine's theological anthropology as it has rejected the body–soul unity. In Chapter 11, we examine the sacramental aspects of secular medicine as it points to its own form of salvation rather than pointing beyond itself, as suggested especially in the Christian tradition. Finally, in Chapter 12, we suggest that, in place of giving honor to God as a gift to humanity, medicine takes glory and credit for itself as the source and genius of healing.

While Boston's Ether Monument and Hopkin's *Christus Consolator* appear to be tributes to bygone theologies, in Part III of our argument we make our case on the impact of secular medicine's spirituality of immanence and why many have good reason to recover and consider how these older traditions may hold power to renew the calling of medicine.[39]

Notes

i. We define the term "theology" in Chapter 8 as "reflection and reasoning that springs out of a relationship and experience of that chief love." Our point is that social forces have embedded or implicit values of what is most important and what it is supposed to serve.

ii. While most healing traditions have been formed in alliance with a spiritual worldview, Hippocratic medicine is unique in that it is a theory and practice that has been easily reframed and adopted by various spiritual worldviews. This flexibility was essential for a positive embrace by the monotheistic communities of Judaism, Christianity, and, later, Islam. Judaism's encounter with shamanistic medicine engendered disapproval of physicians within the

Hebrew Bible (2 Chronicles 16:12) because of its alliance with spiritual mediums and magical remedies (M. L. Brown. *Israel's divine healer*. Grand Rapids, MI: Zondervan; 1995). In contrast, Judaism's encounter with the Hippocratic tradition led to a new posture toward medical practice because the Hippocratic philosophy was easily synthesized with monotheistic beliefs (I. Jakobovits. *Jewish medical ethics: a comparative and historical study of the Jewish religious attitude to medicine and its practice*. New York: Bloch; 1975) that emphasized an axiomatic distinction between Creator and creature and that gave exclusive credit for healing to Yahweh (Exodus 15.26).

Because the Hippocratic concept of health and healing was grounded in material as opposed to spiritual realities, it could easily be conceptualized as part of the material world created by God. Similarly, healing practices associated with Hippocratic medicine could be understood as putting into practice the understanding of God's ordered material world to bring about health—a gift to mankind for which God alone deserved credit as the author of that created order.

iii. Brown argues that the Hebrew Bible should not be interpreted, as suggested by Kee, that "physicians are portrayed in strictly negative terms" (see Brown, *Israel's divine healer*). Rather, it was physicians aligned specifically with pagan deities that received censure. In contrast, Judaism's encounter with the Hippocratic tradition during its Hellenistic period led to an altered viewpoint of medical practice because Greek medical philosophy could be easily synthesized with monotheistic beliefs that emphasized an axiomatic distinction between Creator and creature and which gave exclusive credit of healing to Yahweh (Exodus 15.26) (see also Jakobovits, *Jewish medical ethics*). Because the Hippocratic concept of health and healing is grounded in material biology as opposed to ideas of magic, divination, or pagan worship, it could easily be conceptualized as part of the material world created by God. Similarly, healing practices associated with Hippocratic medicine could be understood as putting into practice the understanding of God's ordered material world to bring about health—a gift to mankind for which God alone deserved credit as the author of that created order.

The disentangling of idolatry from the practice of medicine solved one of two Jewish resistances to Greek medicine. A second objection was based on the biblical assertions (Exodus 15:26, Deuteronomy 32:39, Isaiah 19:22, 57:18–19, Jeremiah 30:17, Hosea 6:1; Psalms 103:2–3, Job 5:18) that God alone occupied the place of healer, indicating "that medicine was an improper human intervention in God's decision to inflict illness."[8] This point may explain why there is an aspect of discontinuity between the Hebrew Bible and later Jewish writers such as Ben Sira and the Mishnah—in that there was no known social office for healers before Jewish Hellenism. The combining of priest and healer, which was widely seen in pagan practice and later in some Christian practice, had no known precedent among Jews before this time. While there is some positive mentioning of physicians (Jeremiah 8:22), healing itself is not occupied by any single social office. "Prior to the Hellenistic period, there is no evidence of a medical profession."[8] Important figures such as Moses, Elijah, Elisha, and Isaiah performed miraculous healings (noting that Isaiah used the medium of a mandrake on Hezekiah) but these would largely appear sporadic in the biblical witness. It is likely that no healing office initially arose in Israel, in part because medical theory preceding Hippocratic medicine was too attached to idolatry, and in part because there was a heightened belief that Yahweh alone held the office of *Rophah* based on Exodus 15:26.

iv. Reflecting the Jewish response during the Second Temple Period is 1 Enoch 8, which suggests that celestial beings, who were generally honored by the Mesopotamians, were the source of various mysteries such as metallurgy for war and plant medicines for healing. Israel believed that the "Watchers" (i.e., celestial beings) were fallen spiritual beings under God's judgment (see how 1 Enoch 7–8 interpreted Genesis 6). Since medical knowledge was first shown to mankind through these evil beings, it created significant resistance among Israelites to participate in the use of plant medicines.

v. But the tradition's naturalism should not be equated with irreligion. Rather, its naturalism was a form of pagan belief in which divinity was immanent in nature. Furthermore, the tradition itself was laden with a "religious aura."[9 [p. 191]] From its inception, Hippocratic medicine was connected to the healing cult of Asclepius that rose within Hellenism and persisted at least through the fifth century A.D. (E. J. Edelstein, Edelstein L. *Asclepius; a collection and interpretation of the testimonies*. Baltimore: Johns Hopkins University Press; 1998). The connection between Hippocratic medicine and the religion of the ancient Greeks is illustrated by the Hippocratic Oath. This oath, pledged by early Greek physicians and persisting in modified form even into recent medical practice, opens with a vow to the Greek gods: "I swear by Apollo the physician, and Asclepius, and Hygieia and Panacea and all the gods and goddesses as my witnesses, that, according to my ability and judgment, I will keep this Oath and this contract."

Greek physicians' connection with the cult of Aesclepius was not simply a "half-hearted concession" (F. Heynick. Jews in medicine. Hoboken, NJ: KTAV Publishing House; 2002, p. 53); rather, Hippocratic physicians generally believed in the power of Asclepius and concluded that he was healer par excellence.[9 [p. 187]] Asclepius was believed to appear in night visions to supplicants sleeping within the temple (a practice known as incubation). Though Asclepius would occasionally perform instantaneous miracles, most patients instead received detailed instructions in their dreams regarding those medical procedures that would result in cure. Patients thus turned to their physicians to carry out the god's recommendations. While Asclepius's advice would occasionally break with Hippocratic norms, causing tension with the physicians, the therapies typically complied with up-to-date Hippocratic practices (Edelstein and Edelstein, *Asclepius*). The relationship between Hippocratic medical practice and Asclepian cultic ritual demonstrates how even a naturalistic approach to medicine can include a carefully constructed social and theological alliance with spiritual beliefs and institutions.

vi. The lexical similarity between Sirach 38.9 (LXX) and the Septuagint rendering of Exodus 15:26 indicates that Ben Sira has the Exodus directly in mind—most likely because Exodus 15:26 was understood to provide a foundational theology for healing. Ben Sira "vigorously opposed any compromise of Jewish values and traditions (cf. 2:12) and pronounced woe to those who forsook Israel's Law (41:8), with which wisdom itself, in his view, was to be identified (24:23)."[2] Consequently, Ben Sira attempted to work out without compromise the tradition of Torah in a Hellenistic-dominated culture, with exposure to a new form of medicine that had not been encountered before by the Jewish tradition.

vii. It is essential to Ben Sira's argument to show how the sick can embody a traditional spiritual piety even when utilizing medical means. This is an important feature to his argument because a traditional Jewish audience, presupposing that faithfulness requires utter dependence on God, will at the very least expect spiritual practices in continuity with Jewish healing preceding the Hellenistic period. Presupposed practices for the sick were based in an unquestioning belief in retribution theology. In its essence, retribution theology is a belief that "Obedience brings divine favor and blessings, including long life, fertility, and health, while disobedience brings divine anger and curses, including premature death, infertility, and disease" (Brown, *Israel's divine healer*). For Ben Sira, "Rewards and punishments in the afterlife were not even considered."[2] Brown shows how God's retributive justice can be found in most books in the Hebrew canon, with Exodus 15.26 serving as the "foundation" and Deuteronomy 32:39 as the "capstone" (Brown, *Israel's divine healer*). Consequently, Ben Sira affirms that reliance upon medicine coincides with retribution theology because the sick person is admonished to "delay not" in prayer, repent from sin, and offer God sacrifices (38:9–11). After beginning these spiritual practices in one's sickness, only thereafter should the person give place to the physician (38.12). The trifold invitation to prayer, repentance, and sacrifice is consistent with the retribution theology found throughout the rest of the book.[2] Likewise, Ben Sira's call to accept Greek medicine does not replace the traditional spiritual practices for the sick but supplements them with a penultimate turn to medical help. But turning to human physicians is not only recommended by Ben Sira, it is "essential to you" (38:1). He pushes this expectation even further, implying that defiance toward the doctor is based in defiance toward God—who created the doctor (38:15). Thus, in a surprising turn of wisdom, not only is it faithful to turn to the physician, it is fundamental to a healthy spiritual practice. Ben Sira's appeal mentions but does not stress (in contrast to modern times) the hope for cure (38:13); the importance of making a place for the physician is primarily based in the argument that the physician is part of God's created order, and the sick need to consent to this order irrespective of outcome.

viii. The physician relies on God because "without Thy help not even the least thing will succeed."[3] The Prayer interpreted sickness in light of the providence of God, who "sendest to man diseases as beneficent messengers to foretell approaching danger and to urge him to avert it." This religious interpretation of the meaning of illness also spurred some Jewish physicians to encourage the sufferer "to ask God's forgiveness through prayer and fasting" (David B. Ruderman. Kabbalah, magic, and science: the cultural universe of a sixteenth-century Jewish physician. Cambridge, Mass.: Harvard University Press; 1988, p. 33). For Maimonides, not unlike Basil, bodily sickness and health were both secondary goods ordered on behalf of the spiritual life. The physician's vocation of aiming for physical health was not a good unto itself, but was, according to Maimonides, "in order that his soul be upright to know the Lord."[7 [p. 53]]

ix. The second and third centuries were marked by reliance upon folk remedies, nursing care, and healing via religious rituals such as anointing with oil and prayer (see A. Porterfield. Healing in the history of Christianity. Oxford/New York: Oxford University Press; 2005). It was during the fourth century and onward that especially monastic communities in both the East and West began to more systematically establish institutions aimed for both care and cure.[10] Monks became proficient in copying and extending medical texts, and some became skilled physicians advancing medical knowledge.[5]

x. By the time Christian communities had developed enough to include organized care for the sick in the third and fourth centuries A.D., Hippocratic medicine and Asclepian cult were more firmly affixed than when Jewish peoples encountered it centuries before (see G. B. Ferngren. Early Christianity as a religion of healing. Bull Hist Med. 1992;66(1):1–15). This resulted in a sharp rejection of the Asclepian healing rite by Christian groups since Asclepius was also considered by pagans as a supreme healing "Savior" and "Great Physician" (see A. Verhey. Reading the Bible in the strange world of medicine. Grand Rapids, MI: W. B. Eerdmans; 2003; and Edelstein and Edelstein, Asclepius). Into the fourth century A.D., Asclepius was a rival healing deity, subsidized politically and financially by Roman authorities, and he socially functioned as a competitor to Jesus as supreme healer (see R. J. Ruttlmann. Asclepius and Jesus: the form, character and status of the Asclepius cult in the second-century CE and its influence on early Christianity. Cambridge: Harvard Divinity School, Harvard University; 1987). Some have argued that, during the second and third centuries, rival religious traditions including Asclepian cult and Christianity were engaged in a fierce competition for patrons, with their powers to heal the sick being a distinctive characteristic for outreach (see H. Avalos. Health care and the rise of Christianity. Peabody, MA: Hendrickson; 1999; R. J. S. Barrett-Lennard. Christian healing after the New Testament: some approaches to illness in the second, third, and fourth centuries. Lanham, MD: University Press of America; 1993; R. Stark. The rise of Christianity: a sociologist reconsiders history. Princeton: Princeton University Press; 1996). One historian, based on a linguistic comparison of writings using terms associated with health and illness during the second and third centuries, found that Christian writing was far more nuanced compared to pagan contemporaries, suggesting a heightened knowledge of disease process and familiarity with care of the sick (Barrett-Lennard. Christian healing after the New Testament). Similarly, Avalos has argued that Christian care of the sick was both cheaper (usually free) and less invasive than other forms of healing cults during the second and third centuries—adding to its popular appeal in contrast to more expensive and potentially invasive procedures (Avalos, Health care and the rise of Christianity). Rodney Stark has argued that the heroic efforts of Christian care, especially in light of epidemics and the fear of infection, became a powerful sociological force partly explaining how Christianity could grow as a religion during a time of periodic state persecution (Stark. The rise of Christianity). While urban populations were decimated by disease during these centuries, Stark suggests that Christians developed immunities. Each of these factors played a decisive role, according to Porterfield, in the relative defeat of pagan healing cults and in the rise of Christianity (Porterfield, *Healing in the history of Christianity*).

xi. *The Rule of St. Benedict*, written in the sixth century as a practical guide to Christian communities, made it incumbent for its ascetic members to "take the greatest care of the sick."[15]

xii. Ferngren argues that, during the first three centuries of occasional persecution, the church had little opportunity to develop healthcare resources sophisticated enough to utilize or systematize Hippocratic practice (G. B. Ferngren. Early Christianity as a religion of healing. *Bull Hist Med*. 1992;66(1):1–15).

xiii. The result was a remarkable alliance that "went beyond anything that the classical world had to offer: institutional health care administered in a spirit of compassion by those whose desire to serve God summoned them to a life of active beneficence" (Ferngren, *Medicine & health care in early Christianity*).

xiv. Basil's principle remarks concerning Hippocratic medicine can be found in his *Long Rules* 55 (and *Short Rules* 315) A critical edition is available in A. Silvas.[13] These were ascetical instructions written principally to monastic communities, but also written with the understanding that the concepts outlined had general application to the whole church.

xv. Within Basil's vision, the use of medicine was paired with those monastic communities that he helped organize and nurture. While initially following a sarabaitic lifestyle marked by individualism, Basil rejected this form of asceticism for a cenobitic, community life. He believed that this more closely followed the biblical and apostolic witness, promoted cohesion and order for the church, and could more easily be implemented with ample examples around him (including a community led by his older sister, Makrina) (see A. Silvas[13]). Having whole ascetic communities participate in the care of the sick had the obvious practical potential of assisting a much larger population of people in need. However, care of the sick and welcoming strangers was also woven into the spiritual ethos of the community life itself. Not only did the sick benefit by having a large cluster of caregivers gathered in a "new city," but also, such activity formed "a centre of religious formation" and education in which life in Christ could be better realized (P. Rousseau. *Basil of Caesarea*. Berkeley: University of California Press; 1994).

xvi. Basil himself was an active caregiver at the institution, "taking the lead in approaching to tend" to the sick (Gregory Nazianzen. (1894). Select Orations of Saint Gregory Nazianzen. In P. Schaff & H. Wace (Eds.), C. G. Browne & J. E. Swallow (Trans.), *S. Cyril of Jerusalem, S. Gregory Nazianzen* (Vol. 7, p. 403). New York: Christian Literature Company.). He greeted the sick with a kiss, treated their physical ailments, and dressed their wounds.[10]

xvii. Basil himself described the purpose of the *Basileias*, later named after the bishop who founded it: "to raise in honor of our God a house of prayer built in magnificent fashion, and, grouped around it, a residence, one portion being a generous home reserved for the head of the community, and the rest subordinate quarters, all in order, for the servants of the divinity—to which there is free access, both for you magistrates and for your retinue. . . . And whom do we wrong when we build hospices for strangers, for those who visit us while on a journey, for those who require some care because of sickness, and when we extend to the latter the necessary comforts, such as nurses, physicians, beasts for traveling, and attendants?" From *Epistle 94*, translated in B. E. Daley.[11]

xviii. Hippocratic medicine was an art that was primarily enjoyed by Roman aristocrats, whereas Christians had few converts from the upper classes before Constantine. This likely created a lack of familiarity with the use of Hippocratic medicine by a poor Roman populace and also meant that there were few Christians trained in Hippocratic medicine during the first three centuries. Basil represents an important shift in this regard, coming from an aristocratic family in the fourth century and trained as a young student in Greek medical practice. Basil brought this background into his Christian conversion and was able, on a sophisticated level, to see how Christian teaching and Hippocratic medicine coalesced.

xix. It was during the fourth century that Eastern regions of the Roman empire, including Asia Minor, underwent population shifts (Miller, The birth of the hospital in the Byzantine Empire). Large populations of people were migrating, with a large influx of primarily a poor populace moving into cities. This process of urbanization was coupled with changes in local governments in which aristocrats were more focused on Rome than on local government. With attention shifted away from local policies, a massive influx of poor peoples with no local ties to ancient cities and worsening economic conditions, including a local famine in Cappadocia in 369 A.D., there was significant but unmet human need (see S. R. Holman. The hungry body: famine, poverty, and identity in Basil's Hom 8. *Journal of Early Christian Studies*. 1999;7(3):337–363).

xx. Such human needs increasingly shifted toward the church and especially toward increasing political power of local bishops. Traditional local governments and their aristocratic families had little desire to assist financially a growing urban poor and willingly shifted this political responsibility to the office of bishops (Miller, The birth of the hospital in the Byzantine Empire). Brown shows how it was especially the bishops who became patrons of the poor, using their influence especially on their behalf (P. R. Brown. *Power and persuasion in late antiquity: towards a Christian empire*. Madison, WI: University of Wisconsin Press; 1992). Leaders such as Basil openly embraced this responsibility and garnered tremendous prestige in part because of it (Miller, The birth of the hospital in the Byzantine Empire). Borrowing Greco-Roman understandings of social responsibility for family members, Holman has shown how Basil made appeals to his citizenship to care for sick and poor strangers based on a new theological vision which redefined the "family" and "household," requiring broad social responsibility and action[14] (see also Holman, The hungry body: famine, poverty, and identity in Basil's Hom 8).

xxi. Miller has argued that there were political dimensions of healthcare policies tied to the Arian controversy in which Basil had been embroiled (see Miller, The birth of the hospital in the Byzantine Empire). Social action and philanthropy played an important role in sensitizing common people and the imperial government to the theological controversy surrounding the second person of the trinity. Basil was very familiar with the hospice care provided by Arian charity, and, by copying aspects of their model, he essentially expanded the scope of this care further than had been accomplished before. By winning the respect and admiration of the people, Basil also aimed to capture them on behalf of Nicene orthodoxy.

xxii. Basil does not use the word "sacrament" but "pattern" and "copy."

xxiii. Basil only alludes to other healing practices apart from medicine. He calls them "invisible" and mentions Jesus who instructed one to wash in the pool of Siloam (John 9) while on another occasion Jesus simply speaks a word of healing (Matthew 8:3). One potential example of an alternative is Basil's older sister, Macrina, who refused to see a physician for a cancerous tumor even when her mother "begged her to accept the doctor's care and implored her many times saying that the art of medicine was given by God to man for his preservation." Macrina refused on the grounds of bodily modesty and instead was healed after praying all night in the sanctuary.[13] [p. 265]

xxiv. The bishop offers a template for disease origin and explains its implications in understanding the purpose of sickness and a patient's proper response. A primary distinction established by Basil is that some diseases have a natural origin caused through improper lifestyle or having some other physical basis and other diseases are spiritually derived, with no natural basis. Basil offers five biblical examples of spiritually derived (or nonnatural) illnesses: (1) Illness caused by sin (at times hidden sin) intended by God as discipline aimed for conversion—the Corinthian church being its example (1 Corinthians 11:30–32). Illness also serving as a physical example of spiritual sins aimed to awaken the sinner who has not examined himself (Luke 15.17) or even acknowledged sin's presence, as in the case of the paralytic (John 5.14). (2) Illness caused by the Evil One, which God allows upon the saints to undermine Satan's boast and manifest the just lives of the saints—exemplified in the life of Job. (3) Physical suffering unto death that brings about eternal life—shown in the story of Lazarus (Luke 16:20–25). (4) Illness aimed to engender spiritual humility, as in the Apostle Paul (2 Corinthians 12:7). (5) Disease having the purpose to manifest the goodness and power of God, as in the case of the man born blind (John 9). According to Basil, illnesses which have a natural origin should be normally addressed using the natural means of medicine. However, those illnesses which are "unnatural"—having only a spiritual cause—require a different response from the sick. For example, those who have discerned that they are being punished by God for sin, according to Basil, must first repent and then "we ought to take it quietly and do without medical attentions and endure whatever comes our way." For Basil, it would appear that his underlying presupposition is that spiritually generated disease should be treated by spiritual remedy, whereas disease generated by natural means should be treated by bodily medicine (interpreted to serve as a pattern for the care of the soul).

xxv. "In your own case medicine is seen, as it were, with two right hands; you enlarge the accepted limits of philanthropy by not confining the application of your skill to men's bodies, but by attending also to the cure of the diseases of their souls. It is not only in accordance with popular report that I thus write. I am moved by the personal experience which I have had on many occasions and to a remarkable degree at the present time, in the midst of the unspeakable wickedness of our enemies, which has flooded our life like a noxious torrent." *To Eustathius the physician* Basil of Caesarea (1895). Letters. In P. Schaff, H. Wace, eds., B. Jackson (trans.), *St. Basil: letters and select works* (vol. 8, p. 228). New York: Christian Literature Company. See also: http://www.newadvent.org/fathers/3202189.htm.

xxvi. It may also be important to recall that few Hippocratic physicians were Christian in Basil's era, implying that the opportunity for coalescing roles was an infrequent opportunity in the fourth century (Ferngren, *Medicine & health care in early Christianity*, pp. 105–106).

xxvii. Richard Baxter (In *Christian directory*; see http://www.ccel.org/ccel/baxter/practical.i.vii.v.html) notes that some physicians may "excuse [them]selves by saying 'It is the pastor's duty.'" He argues, in contrast, that the spiritual obligation of the physician is not theirs "*ex officio*" but "*ex charitate*." It is an obligation of love embedded in the circumstance of illness and the opportunity afforded physicians. In Baxter's view, the physician has a unique opportunity created by the turmoil of sickness to say "a few serious words about the danger of the unregenerate state," an opportunity that many pastors are not given. In addition, the physician carries a level of power over the patient that is to be exercised out of love for the most important thing—the salvation of the soul before death. For a physician to reject this obligation of love is tantamount to the parable in Luke 10 regarding the priest who passed on the other side of road without offering assistance to the half-dead man. Baxter notes that a "few serious words for his conversion" is of utmost importance for a Christian physician to perform since the dying are passing into "the world from which there is no return." Consequently, Baxter stresses the shared and overlapping responsibility that physicians and clergy have regarding spiritual oversight of the sick. A physician who is focused only on the body fails to exercise "compassion and charity to men's souls."

xxviii. Contra Temkin, who concluded that medicine received little in return for the Christian adoption of Hippocratic medicine as an analogue,[9 [p. 177]] here we suggest that Christianity elevated reception of rational medicine through its spiritual endorsement. Without religious authentication, Hippocratic medicine would hardly have gained its monopoly of care in the West in light of its many competitors. In addition to this, Christian endorsement of the medical profession elevated the physician's status to an analogue to divinity. What higher form of authorization or endorsement could possibly be given? Without this endorsement and religious partnership, it is questionable if Western medicine would have enjoyed its privileged position in light of the many other rival healing traditions.

xxix. Within Christian theology, Christ, the Second Person of the Godhead, is grounded in an understanding that God the Son took within his person two natures, divine and human. Within the incarnation, Christ emptied himself of the form of God and took the form of a servant (Philippians 2.6–7). Though fully God in all God's power and glory, Christ temporarily "gave up the independent exercise of divine attributes and powers that constituted his equality with God" (Thomas Oden, *The word of life*, San Francisco: Harper; p. 79). In Jesus' earthly humiliation, he lowered himself to the form of a servant, washing the feet of his disciples and showing hospitality to social outcasts, lepers, and prostitutes. In this fashion, God's power is only matched by God's love, where God is not only desiring to create, but also willing to enter into the creation in order to redeem it. The incarnation was a stooping down, a condensation, motivated by God's love for creatures utterly broken by sin (Thomas Oden, *The word of life*, p. 100). Even so, Christ not only took on human nature, but also allied himself with the lowliest of humanity in order to redeem all. Most Christian thinking has understood Christ's identification with all of humanity as part of an essential component of salvation.

xxx. The language of visitation (ἐπισκέπτομαι) in Matthew 25:36, 43 is also connected to divine visitation both in the Septuagint translation of the Hebrew Bible (Genesis 21:1; Exodus 4:31; Psalm 8:5; 16:3; 64:10; Jeremiah 15:15) and in the New Testament in reference to Christ's incarnation (Luke 1:68, 78; Luke 7:16; Acts 15:14). These latter examples highlight, not only how the divine visits mankind, but also the need to be hospitable toward the divine presence who visits us within the embodiment of the sick person.

xxxi. Although it is not in the focus of our argument, the Christian tradition sees chronic and mental illness and serious illness faced by children in a similar manner. There is obvious tragedy, but every individual tragedy carries within it the possibility of pointing to a greater power and love that imbues meaning and purpose to patient, clinician, and all who look on.

xxxii. William May critiques the philanthropic model of healthcare because he thinks it creates a mentality of condescension rather than obligation by physicians.[37 pp. 119-124] We agree with May that physicians hold a deep debt in caring for the sick. In our use of the term, we simply refer to a deep human compassion and love for the sick, so much so that clinicians are motivated by that love rather than merely by contract, duty, or an external motivation to make money. We agree with May in principle yet still think philanthropy, if rightly understood, is the right word of choice.

References

1. Gary B. Ferngren. *Medicine and religion: a historical introduction.* Baltimore: Johns Hopkins University Press; 2014.
2. Patrick W. Skehan, Di Lella Alexander A. *The wisdom of Ben Sira: a new translation with notes.* Garden City, NY: Doubleday; 1987.
3. David L. Freeman, Abrams Judith Z. *Illness and health in the Jewish tradition: writings from the Bible to today.* Philadelphia: Jewish Publication Society; 1999.
4. Jeffrey S. Levin, Meador Keith G. Healing to all their flesh Jewish and Christian perspectives on spirituality, theology, and health. West Conshohocken, PA: Templeton Press; 2012: http://site.ebrary.com/lib/bostonuniv/docDetail.action?docID=10651481 online book.
5. Gary B. Ferngren. *Medicine & health care in early Christianity.* Baltimore: Johns Hopkins University Press; 2009.
6. Fred Rosner. *The medical legacy of Moses Maimonides.* Hoboken, NJ: KTAV Publishing House; 1998.
7. Fred Rosner. The physician and the patient in Jewish law. In: F. Rosner, Bleich J. D., Brayer M. M., eds. *Jewish bioethics.* New York: Sanhedrin Press; 1979:xix, 424.
8. Elliot Dorff. The Jewish tradition. In: R. L. Numbers, Amundsen D. W., eds. *Caring and curing: health and medicine in the western religious traditions.* Baltimore: Johns Hopkins University Press; 1986:5–39.
9. Owsei Temkin. *Hippocrates in a world of pagans and Christians.* Baltimore: Johns Hopkins University Press; 1991.
10. T. S. Miller. The birth of the hospital in the Byzantine Empire. *Henry E Sigerist Suppl Bull Hist Med.* 1985(10):1–288.
11. Brian E. Daley. Building a new city: The Cappadocian fathers and the rhetoric of philanthropy. *J Early Christian Studies.* 1999;7(3):431–461.
12. Philip LeMasters. The practice of medicine as *theosis. Theol Today.* 2004;61:173–186.
13. Anna Silvas. *The Asketikon of St. Basil the Great.* Oxford/New York: Oxford University Press; 2005.

14. Susan R. Holman. *The hungry are dying: beggars and bishops in Roman Cappadocia*. Oxford/New York: Oxford University Press; 2001.
15. Timothy Fry, ed. *The rule of St. Benedict in English*. Collegeville, MN: Liturgical Press; 1982.
16. Guenter B. Risse. *Mending bodies, saving souls: a history of hospitals*. New York: Oxford University Press; 1999.
17. Fazlur Rahman. *Health and medicine in the Islamic tradition: change and identity*. New York: Crossroad; 1987.
18. Jean-Pierre Poirier. *Ambroise Paré: un urgentiste au XVIe siècle*. Paris: Pygmalion; 2005.
19. Raphael A. Ortega. *Written in granite: an illustrated history of the Ether Monument*. 1st ed. Boston, MA: Plexus Management; 2006.
20. N. McCall. The statue of the Christus Consolator at the Johns Hopkins Hospital: its acquisition and historic origins. *Johns Hopkins Med J.* 1982;151(1):11–19.
21. Randi Henderson, Marek Richard. *Here is my hope: inspirational stories from the Johns Hopkins Hospital: a book of healing and prayer*. 1st ed. New York: Doubleday; 2001.
22. Rasmussen. 'The divine healer' hospital: the representation of Christ the Consoler in the Hopkins lobby still offers hope. *The Baltimore Sun*. October 13, 1996.
23. Jonathan Pitts. Grayson Gilbert's divine strength. *The Baltimore Sun*. May 19, 2011.
24. Daniel P. Sulmasy. *The healer's calling: a spirituality for physicians and other health care professionals*. New York: Paulist Press; 1997.
25. Bret McCarty, Warren Kinghorn. Medicine, religion, and spirituality in theological context. In: John Peteet, Balboni Michael, eds. *Spirituality and religion within the culture of medicine*. New York: Oxford University Press; 2017:341–356.
26. Jonathan B. Imber. *Trusting doctors: the decline of moral authority in American medicine*. Princeton, NJ: Princeton University Press; 2008.
27. R. Baxter, William Orme. *The Practical Works of the Rev. Richard Baxter*. London: James Duncan; 1830;6:109–114.
28. Jean-Claude Larchet. *The theology of illness*. Crestwood, NY: St. Vladimir's Seminary Press; 2002.
29. M. J. Balboni, Bandini J., Mitchell C., Epstein-Peterson Z. D., Amobi A., Cahill J., Enzinger A. C., Peteet J., Balboni T. Religion, spirituality, and the hidden curriculum: medical student and faculty reflections. *J Pain Symptom Manage.* 2015;50(4):507–515.
30. Margaret E. Mohrmann. Professing medicine faithfully: theological resources for trying times. *Theology Today*. 2002(October):355–368.
31. David Novak, Rashkover Randi, Kavka Martin. *Tradition in the public square: a David Novak reader*. Grand Rapids, MI: William B. Eerdmans Pub. 2008.
32. D. Hilfiker. Facing our mistakes. *N Engl J Med.* 1984;310(2):118–122.
33. Talcott Parsons. *The social system*. Glencoe, IL: Free Press; 1951.
34. Allen Verhey. *The Christian art of dying: learning from Jesus*. Grand Rapids, MI: William B. Eerdmans Pub.; 2011.
35. Lydia S. Dugdale. *Dying in the twenty-first century: toward a new ethical framework for the art of dying well*. Cambridge, MA: MIT Press; 2015.
36. John Rawls. *A theory of justice*. Original ed. Cambridge, MA: Belknap Press; 2005.
37. William F. May. *The physician's covenant: images of the healer in medical ethics*. 2nd ed. Lexington, KY: Westminster John Knox Press; 2000.
38. Max Weber, Gerth Hans Heinrich, Mills C. Wright. *From Max Weber: essays in sociology*. New York: Oxford University Press; 1946.
39. Abraham M. Nussbaum. *The finest traditions of my calling: one physician's search for the renewal of medicine*. New Haven, CT: Yale University Press; 2016.

10

Theology Within the Patient–Clinician Relationship

Introduction

Many in Western societies perceive the divide of sacred and secular within medicine as both inevitable and as a change for the better. History is thus perceived as logically marching toward this division, and many approve of it as creating conditions that enable human beings to achieve greater fulfillment. While recognizing that a division between the material and immaterial has enabled human flourishing within multiple realms, our contention is that differentiation, at the cost of deemphasizing a larger unity, has led to many false choices, especially arising in the care of the seriously ill. One important division pervasive throughout medicine, in contrast to the Abrahamic tradition, is the separation of body and soul. Understanding these aspects of personhood in radical separation and independence has led to an imagining of the patient–clinician relationship in nonrelational terms focused predominantly on the material body. There is, of course, no explicitly stated view on these matters. It is not clear if most clinicians even give this issue much conscious thought. What this chapter tries to unearth is that, within practice, are implicit beliefs that are essentially theological concerning the nature of personhood. What are those beliefs? In this chapter, we provide a brief tour of approaches to personhood, concluding that every approach, including those considered secular and neutral, rest on an implicit theology. A theological anthropology lies embedded within the patient-clinician relationship.

The Object–Observer Metaphor

In Chapter 6, we discussed how the plausibility structure of hospitals as institutions of science and technology led to an emphasis on physicians as scientists. This has arguably been the most widespread and enduring metaphor for the role of physicians after the Enlightenment period. As the practice of medicine began to proficiently utilize the scientific method during and after the Enlightenment, "Professional excellence in medicine came to be associated with scientific prowess and laboratory research rather than library-based knowledge and empathetic bedside skills"[1] [p.89]

The idea of physician-as-scientist is directly correlated with an underlying theory of disease and health. This theory underlying the practice of medicine holds three rational principles according to Guenter Risse: (1) materialism that led to a mind–body dualism, (2) reductionism that led to an ontological understanding of disease origin, and (3) empiricism, which has stressed numerical measurements and probabilistic reasoning.[2] A fourth important characteristic informing medical practice, in contrast to premodern and non-Western views of the healer (i.e., Shamanism), is the *objectivity of physicians* whose role does not include innate, therapeutic ability.[3]

How have these principles been formed to shape patient care? The physician-as-scientist is a metaphor that emphasizes the physician as an objective observer. The patient becomes a passive sufferer within his or her illness. The patient's physical body becomes the central focus of observation. The physician, depending primarily on the scientific method, identifies the physical cause(s) for illness and then responds by applying therapies in the forms of medication or surgeries. If left to itself this leads to an impersonal model constructed on a scientific paradigm and emphasizing the observational powers of the physician in diagnosis and therapeutic powers in prognosis and treatment.

Foucault described the shift toward the physician-scientist as part of "two great myths" associated with medicine beginning with the Enlightenment.[4 (p.36)] He stated, "The myth of a nationalized medical profession, organized like the clergy, and invested, at the level of man's bodily health, with powers similar to those exercised by the clergy over men's souls; and the myth of a total disappearance of disease in an untroubled, dispassionate society restored to its original state of health."[4 (p.132)] He described physicians exercising a scientific "gaze," advancing beyond the false rigidity of medical tradition and progress toward real healing:

> The observing gaze refrains from intervening: it is silent and gestureless. Observation leaves things as they are; there is nothing hidden to it in what is given. The correlative of observation is never the invisible, but always the immediately visible, once one has removed the obstacles erected to reason by theories and to the senses by the imagination. In the clinician's catalogue, the purity of the gaze is bound up with a certain silence that enables him to listen. The prolix discourses of systems must be interrupted: "all theory is always silent or vanishes at the patient's bedside."[4 (p.132)]

In Foucault's genealogical account of the rise of modern medicine, the clinic "became medicine's living laboratory," sick people were passive agents, and "doctors were in control."[5 (p.xi)] The physician-scientist emerged with a "practice of power; a form of control; a scientific discourse; a form of applied engineering."[4 (p.132)]

Clearly, this account is a broad description that does not account for all medical approaches. In the mental health field, for example, the therapeutic alliance has been understood to play a central role in the patient's healing process. But the objectivity of the physician as a healer remains broadly an accurate depiction for most clinicians within medical practice, including palliative care. Within patient care, this implies an impersonal model of caregiving, one constructed on the scientific paradigm, in which the physician–patient relationship is transformed into an object–observer relationship.[i]

The object–observer metaphor provides clinicians and patients an influential narrative to follow in the practice and receipt of medicine. It offers both a sense of identity and a social script to follow in their roles as clinician and patient. This metaphor helps explain why the medical profession has been generally resistant to religion and spirituality, especially within the clinicians' role. Most conceive spiritual care as not fitting within this paradigm. The object–observer paradigm does not technically eschew the incorporation of spiritual care into medicine. It can result in a complete rejection of the appropriateness of spiritual care because spirituality and religion are viewed as subjective and nonmaterial and thus unsuited for medical professionals in the course of their practice.[6] Nevertheless, the object–observer paradigm may also identify spiritual care, as others have argued, as another therapeutic instrument within the clinician's arsenal aimed at physical health or cure.[7,8] This approach to spiritual care decreases the importance of the actual substantive content of the patient's spirituality and emphasizes its potential psychological benefits or health outcomes irrespective of content. From this perspective, spirituality and religion are instruments aimed at material ends. The ends become psychological well-being or better health as a system of social control. Under this latter paradigm, the clinician may use the patient's spirituality toward the ends of physical health, cure, and comfort. When spirituality and religion are functionalized for health, then they conform to the object–observer metaphor, which remains the larger framework for its purpose and meaning.[ii]

Tensions with the Object–Observer Metaphor

The object–observer metaphor carries certain weaknesses in tension with the larger aims of healing. These weaknesses by no means negate the enormous benefits yielded by medicine and public health.[9] Nevertheless, if conceptualizing the nature of the patient–clinician relationship from the perspective of an integrated view of science, spirituality, and religion, one begins to see how these point toward compatible systems of knowledge that are needed for the healing of persons to more fully occur. From an integrated understanding of human persons, partnership with science carries enormous benefits proved necessary in the pursuit of healing and the care of the sick. Even so, from an integrated viewpoint, it is an equally enormous mistake to consent to or be silent toward the object–observer metaphor holding pride of place as the guiding metaphor for the practice of medicine. While some clinicians hold the role as scientist, their act as healers in engaging the seriously ill is undermined when their role is chiefly guided by this storyline. The patient's illness is a located within the body but cannot be limited to only the body. When the patient–clinician relationship is informed, acted upon—largely in material-only terms—and advanced within the object–observer metaphor, aspects of healing are clearly marginalized as the patient experience becomes nearly irrelevant.[10]

An integrated view of the person and healing carried by the Abrahamic traditions is not necessarily a critique against anthropologies that advocate for a religious dualism, which understand a human distinction between body and soul. In our estimation, anthropological dualism per se is not the culprit, but rather it is failure to uphold these distinctions within a larger anthropological unity. Among the Abrahamic traditions, there has been a largely consistent embrace of a dualistic perspective of humanity that has recognized the person to comprise both material and immaterial dimensions, or body and soul.[11 [p. 306-349]] This dualistic anthropology has sometimes produced a pessimistic theological account of the body, often thought to be introduced early into the Jewish and Christian traditions through Greek-influenced philosophies such as Platonism and Gnosticism.[12 [pp. 82-83]] For example, Gnosticism in early Christianity concluded that all matter was intrinsically evil, and this consequently led to conclusions that God could not have directly created the world nor that a human Jesus could also be God since both involve the Supreme Deity having direct contact with the material matter of the universe. If matter was tainted with evil, then Ultimate Deity cannot possibly be directly connected to it. The Abrahamic traditions have, as a whole, however, rejected any view that fails to see matter and material things as being intrinsically good. These extremely negative opinions were widely condemned as inconsistent with the biblical narrative in which God created the world "good" and, in the New Testament, where Christ both took on flesh in his incarnation and received a resurrected material body. While slightly different forms of anthropological dualism have dominated the Christian tradition, in its Augustinian and Thomisitic versions there is a general recognition that the body and soul must be held together in unity, despite the recognition of theoretical distinctions between the two. Thus, more recently, Paul Ramsey suggested a unitive understanding of the human as "embodied soul or ensouled body."[13 [p. xiii]] While the Abrahamic traditions have not always consistently theorized about the unity of material and immaterial aspects of persons, leading to problematic diminishments of the body at certain time points, even then a hierarchy of soul over body did not subsequently undermine care for the physically sick. Ironically, it was within ascetic communities where care of the body thrived most consistently.[14-16] So while we would warn against hierarchal or axiological forms of dualism that undermine the importance and sacredness of the human body,[17 [p. 184ff.]] religious practice and compassion for the body have often trumped diminishments of the body within purely theoretical accounts.

This suggests that the problem is less with theories that embrace anthropological dualism and more with the tendency within modern practice to divide and separate body and soul so that they fail to coinhere or mutually penetrate one another as contingent (even if rationally divisible) parts of the person. While some modern theologians blame anthropological dualism *en toto* for current accounts of medicine's exclusive focus on the body,[12] in our view this claim makes an argument of causation but provides little proof beyond correlation.[iii] A simpler and more cautious interpretation should focus on those views that have de-twinned body from soul, to the degree that one sphere has been disproportionally elevated above the other, losing a semblance of mystery and balance between each distinction.[iv] Anthropological dualism has not led to bodily focus, but instead to a willingness to view body and soul as independent of one another. So while the Abrahamic traditions by no means speak with a single voice on this matter, at a minimum there has been recognition and concern about caring for the sick in both body and soul regardless of how philosophically we might understand their particular relationship. Within contemporary medicine, clinicians are socialized to isolate their healing focus to the body only. One of the impacts of this emphasis is that it leads to impersonal ways of thinking about illness and caregiving. Another impact is that it suggests that compartmentalization may be an appropriate way to engage patients as a nurse or physician. Beneath both is a value system about personhood that cannot be proved or disproved by the empirical method. Hence, the object-observer metaphor implicitly rests on a value system or theology of persons.

Human Persons in Relationship

In contrast to the object–observer metaphor, illness includes biological processes but is much more than biology. It is a shattering experience, causing disintegration within the self and within relationships. As Daniel Sulmasy has argued, from an integrated understanding of human persons, we are beings in relationship.[5 (p. 125)] Sulmasy suggests that in order to truly begin to know a person, there is need to understand "the complex sets of relationships that define" the person.[5 (p. 125)] Therefore, rather than defining disease primarily according to a reductionist, scientific model, "disease can be described as a disruption of right relationships" and healing the "restoration of right relationships."[5 (p. 125)] Sulmasy argues that illness and healing are both "intrapersonal," affecting the physical body and the mind, and "extrapersonal," in relationship to the physical environment, other persons, and the transcendent.[5 (p. 126)] Sulmasy called this medical model of healing the "Biopsychosocial-Spiritual" model of care.[18] His proposal is an integrated one that not only attempts to uphold some unity between body and soul, but additionally sees the person as nested within the complexity of multiple relationships. He says, "in this model, the biological, psychological, social, and spiritual are distinct dimensions of the person and no individual aspect can be disaggregated from the whole. Each aspect can be affected differently by a person's history and illness, and each aspect can interact and affect other aspects of the person."[5 (p. 128)] Sulmasy's philosophical anthropology does not in any way reject the scientific method, nor does it deny the use of a reductionist, empirical approach to medicine. Rather, the scientific approach to medicine, in Sulmasy's view, is subsumed under a larger framework based on an anthropology focused on relationships. Consequently, the role of scientist is a subordinate rather than chief role of the clinician.

Sulmasy's presuppositions highlight the fact that, for patients, the experience of illness is not solely a physical or material experience. Illness impacts the body, but it stretches beyond the material to include emotions and relationships. Serious illness raises basic questions about identity, the meaning of life, and what happens after death. It is a disruption of relationships between loved ones, raising existential questions around the permanence of their disruption. These questions are existential and spiritual in character, and, for many, they invite an explicit turn to religion. Because illness frays patients' unifying sense of self and others, there is a natural impulse to seek holism in order to repair integrity, restore order, and reconstitute broken relationships. If illness is an experience that erodes intra- and extrapersonal relationships, fragmenting human aims of order, unity, and coherence, then a structural healing system should self-consciously foster reintegration at all levels of patient relationships. Though the sacred–secular separation operates efficiently within certain aspects of human experience, and while reductionism leads to some insights in disease causation and treatment, in the context of serious illness and according to an integrated model, those ideologies that assume hard divisions of the person amplify the very aspects of illness that patients seek to overcome. Rather than mending the fraying of life caused by illness, an integrated understanding of persons is a critical replacement of body–soul separation, which only exacerbates the feeling of dissolution that patients experience due to their disease.

Within the patient–clinician relationship, the object–observer metaphor removes relationships between the clinician and the patient as a primary human encounter between persons. As scientist, the clinician must be objective and neutral in order to identify and cure the disease and must avoid becoming caught up in her own emotional and subjective feelings. As body, the patient is passively controlled, disconnected from his body, and often reminded that his own subjective experience and agency are less relevant to healing. The metaphor objectifies both clinician and patient and eschews relationship as a necessary dimension of the healing process. In this model, not only is relationship undermined between patient and clinician, but relationship to a larger context is deemed peripheral, a distraction, or an obstacle to the patient's healing.

In contrast to a healing model that is impersonal, Sulmasy's approach demands that understanding of the person, disease, and healing must account for the relational dimension. The genius of this viewpoint is that even among those who deny or are skeptical of the concept of the soul, the relational component of personhood is verifiable on its face. The concept of personhood has theological roots associated with the doctrine of God,[19] and there is growing recognition throughout healthcare that individual bodies cannot be seen or understood in isolation apart from a network of biological, social, and environmental relationships that comprise disease and health.[20–22] Thus, models that are relational in nature and uphold connection remain crucial missing pieces that need to be regained within the patient–clinician relationship. Recapturing a focus on relationships does not eliminate the object–observer dynamic but subjugates it as a secondary lens of understanding that is subservient to relational perspectives.

Ways of Compartmentalization

Chapter 7 explored the plausibility structures that divide life into two overarching, separated domains: the immanent and the transcendent. As illustrated in Table 7.1, the two overarching domains comprise social structures that shape conceptions of human nature, knowledge, and human relationships. The separation of immanence and transcendence cuts across all of life, from the micro level—how we divide an individual's body and soul—to the macro—how we divide socially constructed realities such as fact and value, public and private, or state and church. These social structures have channeled the attention of nurses and physicians away from addressing patients' religion and spirituality within life-threatening illness. Historically, the advance of scientific medicine beginning in the Age of Enlightenment enforced a sacred–secular separation that has ultimately resulted in the current state in which the provision of spiritual care to patients is considered outside medicine's domain.

The sacred–secular divide reflects an underlying understanding of human nature that flattens patient experiences of illness and the nature of caregiving. Though inspiring great discoveries, the primacy of the scientific metaphor undermines the ability of professionals and institutions to care for human persons in their embodied experience of illness and suffering.[10,22] While most readers presumably agree in principle that it is not appropriate to imagine the ill as if they were primarily objects of science, there has been insufficient recognition of this truth in practice. Our claim is that the willingness to compartmentalize sacred and secular lies extremely close to the core reason that gives permission for medical culture to divide body from soul, justifying the object–observer relationship, which in turn inspires less personal social roles for clinicians, patients, and institutions. Impersonal metaphors will continue to dominate patient care until the underlying beliefs supporting it are recognized and addressed.

What lies beneath the sacred–secular divide operating in medicine is an anthropology that claims the possibility of real and actual separation of the human person. The theory behind such a division remains implicit, perhaps unclear within day-to-day practice, yet an implicit theology lurks beneath. One view, often termed *physicalism*, is simply that human persons are material objects, and it is our material selves that produce personality, subjective experience, and other "nonmaterial" dimensions of the person. In this view, there is warrant for medical professionals to focus only on objective dimensions of disease since the subjective dimensions of illness are products of and secondary to the physical. This view rejects the immaterial dimension of persons and complements reductionistic approaches to persons focused on the material body.

On the other end of the spectrum is Platonism and Cartesian dualism, which understands the primary substance of the person to be the immortal soul and the physical body to be a temporary and secondary substance of the person. For Plato, the soul was immortal while the body was its prison.[v] From the view of seventeenth-century philosopher Rene Descartes, the radical distinction between body and soul as separate and divided substances enabled subsequent generations to view the human body in terms of a machine or impersonal thing (*res extensa*).[vi] This latter view does not reject the notion of the soul, but it perceives a radical distinction between body and soul. Herein lies a theological anthropology that understands the material and immaterial dimensions to be radically distinct and able to operate apart from the other. This view of the person lays the groundwork to justify medicine's objectification of the body and its employment of the object–observer metaphor.

Where this understanding of the person becomes theological is in its account of spirituality and religion. Some accounts of physicalism are reductionistic in that they conclude that spirituality and religion are simply neuro- and biochemical processes of the brain. While religion may have a neurochemical basis, the leap in logic occurs when someone claims that religion is *merely* or *only* the result of these processes. When one suggests that spirituality or religion can be fully explained by material processes, then he is not only positing an empirically unverifiable fact about the nature of persons, he is positively claiming to understand the essence of human personhood. It is a conclusion that seems quasi-theological since it renders judgment on the nature of the human soul. Such claims typically result in arguments that reject spirituality and religion as "real," and, consequently, spiritual care is interpreted as irrelevant for the practice of scientific medicine.

Contrastingly, while contemporary accounts of Cartesian dualism acknowledge the immaterial in principle, this form of dualism has come to typically regard religion in terms of private human experience and subjective meaning-making. Here again are theological conclusions in which body and soul are independent entities with no necessary or obvious overlap or interpenetration. Unlike physicalism, the soul is not denied; but like physicalism, Cartesian dualism treats the body as objectified and matter as reducible into its component parts. Because body and soul fall categorically into different realms, it is justifiable for the domestic and personal realms to give expression to the immaterial but equally justifiable for the public to be the realm of the material body, stripped of meaning beyond the mundane and the economic, and exposed to accounts of efficient causation and manipulation through control.[7]

This form of dualism relies upon and proliferates psychological and social compartmentalization. Berger and colleagues described this as a form of consciousness in which persons toggle between multiple relevance structures or forms of consciousness.[23] In their account, they argue that humans are capable of thinking and acting based on a particular set of "relevances" in one social domain and then able to think and act on another set of relevances when operating in a different domain. Thus, the human mind has the capacity to divide itself based on the elevation and devaluation of what is deemed relevant for consciousness related to a set of actions and domains.

For example, among patients, this dualistic form of consciousness may lead many patients to be willing to sacrifice receipt of human compassion in favor of greater technical competence from their physician.[24] The former is viewed by some as less important for the practice of medicine than receiving technically superior medical skills. In this account, patients see physicians as primarily technicians of the body, from whom human compassion may be desired but is not absolutely necessary to the task. Many patients are willing to tolerate being viewed chiefly as bodies, rather than persons, if such a process allows them to ultimately regain physical health. Yet such a division between technical competency and compassion is an unnecessary dichotomy. While many patients are willing, if necessary, to sacrifice compassion but not the physician's technical knowledge and skills, we imagine that few patients desire this division in principle. While this division is possible, it is neither desired nor is it a norm to be sought and instituted. It also fails to account for the role of trust and human connectedness within the patient–clinician relationship as these relate to a therapeutic bond and patient healing. In a similar vein, among medical caregivers, a tendency to dehumanize or objectify patients can lead to derogatory attitudes toward patients, as illustrated by Samuel Shem's disturbing novel about medical residency,[25] corroborated by empirical studies,[26,27] or even occasionally developing into the deeply unethical behaviors described by one recent anonymous author.[28] Because the human mind is capable of compartmentalizing, physicians can be "caring" for the patient's body while performing a medical procedure and yet, ironically, act as devilishly careless and unkind, as Shem and others suggest. Once again, compartmentalization and burnout are risks for all medical professionals, especially when facing a high volume of patients, long work hours, and lack of rest and perspective.[27,29] These tendencies are to be overcome and changed, not accepted as inevitable aspects of human psychology, as Berger and others seem to imply.

What lies at the core of these dichotomies of the person is a belief that it is not a violation or diminishment of personhood to bracket our most core values such as kindness, compassion, love, or spiritual identities when working in certain social contexts. From this perspective, it is warranted to suspend personal human commitments and core values when in certain contexts. These divisions find a home within an ideology of medicine that posits medical professionals primarily as scientists and further justifies that the object of professional medical concern is disease rather than the person who is ill.[22] The dominance of the object–observer metaphor in secular medicine has flowed from an underlying ideology that has divided body and soul as independent entities, and it remains dependent on this division for the object–observer metaphor to hold its sway.

Although humans are clearly capable of compartmentalizing thoughts and actions tailored to specific domains, institutions, and relationships, it is important to also highlight that the human capacity to divide oneself from one's chief values can also lead to a plethora of immoral acts and atrocities.[vii] Against compartmentalization, holistic accounts of personhood aim to pursue integrated forms of consciousness so that what one chiefly loves characterizes all of one's existence, inclusive of every social domain. For example, many traditional religious accounts, especially Abrahamic ones, believe that love for God is "totalizing," proposing that there is no place, time, sphere, or role for an individual to live as if God did not exist. An integrated religious consciousness within the monotheistic traditions expects followers to live *coram deo* ("before the face of God"). In responding to Berger's view, medical oncologist Alan Astrow argued that a Jewish physician most certainly can implicitly integrate her or his identity as a faithful follower of God with identity as a surgeon.[30,viii] Astrow suggests that one need not and should not leave faith aside when entering the operating room. He even suggests that the surgeon's faith-based values can ultimately serve the patient and result in better technical care, further breaking down the dichotomies suggested by Berger's thesis concerning "relevances." Ultimately, human consciousness may indeed be habituated into a form of compartmentalization, but this is not constitutive to the human mind, even in cultures dominated by the sacred–secular division. Suspension of our love—when we act, to use Berger's phrase, "as if God did not exist"—even if performed for a finite period, is a violation of higher human consciousness and the logic of love in relationship. Thus, practices of psychological compartmentalization among physicians reflect, not an intrinsic habit of the mind as suggested by Berger, but an underlying belief system of what it means to be and to act as a human person. Arguments justifying compartmentalization are also quasi-theological as they attempt to partly describe the essence of personhood.

A Theology of Persons

What underlies differences among clinician caregiving patterns is that some theological understandings of the nature of humanity are receptive to and others are resistant to the sacred–secular division. It is not that a subset of American clinicians practice medicine informed by a *theological anthropology*, while clinicians who conform to the sacred–secular social structure are atheological and neutral. Rather, integrated, physicalist, and compartmentalized views rely on unspoken but powerfully influential theological understandings of the essence of human consciousness as well as understandings of how social structures should reflect that consciousness. One group of clinicians believes that human consciousness can be divided or compartmentalized, and thus it is at least somewhat acceptable or perhaps inevitable that clinicians focus on the material realm and leave the immaterial soul of the patient to others. Another set of clinicians believes that human consciousness is integrated, and thus it is unacceptable, even a violation of human personhood, to focus medical care on only the material dimension of illness. Our contention in this chapter is that those who separate body and soul are doing so based implicitly on a theological anthropology and that this overlays a religious-like worldview on all involved in medicine. Many clinicians and patients hold to a variety of spiritual commitments, both traditionally religious and humanistic, which reject compartmentalized beliefs of the person. Instead, many are committed to forms of caregiving and seeing the experience of illness as grounded in a form of consciousness that binds together, integrates, and seeks to make whole. The point is that a theology of persons inheres below all approaches.

What we have argued here is that both an integrated perspective and a model of separation as they pertain to social structures are in fact based on implicit theological presuppositions regarding the nature of the human person as the human relates to ultimate reality. Neither position can prove its position on assumptions concerning the essence of personhood. Neither the integrated or separated views can be proved empirically or demonstrated a posteriori through pure reason. Rather, these are foundational claims about our human constitution that are theological as they relate to what is believed to be ultimate. What this suggests is that our contemporary social structures, which are axiomatic concerning a dichotomy between transcendence and immanence, are socially constructed without basis in an objective reality of personhood. Thus, the sacred–secular distinction is not based in a purely factual reality. Just as separating the material and immaterial dimensions of personhood is a quasi-religious claim, likewise is the bifurcation of social structures illustrated in Table 7.1. These are theological visions of personhood being applied to the social structures of medicine. It is not therefore a question of *if* theology will shape the practices of medicine but *which one*?[ix] Located below the sacred–secular separation of modern medicine are understandings of human consciousness and personhood that are theological rather than, as commonly claimed, neutral and nonspiritual.

These theological understandings of the person also explain spiritual care practice patterns among clinicians. In a nationwide survey, physicians (n = 1,144) were found to be more likely to attend religious services than the general population (90% vs. 81%). However, they were less likely to say that they "try to carry their religious beliefs over into all other dealings in life" (58% vs. 73%), twice as likely to "cope with major problems in life without relying on God" (61% vs. 29%), and twice as likely to describe themselves as spiritual, not religious (20% vs. 9%).[x] This survey indicated that though physicians generally have a *higher frequency* of religious attendance—a finding that surprised many since it had been popularly believed that physicians were similar to other scientists in their irreligion—they tend to privatize religious faith. Many clinicians are in fact attracted to medical careers because of a spiritual sense of calling and an associated desire to care for the most hurting in society.[31] Yet once physicians are duly socialized into the profession, conceptions of their professional roles, responsibilities, and boundaries are more likely to be disconnected from their spiritual impulses and primarily guided by a sacred–secular framework. This framework demands a body–soul dualism and consequently requires clinicians—even those who begin their careers assuming a body–soul integration—to privatize personal faith and calling.

Of course, not all accept these separations in patient care. Curlin reported that high physician religiosity and spirituality predicted a sixfold increase in spiritual care inquiry compared to physicians who reported low levels of religion and spirituality. Yet it would be a misinterpretation of these data to conclude that only religiously oriented physicians are bringing their theology of personhood into the clinical encounter as they see their patients as both body and soul. Its opposite is also accurate: physicians who follow a stark separation of body and soul within personhood are six times more likely to focus on the human body and ignore or avoid spiritual dimensions of illness. Though both approaches rest within implicit theological claims concerning the essence of personhood, it is the object–observer metaphor that currently dominates medicine and helps explain why patients so infrequently receive acknowledgment, discussion, or support of their own spiritual experiences.

Conclusion

The goal of this chapter is to describe distinct theological beliefs about the essence of personhood and explain that these views inform how clinicians inevitably see and engage patients. Dichotomizing the person into immaterial and material is at its root a claim concerning the essence of personhood, and this ultimately implies an underlying religious-like position concerning the presence or absence of a soul. While we grant that the intention of the sacred–secular divide was envisioned to create a neutral and nonreligious sphere, the evidence continues to become clearer that this bifurcated structure is itself based on an unverifiable, religious-like position about human personhood.

Next, our analysis takes an additional important step in our argument as we consider how there is a deep, analogical connection between medicine and religion within medicine's basic structures. The social structures of secular medicine contain sacramental expressions. We will argue that, as secular medicine juxtaposes itself against Western religion, medicine then begins to resemble or appear like a religion itself.

Notes

i. It should also be noted that there is an emerging impersonal metaphor within an industrialized medical environment: the physician–patient relationship as an buyer–seller relationship. We would suggest that this metaphor is emerging in US society, but it currently remains secondary to the object–observer dynamic in most people's imaginations. This metaphor is discussed further in Chapter 16.

ii. Instrumental uses of spirituality and religion are briefly discussed and critiqued in Chapter 3 and then more extensively in Chapter 14.

iii. John Cooper shows how anthropological dualism does not by necessity undermine orthopraxis in chapter 9 of his work.[17]

iv. Monistic understandings of the person, which make essentially no distinction between material and immaterial aspects of personhood, are hardly guaranteed to repair false social dichotomies, but they do risk a continued suppression of the immaterial soul aspect of humanity within medicine since its most extreme view is a materialistic reductionism. Monistic views are heavily weighted toward the material aspect of humans, and one must labor in our current environment to uphold the immaterial or spiritual dimension. It seems to us that there is a knee-jerk rejection of anthropological dualism among some theologians in favor of monism, but we have little confidence that this addresses the true problem that we encounter in medicine. There is a cultural rejection of the reality of the soul or immaterial aspect of humanity, and it is the loss of the soul that is especially in need of recovery in our time.

v. "Every seeker after wisdom knows that up to the time when philosophy takes over his soul is a helpless prisoner, chained hand and foot inside the body, forced to view reality not directly but only through the prison bars, and wallowing in utter ignorance" (Phaedo, 82e).

vi. "Now a very large number of the motions occurring inside us do not depend in any way on the mind. These include heartbeat, digestion, nutrition, respiration when we are asleep, and also such waking actions as walking, singing, and the like, when these occur without the mind attending to them. When people take a fall, and stick out their hands so as to protect their head, it is not reason that instructs them to do this; it is simply that the sight of the impending fall reaches the brain and sends the animal spirits into the nerves in the manner necessary to produce this movement even without any mental volition, just as it would be produced in a machine" (*Treatise on Man* and *Passions*, 7:229–230). See also Drew Leder. *The Absent Body*. Chicago: University of Chicago Press; 1990.

vii. Contrary to what Berger and colleagues have argued, the capacity or even proclivity to compartmentalize is not constitutive to being human. We can deny compartmentalization as an ideal practice of the human mind because, on its face, there continue to be several philosophical value systems and theological anthropologies that argue that compartmentalization reflects human brokenness and should be resisted.

viii. We had the opportunity to engage Peter Berger on these issues in a small working group held at Boston University in 2014, organized by Dr. Jonathan Imber. Respondents engaged and critiqued Peter Berger's views as they applied to medical practice. We thought that Alan Astrow provided the strongest arguments against Berger's dichotomous views regarding secularization applied to medicine. Publications of each presentation, including Berger's argument and Astrow's, were published in *Society*, 2015, 52(5). One of our responses is also in that volume: Everyday religion in hospitals. *Society*. 2015;52(5):413–417.

ix. In the conclusion of Jeffrey Bishop's *The Anticipatory Corpse*, he wonders if "only theology can save medicine?"[7 [p. 313]] What we are arguing here is that medicine already holds to an implicit theology and that this theology undergirds all of contemporary medicine. Medicine is not in need of a turn to theology, but what we take Bishop to really mean is that there is need for both an overt discussion about medicine using theological sources and methods and, moreover, the an acknowledgment of the importance of substantive theological traditions analyzing and reshaping biomedicine.

x. See F. A. Curlin, Lantos J. D., Roach C. J., Sellergren S. A., Chin M. H. Religious characteristics of US physicians: a national survey. *J Gen Intern Med*. 2005;20(7):629–634. This study also found significant differences in religious orientation between religious minority groups in the United States and physician religious affiliation: Jewish (2% vs. 14%), Hindu (0.2% vs. 5.3%), Muslim (0.5% vs. 2.7%), and Buddhist (0.2% vs. 1.2%). Disparity in religious affiliation and spiritual attitudes between physicians and the US population may further exacerbate barriers in providing spiritual care.

References

1. Deborah Lupton. *Medicine as culture: illness, disease and the body in Western societies.* 2nd ed. London: Sage; 2003.
2. Guenter B. Risse. Medical care. In: W. F. Bynum, Porter R., eds. *Companion encyclopedia of the history of medicine.* Vol 1. London: Routledge; 1997:67.
3. M. J. Balboni, T. A. Balboni. Medicine and spirituality in historical perspective. In: John Peteet, D'Ambra Michael, eds. *The soul of medicine: spirituality and world view in clinical practice.* Baltimore: John Hopkins University Press; 2011:3–22.
4. Michel Foucault. *The birth of the clinic.* London: Routledge; 1989.
5. Daniel P. Sulmasy. *The rebirth of the clinic: an introduction to spirituality in health care.* Washington, DC: Georgetown University Press; 2006.
6. Richard P. Sloan. *Blind faith: the unholy alliance of religion and medicine.* 1st ed. New York: St. Martin's Press; 2006.
7. Jeffrey Paul Bishop. *The anticipatory corpse: medicine, power, and the care of the dying.* Notre Dame, IN: University of Notre Dame Press; 2011.
8. Joel James Shuman, Meador Keith G. *Heal thyself: spirituality, medicine, and the distortion of Christianity.* New York: Oxford University Press; 2003.
9. Roy Porter. *The greatest benefit to mankind: a medical history of humanity.* 1st American ed. New York: W. W. Norton; 1998.
10. Arthur Kleinman. *The illness narratives: suffering, healing, and the human condition.* New York: Basic Books; 1988.
11. Veli-Matti Kärkkäinen. *Creation and humanity.* Grand Rapids, MI: W. B. Eerdmans Publishing; 2015.
12. Allen Verhey. *Reading the bible in the strange world of medicine.* Grand Rapids, MI: W. B. Eerdmans Publishing; 2003.
13. Paul Ramsey. *The patient as person; explorations in medical ethics.* New Haven, CT: Yale University Press; 1970.
14. Guenter B. Risse. *Mending bodies, saving souls: a history of hospitals.* New York: Oxford University Press; 1999.
15. G. B. Risse, Balboni M. J. Shifting hospital-hospice boundaries: historical perspective on the institutional care of the dying. *Am J Hosp Palliat Care.* 2013;30(4):325–330.
16. Gary B. Ferngren. *Medicine & health care in early Christianity.* Baltimore: Johns Hopkins University Press; 2009.
17. John W. Cooper. *Body, soul, and life everlasting: biblical anthropology and the monism-dualism debate.* Grand Rapids, MI: W. B. Eerdmans Publishing; 2000.
18. D. P. Sulmasy. A biopsychosocial-spiritual model for the care of patients at the end of life. *Gerontologist.* 2002;42 Spec No 3:24–33.
19. Jean Zizioulas. *Being as communion: studies in personhood and the church.* Crestwood, NY: St. Vladimir's Seminary Press; 1985.
20. Paul Farmer. *Reimagining global health: an introduction.* Berkeley: University of California Press; 2013.
21. Tyler J. VanderWeele. Religion and health: a synthesis. In: Michael Balboni, Peteet John, eds. *Spirituality and religion within the culture of medicine.* New York: Oxford University Press; 2017:357–401.
22. Eric J. Cassell. *The nature of suffering and the goals of medicine.* 2nd ed. New York: Oxford University Press; 2004.
23. Peter L. Berger, Berger Brigitte, Kellner Hansfried. *The homeless mind:modernization and consciousness.* New York: Vintage Books; 1974.
24. C. D. MacLean, Susi B., Phifer N., Schultz L., Bynum D., Franco M., Klioze A., Monroe M., Garrett J., Cykert S. Patient preference for physician discussion and practice of spirituality. *J Gen Intern Med.* 2003;18(1):38–43.
25. Samuel Shem. *The house of God: a novel.* New York: R. Marek Publishers; 1978.

26. C. Feudtner, Christakis D. A., Christakis N. A. Do clinical clerks suffer ethical erosion? Students' perceptions of their ethical environment and personal development. *Acad Med.* 1994;69(8):670–679.

27. L. N. Dyrbye, Varkey P., Boone S. L., Satele D. V., Sloan J. A., Shanafelt T. D. Physician satisfaction and burnout at different career stages. *Mayo Clin Proc.* 2013;88(12):1358–1367.

28. Anonymous. Our family secrets. *Ann Intern Med.* 2015;163(4):321.

29. T. D. Shanafelt, Hasan O., Dyrbye L. N., Sinsky C., Satele D., Sloan J., West C. P. Changes in burnout and satisfaction with work-life balance in physicians and the general US working population between 2011 and 2014. *Mayo Clin Proc.* 2015;90(12):1600–1613.

30. A. B. Astrow. Jewish values, empathy, and the doctor-patient relationship. *Society.* 2015;52(5):418–423.

31. J. D. Yoon, Shin J. H., Nian A. L., Curlin F. A. Religion, sense of calling, and the practice of medicine: findings from a national survey of primary care physicians and psychiatrists. *South Med J.* 2015;108(3):189–195.

11

The Sacramental Nature of Medicine

While the centrality of the patient in medicine has clear connection to certain religious values described in Chapter 9, it has often been observed that key aspects of medicine have strange, even uncanny, similarities with religious phenomena. Renowned nineteenth-century physician and scholar William Osler preached a sermon in 1910 entitled "Man's Redemption of Man" that illustrated these parallels. He upheld the great importance of medical science by interpreting medical progress as a fulfillment of the religious teachings of Christianity. He said that physical disease and pain were the true curse of Adam, passed down as original sin. But with the dawn and "ever-increasing success" of scientific medicine, the promise of the "true gospel" arose. By way of example, Osler suggested that medicine's discovery and employment of ether anesthesia in 1846 was an eschatological fulfillment of the promised Kingdom of God where "neither shall there by any more pain"—a reference to John's Apocalypse as prophesied in the New Testament book of Revelation (21:4) and referenced on the ether monument in Boston described in Chapter 9. He proclaimed that "the leaves of the tree of science have availed for the healing of the nations," alluding to the complete healing foreseen in Revelation 22:2. In Osler's narrative, spiritual salvations originating in God's redemption were symbolic manifestations that ultimately "sink into insignificance" in light of medical science, which carries true power to transform the human condition. For Osler, salvation had arrived through the power of humanity to save others from physical suffering and illness. Reversing the Apostle Paul's words to the Ephesians—"We do not wrestle against flesh and blood but against the principalities, against powers, against the rulers of the darkness of this age, against spiritual hosts of wickedness in the heavenly places" (6:12)—he ended his sermon by calling all medical scientists to "wrestle for [people's] flesh and blood against the principalities and powers" represented by disease and poor public health conditions. As the highly ingenious son of a clergyman, Osler thus reinterpreted these New Testament spiritual concepts and recast Christianity within a narrative of medical science. Osler's view was that the spiritual claims of the old Christian religion were signs and symbols of a greater salvation made available in our grand scientific age that can be accomplished in and through medicine rather than in life after death. Medical science fulfills and eclipses religion.

While Osler's comparison of medicine and Christianity is a good example of Liberal Protestantism's overly realized eschatology, scholars have continued to note important similarities between medicine and religion. For example, consider this observation by the eminent Harvard medical historian Charles Rosenberg: "Most of us harbor a pervasive faith in the world of scientific medicine, a visceral and inarticulate hope of a temporal salvation: modern medicine will extend life, avoid pain, provide a gentle death."[1] [p. 191] Such a sentiment is expanded within a growing literature in medical anthropology that perceives cultural parallels between religiously oriented healing traditions and the religious aura that operates within biomedicine.[2-8] Some anthropologists perceive within biomedicine religious images including a "fundamentalist epistemology" and "salvation . . . present in the technical efficacy of medicine."[9] [pp. 7,86]

Similarly, within the field of sociology, Talcott Parsons suggested parallels between physicians and clergy. He argued that physicians replaced clergy in their function within society by becoming the primary mediators of issues around death. In Parson's view, physicians, as both professional symbols and actors, alleviate social anxiety arising from a fear of death.[10] [p. 444] Parsons suggested that the social function of physicians within modern society carries "very important associations with the realm of the sacred."[10] [p. 445] He did not go so far as to conflate a physician's role with a priest's per se but suggested an affinity in function. Parsons noted that medical students begin their formation into this role through dissection of a cadaver, describing this as "a symbolic act, highly charged with affective significance. It is in a sense the initiatory rite of physician-to-be into his intimate association with death and the dead."[10] [p. 445] Others have similarly reflected on how initiation into medical school can be compared to shamanistic indoctrination and hazing rituals.[11] [pp. 173-174] These are but a few examples of scholars in the fields of history, anthropology, and sociology noting uncanny similarities between medicine and religion.

In this chapter, we argue that the reason that scholars have made comparisons between medicine and religion is that there is an underlying structural bond between biomedicine on the one hand and religious monotheism on the other. There are shared assumptions, values, and institutional structures that create a deep underlying unity between these two spheres. When these two spheres become overtly disconnected from one another as partners, as now is the case in secular medicine, medicine rises perilously to the level of a functional-like religion. While secular medicine attempts to be consciously neutral toward all religions, medicine's internal structures mirror deeper religious concepts.

Medicine and Monotheism

The contention of scholars within anthropology, history, and sociology that aspects of biomedicine are religious-like contrasts with a narrative of secular medicine that explicitly juxtaposes medicine and religion. Suggesting that biomedicine has a religious aura thus may seem on its face nonsensical to those relying on a substantive understanding of religion (see Chapter 8). Yet it is academically plausible to perceive a resemblance between medicine and religion based on functional accounts for religious phenomenon. Based on this analytical perspective, several commentators have argued that, within the United States in the twentieth century, traditional religion has been marginalized to the private realm, and, in its place, science and medicine have arisen as a cultural religion. Scientific medicine now takes the role of religion especially as it pertains to the social function of assuaging human fears associated with illness.[12] Scientific medical knowledge, the social role of physicians, and the hospital as society's healing institution operate in tandem to assuage fear, raise hope, and battle the demons of sickness and death. Together they provide a complex network of beliefs, rituals, and relationships that offer meaning and hope in our secular age.

When adopting a definition of "religion" that does not require belief in the supernatural, medicine can be seen as functionally religion-like.[12–16] For example, upon analyzing scientific medicine through the lens of a functional definition for religion, Vanderpool found that medicine manifests seven of ten religion-like characteristics.[16 [p. 224]] He summarized his analysis by concluding that contemporary medicine is not a religion itself, but, since there are enough shared phenomenological similarities, "The common assumption that scientific medicine is altogether secular and nonreligious is a myth that masks medicine's cultural scaffolding. The religious beams of that scaffolding contribute enormously to medicine's cultural appeal, acceptance, and power."[16 [p. 220]]

The religion-like nature of biomedicine is not a coincidence but rather a sign of the underlying Western cultural context. In fact, Harvard psychiatrist and medical anthropologist Arthur Kleinman has provocatively argued that one of biomedicine's most distinctive features is rooted in its connection to monotheism.[17] He postulated that "the idea of a single god legitimates the idea of a single, underlying, universalizable truth, a unitary paradigm."[17 [p. 16]] Belief in a single Cause in the spiritual realm has produced expectations that the created realm will also be explainable within a frame of single causal chains that explain both pathogenesis and effective therapies. Kleinman argued that no other large-scale cultural healing systems—such as Chinese or Ayurvedic medicine—have this unique characteristic concerning causation precisely because underlying religious presuppositions shape each major healing system. In modern times, Eastern healing approaches have added biomedicine into their arsenal, not because of recognition of some internal insufficiency in Eastern healing, but precisely on the basis of a polytheistic religious context. Polytheistic Asian assumptions of the spiritual realm lead to polytherapeutic acceptance of multiple, non-overlapping healing practices. With the adulation of many gods, one can enthusiastically recognize and incorporate many different healing practices. In Asia, biomedicine has been absorbed as one legitimate type of healing theory among many legitimate choices, whereby polytheism produces an outlook that does not require the ordering of these different medical theories into a single, overarching system of cause and effect. Conversely, in the West, which has been dominated by monotheism, nonempirical forms of healing are viewed suspiciously and accommodated only as inferior forms of healing. They remain on the margins of today's biomedical enterprise, largely incorporated for economic, not theory-based or empirically validated, reasons.

In contrast to the Asian polyideological model, the Abrahamic faiths have concluded that the One God (Deuteronomy 6:4; Mark 12:29–30; Quran 47.19) is the source of healing. God has chosen to regularly provide healing through the mechanisms of the creation governed by divine providence (Ben Sira 38) and in fulfillment of neighborly love and philanthropy. Such theological understandings have justified a material form of healing since the material, finite order is created by God and serves God's purposes.

The demystification of healing practices within Judaism and Christianity has been based within the particular ethos of these faiths' shared understanding of God's nature, providence, and the created realm. Judaism, Christianity, and Islam, in contrast to Eastern religions, have been medicine's principle guardians, institutionalizers, and practitioners for more than two millennia.

Rooted within an Abrahamic axiom that differentiates Creator from creation, the principles of reductionism and positivism are central to the operations of Western biomedicine. Reductionism refers to a manner of description of phenomenon that understands more complex entities as reducible to their simpler and most basic component parts. Positivism assumes that a material object is authentically real (not an illusion) and can be examined through hypothesis testing based on the scientific method. A Creator–creature distinction demystifies creation, enabling an expectation that the creation is rational (made in *imago dei* who is Rationale or *Logos*) and that creation ought to be subdued by nurturing order out of the chaos. It also implies that physical phenomena have a single cause, rather than arising from a complex and often unstable web of influences. From this perspective, the created material order is to be studied, not rejected as an ultimate illusion of mind. Because the created order is finite, the Abrahamic traditions find it inconceivable to worship material objects as an ultimate extension of the divine-self, as in Hindu and other Asian religious systems. A divinization of the created, earthly order calls for its worship, not the making of a scientific mind that seeks to understand finite, non-divine things. Embedded within monotheism are the presuppositions required to approach the material world and its phenomena as real rather than an illusion and as created objects to be studied, rather than as subjects of devotion, worship, or renunciation.[18]

The singularity of objective truth, notwithstanding the role of individual perception, may appear to flow out of monotheistic belief of a single Truth, and it is ultimately this principle which has, over time, mistakenly grown into an impersonal medicine. The subjective aspects of the sick person are believed to be irrelevant to disease processes, and, in fact, the patient's perceptions often get in the way of accurate diagnosis or cure. Eric Cassell lays the fundamental problem of medicine's dualism on the devaluing of subjective knowledge of the sick person and the quest for objective certainty.[19 [p. xii]] Similarly, Kleinman concludes that the radical principles of reductionism and positivism are the ultimate catalyst leading to the dehumanization of the patient.[17 [p. 18]] Cassell and Kleinman have for the past generation been two leading voices providing compelling arguments on how scientific reductionism has problematically mislaid the meaning-making narrative of sick persons.[19-21] In slightly modifying their case, we argue that scientific principles alone do not inherently lead to dehumanization. Instead, medicine's growing disconnection from a larger meaning-making system that was provided by communities within the Abrahamic traditions helps further explain what has happened over time. If monotheism carried forward Western medicine, leaving its imprint on the underlying presuppositions of medicine, then part of the problem has been medicine's eventual independence from these traditions that kept persons at the center of meaning. Jeffrey Bishop's argument seems exact, in that medicine's metaphysical and epistemological approach to the human body has been to disconnect and decontextualize it from the communities and practices that embody purpose and intention.[22 [pp. 297-300]] The scientific approach to reduce, categorize, and test does not in itself lead to dehumanization if incorporated within a larger framework that includes other spiritual values, such as the idea that all persons are created in God's image, that care for the sick is an essential form of neighborly love, and that medical healing is a secondary rather than primary good (as we have seen, the Abrahamic traditions understood health and healing as necessary conditions for seeking and loving God). Likewise, a loss of a larger vision of truth that upholds mystery as provided by the Abrahamic traditions partly explains why medicine might become fixated on certainty.[i] Reductionism and positivism thus only become dehumanizing when they are disconnected from the overt spiritual systems that have served as Western medicine's principle wellspring and guardian. So while monotheism upholds principles that lead to a reductionist method of science, reductionism and positivism are feeble counterfeits as they abandon mystery and dehumanize the patient.

Medicine's Analogical Similarities to Religion

This brief assessment could suggest that an essential problem that ails medicine is that medicine has abandoned religious principles in favor of a too inhuman scientific reductionism. Bishop frames his critique in this way by demonstrating that medicine collectively abandoned formal and final causation and focused on material and efficient causation.[22 [p. 20]] In our view, there is an additional level of analysis that is needed. It is that medicine's preference for function of disease and its amelioration over against human purpose in care and suffering operates in a religious-like manner. In other words, contemporary medicine did not abandon religion for the pursuit of science (as the story is often told), but rather secular medicine retains religious structures in its collective practice as it seeks a different final end (or *telos*).

There are five broadly shared connections between secular medicine and the monotheisitic religions—especially akin to Jewish and Christian traditions[ii]—where medicine and religion mirror one another in values and structures. These five points of connection include sickness/sin, the role of the healing mediator, therapy, patient disposition, and the healing milieu.

Sickness/Sin

In Judaism and Christianity, the problem is sin or a broken relationship with God. In biomedicine, illness is seen as abnormal, undesired, and a form of social deviancy,[10] [pp. 437–439] provoking basic human anxieties concerning vulnerability and finitude. In Judaism and Christianity, sin, as a disconnection from God, is a distortion of our original nature and a destructive force within relationships that gives rise to fear and pride. Within biomedicine, disease has multiple potential causes both from within the body (e.g., autoimmune disorders) and from outside it (e.g., environmental factors). Likewise, sin is an internal moral corruption of the soul but can be enflamed by persons, social structures, and circumstances from the outside.

Beyond these similarities, Judaism and Christianity also explicitly see an organic link between sin and sickness.[23 [pp. 33–39]] This is not to say that the etiology of disease is related to an individual's moral actions (the idea of unjust or innocent suffering is highlighted in the book of Job and in the teachings of Jesus), save for the sense that physical disease can at times be causatively linked to unhealthy or immoral actions (e.g., cigarette smoking leading to lung cancer).[24 [pp. 42–63]] Nevertheless, Judaism and Christianity both understand that the consequences of human sin (in the sense of original sin beginning in Genesis 3) result in human disease and physical death. This has steered many on the side of medicine to observe how sickness raises spiritual questions and issues.[25] It has also directed many in the Christian tradition to understand the relationship between physical disease and moral sin as involving a figurative analogy, but also being intrinsically related—as an object may be reflected in a mirror.[23] Physical sickness can thus be seen both as a metaphorical sign of human brokenness with God (the physical reflecting the spiritual) and as etiologically rooted in spiritual disconnection from God.

Healing Mediator

In biomedicine, physicians are clothed in authority because of their role in diagnosing disease, prescribing medicines, and performing surgery. Their authority is grounded in exclusive professional knowledge and experience, exercised through technical skills and safeguarded on the basis of the physician's moral virtue and calling. The symbols of this authority include the white coat and the stethoscope.[15,26] The white coat symbolizes their authority drawn from science and its laboratory of knowledge,[15] whereas the stethoscope hints at the "power to enter the secret world of interior knowledge."[15] Many have interpreted physicians to be akin to a modern-day priesthood.[13,27,28]

Similarly, in their roles as priests and pastors, clergy serve as authoritative mediators in diagnosing the sin-sick soul and administering spiritual therapy. They evaluate and discern the specific manifestations of sin, observing its symptoms, its root causes, and its varied manifestations in order to identify a path of spiritual healing. Often vested in symbolic clothing, clergy hold unique positions of authority further grounded within their training and ordination, their generally higher level of knowledge of sacred texts and tradition, and, especially within sacerdotal traditions, the exclusive priestly authority to preside over sacramental and community rites. These rites, mediated by clergy in all the major branches of Christianity, hold a unique therapeutic position in succoring and restoring the soul. Although most Christians have differentiated the effect of a sacrament from the moral agency of the priest, it still remains the case that ministers are moral and spiritual examples of the faith as well as conduits of spiritual healing.

For example, in the Christian tradition, the connection is reinforced by the similarities between Jesus' own ministry and the work of a physician (Mark 2:17; Luke 5:31). In fact, by the second century A.D., Jesus was commonly given the title *Christus medicus* or "Christ the physician."[24 [p. 30]] As the Great Physician, Christ was not only the healer of souls but would also resurrect *the body* in the consummation of His coming Kingdom at the end of the age. With this eschatological hope, comparing Christ to a physician goes beyond mere analogy because, in the bodily resurrection of the righteous (Matthew 25), the ultimate physician heals both soul and body.

The moral roles of physicians and clergy are unique: people trust their naked and sometimes unconscious bodies to physicians and their confused and searching souls to ministers.[iii] The moral agency of both physicians and clergy is thus constitutive of their profession. For example, in the Christian tradition, while Christian clergy most clearly mirror the work of Christ by directing Christ's healing of the soul, physicians reflect the work of Christ's promised resurrection through temporary and finite physical healing of the body. The roles of clergy and physicians therefore imitate one another in the form of an analogy as well as reflect the different dimensions of Christ's work regarding the body and soul.

Therapy

In biomedicine, the physician responds to disease processes by applying the appropriate therapies in the form of medicines or surgical procedures. In their ideal form, the therapies reverse a path of activity within the body that created symptoms and dysfunction, potentially threatening life itself. The act of therapy restores physical health. In the spiritual domain, clergy respond to sin by applying the appropriate therapies aimed at healing the soul; these might include spiritual practices such as prayer, framing beliefs in Scripture, receipt of confession, facilitating forgiveness, and offering spiritual direction and discernment as a person encounters difficult emotions, troubled relationships, or challenging circumstances. Spiritual therapy restores spiritual health. However, the line between physical and spiritual health is often blurred. The Hebrew term shalom (שָׁלוֹם) and Christian vocabulary (θεραπεύω, σώζω, ἰάομαι) utilize single terms to denote both physical healing and spiritual salvation. For example, the semantic range of the New Testament use of the verb "to save" (σώζω), can refer to both physical restoration (Matthew 9:22; Mark 10:52) or spiritual salvation (Mark 8:35; Luke 19:10).[iv] Additionally, in several New Testament texts, physical and spiritual healing appear to be conceptualized simultaneously as overlapping constructs (e.g., Luke 5:17–26; James 5:15–16). These examples demonstrate how physical and spiritual therapies can be patterned after one another and ultimately be part of the same therapeutic processes.

In like fashion, Basil of Caesarea stressed that medicine was a "pattern for the healing of the soul."[29] Seen from this theological perspective, medicine's primary purpose is to illustrate spiritual realities and truths, especially among the sick. For example, he suggested that chronic diseases teach that spiritual healing may take a long time and require "sustained prayer and prolonged repentance and a more laborious struggle than reason would suggest to us is sufficient for our healing." Basil identified spiritual meaning in medicine and disease not merely to justify medicine's acceptance but as a governing principle that orders medicine's proper and faithful use. When medicine is not allowed to direct and form the soul toward salvation, then its purpose diminishes. For Basil, physical health and healing were secondary and temporal activities, subject to the pursuit of a never-ending salvation. Physical disease and healing thus provided a manner for comprehending and experiencing spiritual truths.

In these ways, medicine holds a sacramental-like character[v] pointing beyond its own physical dimension toward spiritual and redemptive realities. As a sacramental, medicine is perceived as a visible sign representing invisible, salvific realities. Basil concluded that when medicine is practiced by physicians or received by patients without this spiritual signification in view, then an adequate justification for using medicine is absent since there is no spiritual lesson being underscored. While Basil acknowledged that medicine was originally established in God's creative order, in his account, followed by others,[23] medicine can only be rightly understood as a divinely created sign ultimately pointing to the story of redemption culminating in Jesus Christ. This is not to suggest that the physical dimension is inconsequential to the spiritual dimension, but rather that both are closely held together as each points to and affects the other.

The Sick Role and Patient Trust

In biomedicine, the sick role typically requires the patient to recognize a physical lack or need that cannot be addressed without outside assistance and intervention. The patient must call upon a physician who has special knowledge and skills in healing and then submit to the physician in a disposition of trust and faith in his or her healing ability, medical knowledge, and moral good will.[30] The patient is also responsible for listening to and following through on the therapeutic advice of his or her physicians.[10] On the spiritual side of the analogy, this is mirrored in the need for an underlying trust in God. The ill soul recognizes a fundamental moral and spiritual lack and thus the need to turn to outside interventions for spiritual healing. Just like the patient offers faith in the physician to bring physical healing, a person must trust in God to find spiritual healing.

While the sick role has been understandably criticized for affirming medical paternalism and relegating the patient to a state of passivity, and while significant corrective steps have been taken to reempower patients by emphasizing their autonomy, biomedicine will always require patients to fundamentally yield trust to medical caregivers if they desire to get well. The analogy between religion and medicine can help illuminate the complexity of this dynamic because religion makes it clear that faith is both active and passive—active because it requires the conscious decision to admit helplessness and to ask for help, but passive in the sense that it recognizes that the source of healing resides outside of one's self, requiring trust not in one's self for healing but in an outside power. The disposition of faith and patience is required of both the physically sick in biomedicine and of sinners in the Jewish and Christian traditions.

In the patient's experience, these two objects of trust—one in the physician regarding medicine and the other in God pertaining to the soul—coexist but are also ordered in reference to one another. Both Judaism and Christianity censure faith in human physicians when such faith displaces trust in God (2 Chronicles 16:12). According to Ben Sira, a Jewish scribe writing around 180 B.C.,[31] trust in physicians is warranted only to the extent that they are understood to be divinely appointed means to receiving God's healing. He instructed his Jewish readers to "Make friends with the physician for . . . him also God has established in his profession" (38:1).[31] In fact, he stressed that turning to human physicians is "essential to you" (38:1) and that defiance toward the doctor can be considered defiance toward God as the Creator of the doctor (38:15). Ben Sira's argument for making a place for the physician is primarily based on the idea that the physician is part of God's created order, and therefore the sick need to consent to this order irrespective of outcome. In addition, one can faithfully turn to the physician within illness because the physician also has faith in God who alone heals. Thus, faith in medicine or the physician runs parallel to faith in God; nor are these two types of faith inconsistent with each other. Rather, Ben Sira argues that putting one's faith in medicine and the physician can be an act of faith in God who made both. Hence, to resist reliance on medicine and the physician amounts to a rejection of God's wisdom and providence, who has included within the creation sources of healing that are from the fount of God.

As the Western tradition historically developed, the conceptual background of the ill person was bound up in the Latin concepts of the "sufferer" (*patiens*) and the virtue of "patience" (*patientia*). So, in the experience of illness, the moral calling was for the sufferer to endure his illness by allowing the virtue of patience to be formed within the soul. This was not a romanticism of suffering, but rather recognition that within illness one can be more perfectly formed into a person of courage and strength. In illness, one may resist evil by learning self-restraint more deeply in the greatest trials of living, waiting patiently upon one's medical caregivers to diagnose and appropriately intervene, waiting on God's providence to cure, and patiently accepting the possibility of death at one's appointed time. This model for suffering and patience within illness does not need to lead to a view that patience is "redolent with the sights and smells of the clinic and which leaves an afterimage of a compliant, passive object of medical care.[20] [pp. 3-4]" A more sympathetic depiction of the virtue of patience gives meaning to the sufferer not as primarily passive or as an objectified body, but predominantly as a moral and spiritual agent invited to courageously defy evil through endurance[32] [pp. 143-144] and to act with faith by trusting both God and human caregivers.

In summary, the very terminology of the "patient" identifies the moral agency and spiritual meanings that are intrinsically at work in the sick role. In these ways concerning the sick role, biomedicine and the monotheistic religions have reflected within one another a shared understanding of the patient's experience and the patient's moral and spiritual responsibilities. Both medical and spiritual realms have historically affirmed that sick persons must actively call upon others for help and, in so doing, must passively trust in external support. This faith in its active and passive forms is true of faith both in doctors and in God. Faith in medicine and God directly inhere within the patient's experience as the spiritual struggle to be formed by the virtue of patience plays out within the patient's interactions with his physicians and health caregivers. In other words, trust in God is mediated through actions and intentions regarding faith in medical caregivers. In order to trust in God, patients should trust in their medical caregivers, who are themselves called to reflect the highest standards of morality, compassion, and practical wisdom.

Healing Milieu

Beyond the patient–clinician relationship, healing takes place within a social and institutional healing context. The environmental milieu is critical to both mending bodies and saving souls.[33] [p. 680] In biomedicine, healing proceeds quintessentially in hospitals, which are highly structured organizations with a mission to cure and care for the seriously ill. Hospitals, especially teaching hospitals, are social locations for healing converging into a thickly organized community. Hospitals are the prototypical place where medical professionals practice and act. They are the places where healing knowledge is produced, safeguarded, and incorporated in caring for the ill. They are necessary for education and clerkship to be passed on to the next generation of clinicians. In the United States, hospitals have generally been (with varying and fluctuating patterns of use) associated symbolically with major human transitions including birth, illness, and dying.

In light of these transitions, hospitals are places of anxiety and expectation within serious illness. They are also places where the language of "miracle" finds ongoing usage among patients, medical staff, and hospital administration and within public relations. In a culture that has grown deeply suspicious of organizations of power, hospitals continue to receive overwhelmingly strong patient reviews.[vi] From a social and political perspective, hospitals remain organizations guided first by charity, where the poor cannot legally be turned away in an emergency and where motives of profit are subjugated to social benefit. But hospitals are also financial powerhouses, receiving approximately one-third ($1 trillion) of the total 17% of gross domestic product that goes toward national health expenditures.[vii] The sheer quantity of money that the United States puts toward healthcare is a reminder that our society upholds physical health and cure as a central cultural concern.

As hospitals are to biomedical healing so are religious communities to spiritual salvation. Religious communities do not themselves produce salvation, but they carry out the mission of salvation to sin-sick souls. Like modern hospitals, most religious communities are highly organized social structures with varying levels of hierarchy. Many people turn to religious communities to find comforting answers to life's deepest mysteries and to channel their anxieties, expectations, and hopes for spiritual and physical miracles and healing.

Religious communities are also places that celebrate and ritualize significant life transitions such as birth, marriage, and death. Similar to hospitals, religious communities are charitable organizations that exist to support the physically and spiritually destitute. In the United States, more than $100 billion are donated to religious communities each year, signaling their importance within American culture.

Because religious communities created the original concept of the hospital, as discussed in Chapter 2, and have continued to deeply influence the hospital into modern times, it should not be surprising that modern hospitals and religious communities have deeply similar organizational structures. Indeed, there is an ancient tradition of referring to the Christian church as a "spiritual hospital." Even the origin of the term "hospital" is rooted in a Christian philanthropy in which showing compassion to strangers (*hospitalis* in Latin) was a core Christian value.[24,33,34] But though one structure has grown from the other, some commentators have described an eclipsing of religious communities in favor of medical hospitals within modern culture. Rieff described the hospital as "heir to the church as the central institution of Western culture,"[35 [p. 355]] and others have described a "societal deification of health" in which hospitals now function as modern sacred temples with health as "the highest aim and greatest good of life, i.e., it becomes a kind of quasi-religion."[36 [p. 215]]

Modern hospitals have partially replaced religious temples as the chief place for cultural expectation of hope and temporal salvation. Like religious temples, modern hospitals are cultural symbols of what Americans chiefly hope for, particularly in times of trouble when awareness of our own mortality rushes upon the psyche. As institutions, hospitals continue to reflect the deep structural values of religious communities, including an entrenched social hierarchy and a commission aimed toward philanthropy and human well-being. They are cultural symbols of mystery and blood, where death is averted and life is restored. Like the Christian eschatological vision of bodily new life, the technological prowess of today's hospital holds out to all its weary comers hope of (temporary) bodily salvation.

In summary, these five domains contain striking similarities between today's medicine and Western religion. In the next section, we consider why these analogies exist and their potential implications.

Medicine as a Sign and Symbol of Spiritual Realities

Why do medicine and monotheistic religions share such similarities on a foundational level? Medicine and religion are autonomous spheres of human engagement and distinct human realities. Medicine is not a religion and most religions—at least Judaism, Christianity, and the other major world religions—are only *secondarily* concerned with temporary physical healing.

One plausible explanation for these similarities described here is that the analogical structures of medicine and religion reflect a third, nonmaterial transcendent reality (Figure 11.1). The difference is that while religion explicitly or overtly points beyond itself by signaling its sacramental nature, medicine's underlying structures

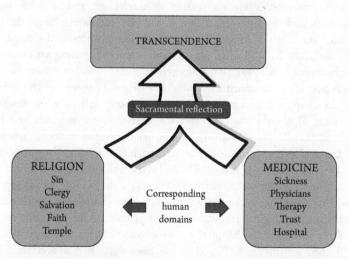

Figure 11.1 An explanatory model of the independence and mirroring of medicine and religion, reflecting both their distinction as human spheres and their sacramental character, pointing to hidden and invisible realities of the Transcendent.

can be discerned only by way of inference. Just as monotheistic religions point to a transcendent reality that is chiefly loved, even so medicine, as a gift of God, points to a transcendent object. Both religion and medicine in their unique manifestations reflect these invisible realities by their forms and structures. While medicine is obviously centered on material illness and care of the body, its social structures are extraordinarily similar to those of monotheistic religion. Biomedicine and its practitioners have taken many steps to distance the field from religion in the United States, including pursuing a closer identification with science for the past two centuries. Nevertheless, medicine's continuing analogical connection with monotheistic religion suggests a deeper pattern: medicine is a sacramental sign reflecting an immaterial, invisible reality.

In the words of the *Book of Common Prayer*, a sacrament is defined as an "outward and visible sign of an inward and spiritual grace."[viii] The adjectival form of sacrament is *sacramental*, which suggests that an entity may not explicitly be considered a sacrament but that it does have a sacrament-like character that functions implicitly like the formally recognized sacraments. Roman Catholic theology recognizes that embedded within the material universe created by God are "sacramentals," defined as "sacred signs" that "prepare us to receive grace and dispose us to cooperate with it."[ix] The Catholic Catechism suggests that sacramentals can include a broad array of material entities, presumably including biomedicine. Similarly, in Protestant theology, there has been recognition of both a wide and narrow sense of the meaning of sacraments. While the narrow meaning typically focuses on liturgical rites, especially baptism and Eucharist in the Christian tradition, the broader meaning references how the entire created realm points to God and spiritual realities.[x] A broad understanding of "sacrament" is similar to what Eastern Orthodox theologian Alexander Schmemann has called "the sacramental potentiality of creation in its totality."[37 [p. 132]] Any created, finite material object can point as a sign and symbol to infinite, invisible, and mysterious reality. In this broader sense of the term, a material object in the created order can hold sacramental significance but not be explicitly liturgical or sacerdotal so that it requires attendance from a specific class of ordained clergy. Thus, a sacramental in its general theological meaning refers to any material object that has embedded within it structures which point beyond the object to hidden and invisible realities seen in the physical object. However, sacramental signs are most effectively received if accompanied by verbal communication that signals to participants the nature of that sign as it points beyond itself to the spiritual realm. Sacramental-like entities inherently require human interpretation and verbal communication in order for material participation to effectively signify symbolic meaning to those experiencing the physical reality.[xi] Yet, even without words, the object holds implicit capacity as an outward and visible sign pointing toward inward and invisible grace.

As Figure 11.1 illustrates, the domains of religion and medicine share embedded structures that mirror one another in concept and ultimately connect in the reality of experience. Religion is by type revelatory, birthed through illumination, prophecy, and charisma, whereas medicine is an example of natural theology.[xii] Recognizing the parallels between religion and medicine is not merely a literary analogy but also finds interconnection between the two in human death and healing. Physical death is a result of a spiritual disease in a broken connection with God.

Spiritual salvation, in which God and humans are reconnected, yields physical health in terms of bodily resurrection into eternal life. Likewise, when most persons become physically sick, they correspondingly ask spiritual questions and seek spiritual direction. Thus, religion is ultimately about the body (its healing restoration), and medicine turns the heart toward the soul. As the figure suggests, a call to faith should be placed in the Transcendent God, not in, on the one hand, religion, clergy, or spiritual practices, or, on the other hand, medicine, physicians, or technology. The touchpoints are both theological in content as well as empirically notable in patient experience (as discussed in Chapter 2).

Does religion hold power over medicine, or does medicine rule religion? We think that, most consistent with the sacramental view depicted in Figure 11.1, neither domain holds power over the other. This perspective depicts religion and medicine as being sufficiently stratified from each other so that each sphere calls for its own distinctive methods according to the phenomena of engagement. Thus, theology does not dominate medicine, nor does medicine rule over religion. From a historical perspective, Amundsen suggested a typology for potential relationships of religion and medicine as either partial or complete separation or in terms of one sphere dominating the other.[38 (pp. 2–4)] His typology may historically describe the tensions between the two domains. However, from a sacramental perspective, the intrinsic analogy between religion and medicine suggests a partnership in terms of a symphony.[39 (p. 71),xiii] Within the symphonic sounds of religion and medicine, neither one dominates, confuses, or separates from the other, but both uphold mutual respect and seek to create a unity and synthesis on behalf of patients who are both body and soul. In terms of a symphony, each sphere is not "subject to the other, but both were united in common faith and shared service; each was responsible for different aspects of the life of the people."[39 (p. 71)] In reflecting a transcendent reality, both spheres join together in a mutually beneficial partnership.

But is this sacramental-like connection metaphysically real or merely constructed and imaginative? Does this superimpose a narrative upon medicine that is wishful theological thinking? Believers may look at the similarities between medicine and religion and conclude that a broader sacramental relationship exists between medicine and religion. After all, the believer argues, God is the source of both religion and medicine (as Ben Sira concluded in the second century B.C.). If God is the true source of healing, then it would not be a surprise that the same underlying rationality and structures exist in both the material and immaterial realms. Conversely, skeptics may look at the underlying similarities between medicine and religion and deny any similarity, or perhaps conclude that they are merely coincidental, a contingency of history or a by-product of an intertwined social relationship. After all, Hippocratic medicine influenced Western religion, and Western religion formed biomedicine.[40] Others may argue that the similarity is based within the biological and psychological makeup of being human; all maladies—physical, relational, existential, and cosmic—are products of our evolutionary and social nature and consequently take similar social forms.

There are multiple possible interpretations, none of which can be absolutely ruled out. Presuppositions about the material and spiritual realms will influence interpretation in distinct directions, and *neither believers nor skeptics can prove or disprove* whether the relationship is metaphysically real, accidental, or simply the result of many confounding factors embedded within human makeup. While settling this question does not appear possible, the more immediate issue is not if the analogy is metaphysically real but whether the structure of the relationship between medicine and religion should be conceived as a partnership or in terms of separation.[xiv]

Medicine and Religion as Partners

For most of Western history, medicine and religion were approached in terms of structural partners. In the context of this partnership, medicine was practiced as a secondary good pointing beyond itself to infinite and final ends—acknowledging that the experience of illness has always raised fundamental questions of human meaning and existence. When structured in the form of a partnership, the relationship between medicine and religion achieves two simultaneous goods. First, medicine is freed to center its activities on advancing bodily health, seeking physical cure, prolonging life, and alleviating pain. Circumscribing medicine around physical health and the material body unburdens it from needing to solve the many problems of the human condition.[41] A more humble medicine that resists medicalizing every dimension of the human condition will lead to a better and more balanced medical practice.[42] Second, a partnership enables spiritual care of patients to remain a central dimension of care to those facing physical illness. Serious illness arouses immense spiritual questions and concerns that must be adequately engaged to alleviate human fears and anxieties that are interwoven with illness, finitude, and the possibility of death. In limiting itself to the pursuit of physical health and cure within the partnership model, medicine simultaneously perceives the human soul and spiritual ends as holding primacy. In prior generations, this partnership allowed medicine to provide physical care within its own institutions and professions while recognizing, encouraging, and giving place and priority to spiritual issues. As medicine served the body in its actions and purposes, it self-consciously circumscribed physical cure and bodily care as secondary goods subservient to the spiritual dimensions of illness. The practice of medicine was not indifferent to spiritual concerns but was self-consciously focused on the body with the purpose of serving ultimate ends related to the spiritual.

In the United States, medicine has historically signaled its orientation toward a spiritual reality—and its partnership with religion—through symbols, positions of governance, and physician practices. For example, the use of religious statues in prominent locations in hospitals communicated medicine's sacramental-like nature. The Jesus statue in the main lobby of the secular John Hopkins Hospital serves as one preeminent example (see Chapter 9). In similar fashion, the Bulfinch Building of the Massachusetts General Hospital, home of its famed Ether Dome, which was completed in 1823, was designed in the form of a crucifix. Likewise, religiously affiliated persons have held prominent roles within Catholic, Jewish, and Adventist medical institutions. For example, at the Mayo Clinic in Rochester, Minnesota, Franciscan sisters have continually held prominent positions of hospital governance up until the past decade. Finally, physicians long considered it a normal part of their role not to explicitly act as priests, but to offer, as Richard Baxter suggested in the seventeenth century, "a few gentle words" to facilitate the patient's spiritual mindset as part of their care of the sick.[43] This allowed and encouraged patients to consider and engage the spiritual implications of their illness.

In maintaining a positive and overt partnership with religion, medicine circumscribed itself to the physical. In remaining focused on the material aspects of illness, it maintained a partnership with religious entities that focused on the soul. Such uses of symbols, authoritative positions, and professional practices tilled the soil for clergy, chaplains, and religious communities to directly intervene in the form of prayer, spiritual counsel, and religious rites. Unlike a bureaucratically envisioned division of labor, which emphasizes clear roles and non-overlapping responsibilities aimed toward efficiency,[44] a partnership authorizes overlapping professional boundaries and roles.[45] An overlap or slightly blurred boundaries does not eliminate professional specialization, but instead guarantees that patients' material and spiritual concerns are adequately engaged rather than overlooked, as they are mostly today. Partnership supports a medical context that both recognizes professional specialization while also enabling a deeper unitive vision, organizational interconnection, and public signals of transcendence. The analogical connection between religion and medicine calls for symphonic partnership.

Medicine and Religion as Non-Overlapping

As secular perspectives have expanded in the United States, partnership between medicine and religion has eroded. Under the banner of the secular, medicine now generally conceives itself to be neutral and non-overlapping as it pertains to spirituality or religion.[46] Though its institutions and professions continue to focus on the material or physical realm, it now claims to withhold judgment on and be indifferent toward issues pertaining to the soul and the immaterial realm.

By no longer recognizing its analogical relationship with religious structures or its sacramental-like form, which points to transcendent realties, medicine is left with the options of denial or indifference. The problem with indifference is that this approach can at best be applied on an individual rather than a corporate level. At the corporate level, which includes medicine's institutions, professions, and related social structures, the intentional absence of religion or spirituality amounts to a *functional denial*. Furthermore, denial of this relationship amounts to a *theologically grounded* decision because it is a claim grounded on presupposed dualisms between the material and immaterial worlds. This dualistic view of the material and immaterial is a metaphysical claim, and its division cannot be proved a priori or through an appeal to empirical evidence. It is an entire social system built on a problematic conception of religion (see Chapter 8), one that appears to mimic the underlying structures derived from the Abrahamic traditions.

As a result of these rejections, hospital spaces are mostly stripped of traditional spiritual symbols, institutions seldom include religious voices on their boards of trustees, and the spiritual formation of medical trainees is disregarded as unnecessary to either the formation of physician morality or to addressing the spiritual dimensions of illness. Ironically, certain integrative medical practices such as yoga, reiki, and meditation, all of which have their roots in Eastern spirituality, have become increasingly accepted within secular medical contexts as long as their underlying religious roots remain muted. However, these maneuvers to secularize spiritual practices do not account for embedded theological assumptions that are impossible to remove from the internal logic of a spiritual practice.[47] This has resulted in traditional Western religious symbols and practices being stripped from medical care, while Eastern religious practices have become increasingly acceptable—under conceptually problematic claims that they are not defined as religious.

When social structures are stripped of signals of religious transcendence,[48] it suggests to individual patients and clinicians that these are secondary, optional, and aesthetic concerns. This viewpoint undermines the individual clinician's likelihood to either partner with religion or point the patient to consider spiritual realities. Thus, even when officially intending to be neutral toward religion and spirituality, a secular medicine not only functionally repudiates a partnership with religion but also leads to a silencing of transcendent meanings. Secularism, then, is not neutral—it is an internally consistent worldview comparable with religion. When medicine's own underlying structures so closely parallel forms of religion seen in Western religion, the claim of religious neutrality is perplexing. How can medicine be neutral toward all religious faiths if its underlying professional and institutional structures continue to mimic the deep structure of beliefs provided by Western religion?

Conclusion

In summary, we have argued that the Abrahamic traditions have shaped the structures of medicine and that these structures are reflective of the underlying religious systems that have produced them. As medicine has attempted to distance itself from the Abrahamic traditions in more recent times, its unwillingness to partner with religion has nonetheless not eliminated its underlying, religious-like structures. In the next chapter, we will bring our theological description to a finale by suggesting that secular medicine is not neutral toward spirituality or religion. Instead, we will argue that a spirituality of immanence is latent to secular medicine, not only in structural form, but also in the faith and hope it engenders.

Notes

i. A certainty of God as One seen in the Abrahamic traditions does not eclipse how these traditions have also emphasized the mystery and unknowability of the divine, where certain ultimate truths remain hidden from human knowledge or where even what is believed to be known about God is at best inadequate (sometimes called *apophatic* or *negative theology*). Even as an infinite God lies within the darkness of mystery, likewise, a finite creation that reflects the divine nature also holds mysteries and uncertainty. Medicine has gone in the direction of pursing absolute certainty, not because of a monotheistic imprint, but because of a collective movement away from the Abrahamic traditions that have recognized that God is both certain and unknowable. The spurning of religion has allowed medicine to become imbalanced in this way.

ii. Judaism and Christianity have both similarities and differences in their interpretations of medicine. As a partner to and guardian of biomedicine, Christianity has interpreted medicine as a secondary good, not only because physical health and healing are preconditions to seeking and loving God, as stressed by Judaism, but because of its analogical and sacramental relationship. Both religions have maintained that medicine is a gift of God's providence, embedded within the created order, made available to mankind to alleviate suffering, and a secondary good serving the soul. However, Christianity, using a deep, organic analogy, has also emphasized that medicine is a spiritual tutor. Such an understanding also existed within Greek philosophy, which used a body–soul analogy to compare physical healing and the cure of the soul (Gary Ferngren, Medicine and Health care in *Early Christianity*. Baltimore: John Hopkins University Press; 2009, p. 29). These well-known figurative connections involving Hippocratic medicine likely enabled the Christian tradition to quickly absorb medicine into its narrative and practices, not only because it assisted philanthropy or the love of neighbor, but because medicine also analogically reflected its own underlying structures and beliefs.

As shown in Ben Sira (38), Judaism emphasized how medicine is part of God's created order. Medicine is rightly used to restore physical health, which is considered a necessary secondary good aimed at serving the soul. The Prayer of Maimonides, falsely attributed to prominent physician-rabbi Moses Maimonides (Fred Rosner. The Medical Legacy of Moses Maimonides. Hoboken, NJ: KTAV Publishing House; 1998), provided a compelling eighteenth-century portrait of how Jewish faith informs medical practice as a divine vocation. The physician prays to rely on God because "without Thy help not even the least thing will succeed" (David L. Freeman, Abrams Judith Z. Illness and health in the Jewish tradition : writings from the Bible to today. Philadelphia: Jewish Publication Society; 1999). The Prayer interpreted sickness in the light of the providence of God, who "sendest to man diseases as beneficent messengers to foretell approaching danger and to urge him to avert it." This religious interpretation of the meaning of illness also spurred some Jewish physicians to encourage the sufferer "to ask God's forgiveness through prayer and fasting" (David B. Ruderman. Kabbalah, magic, and science : the cultural universe of a sixteenth-century Jewish physician. Cambridge, Mass.: Harvard University Press; 1988).

While Christianity also emphasized that medicine and physical cure serve the soul and right relations with God, the emphasis fell not primarily on medicine's established created order (although this theme also exists, as apparent in Basil's *Long Rules*), but on how medicine points to redemption in Christ. Within Judaism, medicine is justified as bringing physical health that is a necessary condition for the soul to worship God. Within Christianity, medicine is justified because, embedded within its practice, are signs and symbols pointing to redemption in Christ. Judaism points back in history to creation for its primary rationale in justifying medicine. Christianity points forward in history to redemption and resurrection as its primary justification of medicine. Christianity includes the rationale of creation but goes beyond it to the "new creation" established through the resurrection of Christ.

iii. Moral agency in other careers is of course preferred, as most in society do not want corrupt politicians, accountants, or lawyers. But the existential threat is arguably most notable and has its greatest impact among those professions that directly interface with vulnerable and defenseless persons. The morality of the physician or minister is constitutive to their profession, whereas in certain instances a lack of morality may seemingly benefit persons within certain professions operating on their behalf (e.g., a lawyer).

iv. See W. Arndt, Danker F. W., Bauer W., and Gingrich F. W. (2000). *A Greek-English lexicon of the New Testament and other early Christian literature* (3rd ed., p. 982). Chicago: University of Chicago Press.

v. See Chapter 10 (endnote 27) for a definition of sacrament.

vi. These data can be explored at https://data.medicare.gov/Hospital-Compare/Data-Updates/bzsr-4my4

vii. See http://www.cdc.gov/nchs/fastats/health-expenditures.htm

viii. In defining a sacrament, the Anglican catechesis says, "I mean by this word Sacrament an outward and visible sign of an inward and spiritual grace given unto us; ordained by Christ himself, as a means whereby we receive this grace, and a pledge to assure us thereof." (The Protestant Episcopal Church in the United States of America. (1976). *The book of common prayer and administration of the sacraments and other rites and ceremonies of the church* (p. 292). New York: Seabury Press).

ix. See *Catechism of the Catholic Church*, Part II, section 2, chapter 4, article 1, 1667, 1670).

x. In the Protestant Reformed tradition, John Calvin discusses a general meaning of sacraments found outside "ordinary" ecclesiastical use in the *Institutes of the Christian Religion*, book IV, chapter XIV, 18.

xi. Both Catholic and Protestants agree that sacramentals require faith and recognition on the part of the recipient in order to have their divine effect. A sacramental is not *ex opera operato* but has its effect only as the sign directs the heart to the thing signified.

xii. This view would be consistent, for example, with Aquinas: "By the understanding of natural substances we can be led, according to true philosophical principles, to the knowledge of immaterial substances. . . . From material things we can rise to some kind of knowledge of immaterial things, but not to the perfect knowledge thereof; for there is no proper and adequate proportion between material and immaterial things, and the likenesses drawn from material things for the understanding of immaterial things are very dissimilar therefrom" (Thomas Aquinas. [n.d.]. STh., I q.88 a.2 resp. *Summa theologica*. [Fathers of the English Dominican Province, Trans.]. London: Burns Oates & Washbourne). Within the Reformed tradition, Calvin also discussed the nature of medicine and bodily anatomy as holding a "seed of religion" that points to immaterial realities (*Institutes of the Christian Religion*, I, v. 2). Similar to Aquinas, Calvin argued that the human mind was like a "labyrinth" making man incapable of arriving to clarity about God or spiritual truths without the aid of special revelation. He says, "For it must be concluded, that the light of the Divine countenance, which even the Apostle says 'no man can approach unto,' is like an inexplicable labyrinth to us, unless we are directed by the line of the word: so that it were better to halt in this way, than to run with the greatest rapidity out of it" (*Institutes of the Christian Religion* I, vi, 3).

xiii. In the Eastern Orthodox tradition, church–state relations have been cast in terms of "symphonia," whereas the church is responsible for spiritual concerns and the state is responsible for material ones. For a recent overview, see Lucian N. Leustean. The concept of symphonia in contemporary European Orthodoxy. *International Journal for the Study of the Christian Church* 2011;11(2–3): 188–202.

xiv. In this discussion, it is important to not only hear the accounts of patients who overwhelming acknowledge the spiritual and religious components of their physical disease (see Chapter 2); in addition, it is critical to weigh the import and implications of human interpretations of medicine that so closely parallel the function of spiritual and religious claims.

References

1. Charles E. Rosenberg. *Our present complaint: American medicine, then and now.* Baltimore: Johns Hopkins University Press; 2007.
2. S. van der Geest. Christ as a pharmacist: medical symbols in German devotion. *Soc Sci Med.* 1994;39(5):727–732.
3. S. van der Geest. 'Sacraments' in the hospital: exploring the magic and religion of recovery. *Anthropol Med.* 2005;12(2):135–150.
4. S. J. Vellenga. Longing for health. A practice of religious healing and biomedicine compared. *J Relig Health.* 2008;47(3):326–337.
5. J. S. Welch. Ritual in western medicine and its role in placebo healing. *J Relig Healing.* 2003;42(1):21–33.
6. P. Katz. Ritual in the operating room. *Ethnology.* 1981;20:335–350.
7. D. E. Moerman. Anthropology of symbolic healing. *Curr Anthropol.* 1979;20(1):59–80.
8. J. Dow. Universal aspects of symbolic healing: a theoretical synthesis. *Am Anthropol.* 1986;88:56–69.
9. Byron Good. *Medicine, rationality, and experience: an anthropological perspective.* Cambridge/New York: Cambridge University Press; 1994.

10. Talcott Parsons. *The social system*. Glencoe, IL: Free Press; 1951.

11. Melvin Konner. *Becoming a doctor: a journey of initiation in medical school*. New York: Penguin Books; 1988.

12. Joel James Shuman, Volck Brian. *Reclaiming the body: Christians and the faithful use of modern medicine*. Grand Rapids, MI: Brazos Press; 2006.

13. D. Barnard. The physician as priest, revisited. *J Relig Health*. 1985;24(4):272–286.

14. R. Branson. The secularization of American medicine. *Stud Hastings Cent*. 1973;1(2):17–28.

15. M. P. Wardlaw. American medicine as religious practice: care of the sick as a sacred obligation and the unholy descent into secularization. *J Relig Health*. 2011;50(1):62–74.

16. H. Y. Vanderpool. The religious features of scientific medicine. *Kennedy Inst Ethics J*. 2008;18(3):203–234.

17. Arthur Kleinman. What is specific to Western medicine? In: W. F. Bynum, ed. *Companion encyclopedia of the history of medicine*. Vol 1. London: Routledge; 1994:15–23.

18. Lesslie Newbigin. *Foolishness to the Greeks: the Gospel and Western culture*. Grand Rapids, MI: W. B. Eerdmans Pub.; 1986.

19. Eric J. Cassell. *The nature of suffering and the goals of medicine*. 2nd ed. New York: Oxford University Press; 2004.

20. Arthur Kleinman. *The illness narratives: suffering, healing, and the human condition*. New York: Basic Books; 1988.

21. Arthur Kleinman. *What really matters: living a moral life amidst uncertainty and danger*. New York: Oxford University Press,; 2006.

22. Jeffrey Paul Bishop. *The anticipatory corpse: medicine, power, and the care of the dying*. Notre Dame, IN: University of Notre Dame Press; 2011.

23. Jean-Claude Larchet. *The theology of illness*. Crestwood, NY: St. Vladimir's Seminary Press; 2002.

24. Gary B. Ferngren. *Medicine & health care in early Christianity*. Baltimore: Johns Hopkins University Press; 2009.

25. Daniel P. Sulmasy. *The rebirth of the clinic: an introduction to spirituality in health care*. Washington, DC: Georgetown University Press; 2006.

26. V. A. Jones. The white coat: why not follow suit? *JAMA*. 1999;281(5):478.

27. Robert S. Mendelsohn. *Confessions of a medical heretic*. Chicago: Contemporary Books; 1979.

28. D. E. Hall. Altar and table: a phenomenology of the surgeon-priest. *Yale J Biol Med*. 2008;81(4):193–198.

29. Anna Silvas. *The Asketikon of St Basil the Great*. Oxford/New York: Oxford University Press; 2005.

30. E. D. Pellegrino. Toward a reconstruction of medical morality. *Am J Bioeth*. 2006;6(2):65–71.

31. Patrick W. Skehan, Di Lella Alexander A. *The wisdom of Ben Sira: a new translation with notes*. Garden City, NY: Doubleday; 1987.

32. William Barclay. *New Testament words*. Philadelphia: Westminster Press; 1974.

33. Guenter B. Risse. *Mending bodies, saving souls: a history of hospitals*. New York: Oxford University Press; 1999.

34. Andrew T. Crislip. *From monastery to hospital: Christian monasticism & the transformation of health care in late antiquity*. Ann Arbor: University of Michigan Press; 2005.

35. Philip Rieff. *Freud, the mind of the moralist*. 3rd ed. Chicago: University of Chicago Press; 1979.

36. Paulina Taboada, Cuddeback Kateryna Fedoryka, Donohue-White Patricia. *Person, society, and value: towards a personalist concept of health*. Dordrecht/Boston: Kluwer Academic Pub.; 2002.

37. Aleksandr Shmeman. *For the life of the world: sacraments and orthodoxy*. Crestwood, NY: St. Vladimir's Seminary Press; 2004.

38. Darrel W. Amundsen. *Medicine, society, and faith in the ancient and medieval worlds*. Baltimore: Johns Hopkins University Press; 1996.

39. Stanley S. Harakas. *Health and medicine in the Eastern Orthodox tradition: faith, liturgy, and wholeness*. New York: Crossroad; 1990.

40. Gary B. Ferngren. *Medicine and religion: a historical introduction*. Baltimore: Johns Hopkins University Press; 2014.

41. Leon R. Kass. Regarding the end of medicine and the pursuit of health. *Interest.* 1975;40:11–42.

42. Margaret E. Mohrmann. Professing medicine faithfully: theological resources for trying times. *Theol Today.* 2002(October):355–368.

43. M. J. Balboni, T. A. Balboni. Medicine and spirituality in historical perspective. In: John Peteet, D'Ambra Michael, eds. *The soul of medicine: spirituality and world view in clinical practice.* Baltimore: John Hopkins University Press; 2011:3–22.

44. Max Weber, Gerth Hans Heinrich, Mills C. Wright. *From Max Weber: essays in sociology.* New York: Oxford University Press; 1946.

45. M. J. Balboni, Balboni T. A. Reintegrating care for the dying, body and soul. *Harvard Theol Rev.* 2010;103(3):351–364.

46. D. E. Hall, Curlin F. Can physicians' care be neutral regarding religion? *Acad Med.* 2004;79(7):677–679.

47. Candy Gunther Brown. *The healing gods: complementary and alternative medicine in Christian America.* New York: Oxford University Press; 2013.

48. Peter L. Berger. *A rumor of angels: modern society and the rediscovery of the supernatural.* Exp., with a new introd. by the author. ed. New York: Anchor Books; 1990.

12

A Spirituality of Immanence

In an exploratory fashion, Part II engages how the Abrahamic religions have shaped medicine and the impact that religion continues to have within secular medicine. Contrary to the contemporary views on the separation of the two spheres, these religious traditions have embedded themselves within the presuppositions and structures of medicine, which carry them forward into contemporary medicine. Without the influence of the Abrahamic traditions, it is difficult to imagine that medicine would have such a large role in American life today. Perhaps most importantly, the emphasis on care of the patient has flowed from the theological premises that persons are made in the *imago dei* and deserving of compassion and that to care for the patient is itself a sacred and holy act. It is difficult to justify and mobilize care of the weak and suffering without also entering into the realm of human values. For most, discussion around values is based on human norms and standards that are either overtly religious or at least religious-like in justification and perspective.[1]

As the final theological chapter in our argument, we will thread together our prior claims about the shared presuppositions of Western religion and how these play out in secular medicine. In this chapter, we argue that by secular medicine's repudiation of religious partners, it ironically establishes itself as a religious-like phenomenon. In addition to the empirical and sociological reasons provided in Part I, the infrequency of spiritual care provision by medical professionals appears to have links to religious-like dynamics operating within secular medicine itself. Medicine is dangerously close to aligning itself with a spirituality of immanence that is centered on the body. This realignment away from Western religions and toward a spirituality of immanence monopolizes the structures of medicine, marginalizing the Abrahamic religious traditions, and animating a rival spiritual power. Contemporary medicine is not freed from spirituality or religion but rather is emboldened to exalt itself, not as a sacramental sign, as discussed in Chapter 11, but to the "thing" signified. To begin, however, we return to the issue of definitions since this remains important to this analysis.

Substantive and Functional Approaches to Spirituality and Religion

The claim that religion still has some underlying, if hidden, relationship with medicine is flatly denied by those committed to a secular medicine. This view argues that medicine has no real or necessary dependence on religion to function well and that these two spheres are consequently best kept separate. However, the secular argument for separation assumes conceptually problematic definitions for spirituality and religion. The secular approach described in Chapter 7, which broadly dichotomizes immanence and transcendence, relies on substantive understandings of religion. As shown in Chapter 8, substantive definitions inevitably locate religion around ideas of the supernatural, superhuman, or some invisible realm of the immaterial. Correspondingly, the secular realm refers to the human sphere oriented around the non-supernatural, temporal order of material and social realities.

The tendency to define religion in this way is illustrated in Richard Sloan's work *Blind Faith*,[2] in which he forcefully argues that medicine and religion must remain separate. A fundamental shortcoming in Sloan's overall argument, however, is his failure to define the concept of religion. Throughout his book-length project and other journal publications, Sloan assumes that religion is roughly akin to the supernatural, demons, magic, and the god(s), all of which can be contrasted with "rational medicine."[2 (pp. 18–19)] Medicine is on the side of the "natural," whereas religion is on the side of the supernatural.[2 (p. 26),i] While there is no consensus on this issue among scholars, we follow Cavanaugh, who says that substantive conceptions of religion mask the socially constructed human perception of what religion is or what it is not.[3 (p. 119)] The meanings of spirituality and religion are tethered to perspectives and to underlying motives of power and social control. Thus, by circumscribing religion to substantive concepts oriented around god(s), superhuman, or the supernatural, the question is nearly settled before real dialogue can take place between medicine and religion. If religion pertains only to the supernatural or superhuman, and medicine refers to the rational and material, then Sloan's conclusions are nearly a foregone conclusion. However, even to those who might still prefer substantive definitions of religion, there may be some recognition that there does appear to be phenomena operating within medicine that is "religious-like." This means that it is not technically religious in substance but that it follows similar religious-like patterns.[ii] Either way, readers should appreciate how approaches to spirituality and religion cannot be easily settled but are tied closely within interpretations in what we are able and choose to see and the presuppositions that influence our description. Thus, power dynamics are laden in our definitions and impact how we describe the nature of medicine.

Power Dynamics

Substantive definitions for religion can especially be problematic because they pertain to a larger social struggle with Western religion, especially Christianity. Substantive definitions struggle to adequately account for nontheistic religious-like systems, such as Buddhism and Confucianism, or dynamics such as civil religion.[4] Identifying religion based on whether groups self-identify (anthropologists call these "emic" approaches) as religious can also struggle when certain proponents or ideologues within Marxism, such as Antonio Gramsci, described Marxism in "religious" ways.[3 (p. 111)] Elsewhere, Cavanaugh describes how the Japanese government strongly denied that Shinto was a religion, not because of sound conceptual reasons, but for political and social ones.[5 (p. 119)] Other religious groups, such as Evangelical

Christians following Billy Graham, have sometimes argued that the Christian gospel is not a religion but a relationship. Dietrich Bonhoeffer wrote concerning a "religion-less Christianity." [6 [pp. 280–282]] Cavanaugh points out a number of recent books[5 [p. 120]] that have repeatedly attempted to identify the inconsistencies and inaccuracies of the popular definition of "religion," including *The Invention of World Religions*,[7] *The Western Construction of Religion*,[8] and *The Invention of Religion*.[9] The point here is that the concept of religion is at least a partly constructed concept, proscribing the nature of religious phenomena as much as describing it.

Substantive definitions have been forged within sociopolitical agendas that arose during the time of the Enlightenment, tailored to control and limit Western religion, especially Christianity, in its influence on social structures in Europe and the United States.[3,10] These definitions arbitrarily apply to Western religious forms and ideas, but they are less likely to account for Eastern religions or religious-like phenomenon such as the occasional tendency of patients to functionally divinize their physicians, or trust in energy waves for healing, or place enormous hope in complementary and alternative medical (CAM) practices such as yoga or mindfulness meditation. In regards to CAM, others have pointed out that CAM includes spiritual practices, which, though advertised as being secular and natural,[11] are theory-laden with implicit theologies.[iii] Similarly, substantive approaches to religion reject authority structures that are overtly religious but then fail to recognize that alternative claims of authority such as scientific knowledge, the powers of clinical techniques, or contemporary emphasis on patient autonomy are equally religious-like commitments.[iv]

At stake is not a purely academic debate about definitions, as if religion is known on its face as a brute fact whenever encountered. Rather, underneath substantive definitions of religion lie agendas for our social and political worlds and assumptions that circumscribe only particular types of religious phenomena. It is a problematic way of conceptualizing the nature of religion since it creates circumstances in which only certain religious phenomenon are identified as religious and other religion-like phenomena are described in nonreligious terms. Such an approach creates synthetic divisions which marginalize certain religions but empower others with dominance over the sphere of healthcare. These concerns create conceptual problems by defining religion using substantive criteria, and we therefore suggest that a functional approach to characterizing religion avoids these pitfalls.[v]

It is also worth considering abandonment of the term "religion" altogether in order to move beyond these power dynamics of imagining and constructing a larger social order. The tension that exists concerns popular usages of terms that, upon examination, are conceptually inexact or flawed, though they are regularly employed throughout the culture. Western social order is largely based on these constructs of religion and the secular, which are thoroughly embedded within our legal system and cultural imagination. The religion–secular binary is presumed by many to be transcultural and transhistorical.[5 [pp. 105–121]] This may also partly explain the rise of the term "spirituality" as it is an attempt to convey a broader construct than organized religion while still pointing to what is most preeminent and ultimate. Curiously, the term "spirituality" is often used in the wider culture on the popular level to differentiate certain practices from religion. While people in traditional religions have remained comfortable with religious and spiritual terms, those who personally reject traditional religion for themselves, especially the Abrahamic traditions, sometimes employ spirituality to differentiate themselves from religion. The dynamics that lie behind these word games at a minimum include into what place and position these concepts in their actual practices and beliefs can be appropriately included in the secular sphere. If spirituality is not religion, then it goes to reason that it may be included in the secular sphere, including secular medicine. If it is religion, then our social norms and laws attempt to regulate how it is expressed within the secular realm. If something is secular, then it may of course be included and expressed without challenge, even if that secular matter appears and functions in a religious-like way. Thus, how we define and conceptualize religion and spirituality is entwined within social power and control over the structures of medicine. We are suggesting that, although employing these terms is inescapable, everyone is suspect (including ourselves) in the definitions opted for and the motives behind those choices. We believe this is exactly what has been taking place for several hundred years concerning these terms; it is what lies behind our culture's current usage of terms such as "religion," "spirituality," and "secular." These are a manifestation of our culture wars, this time surrounding the care of the sick in medicine. We favor a functional approach to religion because it exposes these power dynamics and levels the playing field and because adoption of this approach provides a compromise that we will argue for in Part III.

Traditional Religion Remains Under the Surface

Secular medicine has conceptualized itself as being nonreligious in its underlying aims primarily based on a substantive understanding of religion. However, even when medicine does not mention or recognize God or the superhuman in its social structures, ultimate concern rests just under the surface within contemporary medical practice. For example, contemporary medicine provides a remarkably thin account for why humans should expend enormous time, energy, and finances on the sick and dying. By leaving deep motivations unstated, it enables many different reasons for doing healthcare, some of which are religious or religious-like, including reasons identified to be operative within the Abrahamic traditions. While there appears to be a large consensus within the West that caring for the sick and dying is a basic human good and responsibility, the actual motives and rationales for such a good are seldom explicitly stated.

The motives grounding and energizing caregiving are largely based on human values, not empirical reasons. Where are these values derived from? Certainly, philosophers have provided rational arguments,[12] not based on traditional religious stories and rationales, aimed to guide a society's responsibility of justice and extrapolated to issues around human care of the sick and dying. Yet how many people are motivated to care based on rational, philosophical arguments? We imagine that far fewer are motivated or energized by philosophical arguments in comparison to rationales that flow out of traditional religions. Many caregivers and systems of care are galvanized and sustained by a matrix of highly personal, emotive, and overtly religious rationales, as suggested in data discussed in Chapter 5. Similarly, nearly half of contemporary American physicians report that they are "called" into medicine.[13-15] Although it is not the case for all, most presume a "Caller" if called.[16] This is a reminder of the ongoing influence of religious motivations within the practice of medicine and caregiving. Some of the strongest reasons for care of the sick and dying vary widely between Humanists, Buddhists, Jews, Muslims, and Christians, but their reasons for offering care are not based on empirical science or brute fact. There are religious and religious-like values energizing and undergirding the care of patients by clinicians, and these values highlight what is considered most important and most deeply concerning to the nature of being human. While the motive *to act* on behalf of the sick and dying appears to remain a large consensus, any actual discussion about the substantive core *reasons* for these actions exposes enormous difference and disagreement between caregivers. These differences may justify suppression of our deepest motives in caring, since doing so would expose professional differences and threaten the existing consensus of action on behalf of the patient.

This predicament highlights an important irony that is often missed within discussions around the relationship of medicine and religion. Omitting our deepest reasons for caring for the sick disguises how religion and religious-like energies continue to animate medicine. The privatization of traditional religious motives within medicine does not remove those motives but simply hides them as unspoken motives, suppressed because they are publicly inappropriate to express. Silence pertaining to our deepest motives for caring can also give the impression that traditional religion is not actually operative or holding an influential role within medical values of cure and care. Yet in this public silence is "everyday religion" where religious motivations guide conversations and interactions throughout medicine.[17] This silence may bias nurses and physicians in appealing to religion since a secular narrative holds that a secular and scientific endeavor should remain separate from religious concerns.[18,19] Yet the individuals and collective forces that come together to care for the sick are thoroughly infused with clear, though privatized, religious rationales or religious-like humanistic values. Without these religious and religious-like motivations undergirding medical care, it would be hard to imagine contemporary medicine growing into the behemoth that it is.

Reconsidering the Secular

In adopting a functional understanding of religion informed by Tillich's concept of ultimate concern[20 [p. 8]] (or our preferred emphasis on "chief affection"), readers may anticipate that it challenges the meaning of the "secular." If spirituality is the ultimate concern or what one chiefly loves, and if religion refers to the social structures that collectively support pursuit of that ultimate concern or chief love, then to what does the secular refer? From a substantive and status quo understanding of religion, the secular refers to all those cultural spheres that are not in direct reference to the supernatural or superhuman. The secular refers to both institutions and spheres that do not operate in reference to the gods or superhuman. From this viewpoint, medicine is secular in its knowledge, professions, institutions, and practices because it deals with the human body and processes around care for the body. On these grounds medicine, appears to have little to do with religion, transcendence, the supernatural, or the gods.

From a functional conception of religion, however, the secular refers to all that which is not the ultimate concern or chief love. This means that, like the religious, the secular cannot be identified primarily by institutional affiliation, spatial location, professional activity, or the substantive absence of the supernatural or superhuman as core ideas. *Rather, the secular refers to any matter that is a second-order, nonultimate concern or an ancillary affection and desire.* The secular is not the antithesis of institutional religion or creedal beliefs about the supernatural, nor is it grounded, as Taylor suggests, in an immanent human flourishing without reference to God.[21] From a functional perspective of religion, the secular refers to all second-order loves that are not final ends or our deepest human ambitions. From this perspective, many relationships, practices, institutions, and beliefs that may traditionally be located under the category of religion are "secular" if defined as second-order concerns that do not support or enable a chief affection. Likewise, other relationships that are often considered secular in their popular meanings are functionally religious or religious-like because they are concerned with and love that which is primary and chief.

Conceptualizing medicine and religion from a functional viewpoint alters how to conceive of the relationship between these two realms. From a functional standpoint, medicine can be both religious or secular, considered both from an individual and a collective outlook.

For individual patients and clinicians, whether medicine is secular or not depends on their underlying affections and deepest loves. Patients may approach their medical care as an ultimate good and place their entire hope in medicine's power to cure and alter their health situation. Functionally, this turns the use of medicine into a religious-like sphere for those patients who approach medicine in this manner. This is certainly not a hypothetical position because it is often the case that patients and patients' families look to and rely on their physicians and medicine with a religious level of faith and trust with the hope of healing. On a substantive level, patients would not conceive of their cure through medicine as holding their deepest level of love or ultimate concern, but functionally the drive to be healed through medicine operates in a religious-like manner. In a similar fashion, physicians and clinical scientists can approach their research and practice as if it were the most important and central aspect of their lives. Clinicians may be motivated at the deepest level by power, greed, or care—or some combination of these—and, within their professional roles, clinicians may think or act as if they were mediators of a godlike power to cure or stave off death. On an individual level, these attitudes and beliefs operate frequently and have a religious-like quality since they carry meanings of ultimacy and deepest hopes.

On the collective level, we also *sense* that medicine is captivated by a certain zeitgeist that has a religious-like *feel*. We use the terms "sense" and "feel" because these are not overt claims within medicine but an unconscious effluence of ideas and attitudes operating underneath the surface. One way that this zeitgeist expresses itself within medicine is shown in the slogans of medicines and healthcare. For example, a prominent medical school announces in a large banner across its campus, "The World Is Waiting." Some local Boston hospitals make their appeals to potential donors: "With your help, there is no limit to what we can accomplish," "Miracles Happen Here," and "Until Every Child Is Well." But it is not only Boston hospitals that endorse these slogans. In contrast to the kind of humility that is advocated by the Abrahamic traditions that uphold the patient as sacred, many hospitals in the United States flatter themselves with god-like slogans: "First. Best. Always," "Depend On Us for Life," "In Love with Health," "The Power to Heal," and "More Science. Less Fear."

Ironically, one of the main teaching hospitals associated with Columbia University Medical Center, the academic home of Richard Sloan,[2] has as one of its slogans, "Amazing Things Are Happening Here." At the time of this writing, there is a picture on the front page of the hospital website of Andree Brown, a patient of the hospital, saying, "It made all the difference to hand myself over to the New York-Presbyterian team with total and unconditional trust."[vi] Total and unconditional trust? While substantive definitions of religion and the secular blind us in seeing religious-like phenomena, a functional conceptualization suggests that there is a lot more going on in our hospitals than hard science and clinical medicine.

Are these merely slick slogans aimed to appeal to desperate patients or potential philanthropists, or do these also convey a deeper zeitgeist, in fact, even an underlying theology? The irony of these mantras is that they are perpetuated by institutions and professions that portray themselves as self-consciously irreligious and secular. Yet these slogans betray attitudes that are inculcated by patients, clinicians, and administrators and point to underlying theological beliefs. What other than a god would be willing to call itself *first, best, and always*? Who is it that deserves one's *total and unconditional trust*? For whom is the world waiting? Such mottos convey a message that the institutions and professions of medicine are new incarnations of divine-like power and hope. They appear strangely like a call to faith. Can any human institution claim a legitimate mission *until every child is well*? Such mantras resemble eschatological perspectives of salvation for the world. Similarly, what is the meaning of being *in love with health*, other than it discloses what is functionally an ultimate concern and deepest affection? Rather than being the exception, these slogans can be found throughout American medicine. From a functional perspective of religion, how are these mottos distinct from what religions claim about God, salvation, or the object of worship?

On a substantive level, these are merely consumerist pitches and glossy mottos from hospital and medical school development offices. But functionally, it is a language that suggests a spirit that lies deeper, a spirit that resembles what religion at its deepest levels claims to accomplish and perform. While medicine and healthcare seem utterly irreligious according to Enlightenment categories for the secular sphere, a deeper zeitgeist appears to be at work within the practical ways that medicine conceptualizes and portrays itself. While we agree with many of the critical points put forward in *Blind Faith*[2] pertaining to empirical research of spirituality and health, there is a larger cultural blindness that results from failing to recognize how medicine and science have come to hold a religious-like aura within the social imagination. The underlying spirituality that drives patients to hospitals, the money that pours in from taxpayers and the prestige associated with being a scientist in healthcare, are all anthropological signals that a prevailing spirit dominates medicine and healthcare. In our view, there is a great deal of irony in that Sloan[vii] simultaneously rejects the "unholy alliance of religion and medicine" yet fails to take notice that the culture of medicine acts far too closely in a religious-like manner. A functional understanding of both the nature of religion and its twin—the meaning of the secular—exposes this as a double standard and calls for a provocative line of additional inquiry that goes beyond problematic and potentially passé categories that conceal rather than reveal.

A Spirituality of Immanence

What are the implications when secular medicine overtly rejects any spiritual or religious relationship and yet acts like a religion in certain ways? What conclusions should be drawn if medicine no longer recognizes its analogical or sacramental relationship (as argued in Chapter 11) with Abrahamic religious traditions? Or when it embraces neutrality toward religion rather than partnership, and when it no longer identifies its social role in terms of secondary human goods and benefits but is prone to describe itself with latent theological praise ("First. Best. Always.")?

When medicine no longer recognizes its analogical design or partnership with religion, it suggests that, within our cultural imagination, medicine itself operates in a religious-like manner. When medicine claims indifference or neutrality concerning the spiritual dimensions of illness, medicine's own deep structures as described in Chapter 11—the mediatorial role of the physician, the need of patients to extend trust, the power of therapy to overturn death, or the hospital as a type of temple—emerge as chief ends in themselves. Or, simply, medicine risks divinizing its own primary physical ends as chief loves when it no longer overtly points to greater spiritual realities beyond its own immanent concerns. The structures of medicine are so implicitly potent with basic human meanings of finitude, death, and salvation that medicine must overtly point to that which is greater than itself, which it consequently serves as a second-order good. Such an alliance has been described here ("symphony") and in other sources,[22] in which medicine was not conceived either in terms of independent or dependent from religion, but pointing beyond to greater transcendent realities. Failure to preserve this constructive alliance risks elevating medicine and healthcare to a religious-like level since medicine serves those facing the difficult existential challenge of life-threatening illness. Perhaps other spheres of life, such as education or business, can function without risking the appearance of being religious-like since less than life and death is at stake in those arenas. Such spheres of life we leave to others to describe and discern. But medicine deals with the most vulnerable, the shaken, and fearful. It is part of a dangerous and uncertain journey.[23] Thus, by its nature, failure to reference ultimate human concerns and our deepest affections elevates medicine to a religious-like status when traditional spiritualities and religious forms remain outside the purview of the collective structures of medicine.

This theological perspective brings together multiple issues that we have raised during the course of this argument. We conclude here in Part II that secular medicine exudes a functional spirituality in its deepest structures. This underlying spirituality elucidates why American culture places inordinate faith in medicine's ability to stave off death. By no longer recognizing a partnership with religion or pointing to transcendent realities, the analogical structures of medicine inadvertently point back upon themselves as their own chief ends, rather than beyond themselves to something more enduring or deserving of our deepest affections (as illustrated in Figure 11.1).

Socialization Within Immanent Spirituality

If medicine has unconsciously received our deepest human aims, loves, and aspirations, then our nurses and physicians are socialized into this immanence and formed by an immanent spirituality. This socialization can be described using at least four distinct levels of analysis: institutional, professional, philosophical, and theological.

Institutional Aspects of Socialization

Medical historian Guenter Risse profiles the evolutionary changes of medical hospitals.[24,viii] In Byzantium, hospitals were houses of "mercy, refuge, and dying."[24 (p. 675)] Emphasis was placed on the spiritual comfort of the sick and dying, with Hippocratic medicine subservient to the larger meanings of Christian compassion. With the Enlightenment, the purpose of hospitals had further shifted by the eighteenth century, so that they became "houses of cure" in which physicians controlled the processes of admission and discharge. If a patient was not considered curable, he was not typically admitted. This then transformed the purpose of a hospital within and after the rise of the Enlightenment into a "house of teaching and research" and a "house of dissection."[24 (p. 676)] By the mid-nineteenth century, the continuing medicalization of the hospital transformed it into a "house of surgery,"[24 (p. 676)] and, by the early twentieth century, into a "house of science."[24 (p. 677)] It was at this point that hospitals became acute facilities that had "shed their convalescent and dying functions."[24 (p. 677)] Risse concludes by describing the postmodern hospital as a "house of high technology, providing mostly intensive patient care with the aid of a wide array of powerful and complex diagnostic and therapeutic devices."[24 (p. 677)]

Risse's historical method focuses on six characteristics of hospital life: "mission, patronage, organization, staff, patients, and ritualized caring activities."[24 (p. 4)] These characteristics construct a "milieu" in which "the early Christian shelters provided great spiritual solace but minimal physical comforts. The accent was on holism and communal life at the expense of individual privacy. Modern hospitals, by contrast, have reversed this emphasis and now focus primarily on individual physical rehabilitation in more fragmented and depersonalized environments."[24 (p. 680)] Risse's analysis leads to a preliminary conclusion that the postmodern hospital has become a secular context, not because it overtly rejected traditional religion per se, but because of the decentralized role that religion holds among each of the six institutional characteristics. On an institutional level, religion and traditional spirituality have been decentralized so that they hold no explicit role or purpose in the structures of modern hospitals. The marginalized role of religion plays a pivotal role in making these academic medical contexts "secular."

The displacement of religion on an institutional level in postmodern hospitals has a socializing effect on clinicians. As physicians and nurses work within the structures of academic hospitals, the institutional structures have been stripped of traditional religion in each of the six characteristics of hospital life. The absence of religion within the institutional structures socializes clinicians to accept that religion and traditional spirituality have no formal or institutional role within medicine. At the same time, however, the structures of hospital life are infused with immanent sensibilities. The mission of a secular hospital is focused on physical cure and health, leaving transcendent dimensions of mission absent. Religious and ethnic identities are no longer considered welcoming, and thus patrons are not encouraged to engage the hospital based on their religious and ethnic identities. This socializes clinicians to not see their patients in these terms. Hospital staff and organizational structures give no place to clinicians' religious identity or personal characteristics as these are considered private and personal. In place of religion, immanent identities oriented around professional roles and technical competencies replace these personal aspects. Clinicians become part of a bureaucratic organization, depersonalized from their own primary socializations, and expected to identify and represent hospital and medical structures focused on the immanent. These are finally reinforced in the ritualized caring activities that are simultaneously disconnected from traditional spiritual practices (e.g., collective prayers) and highly focused on narrow and pressing needs driven by the medical bureaucracy of emails, schedules, consent forms, and medical records, constant technological concerns ensuring that machines operate and therapies are properly executed. In the absence of institutional practices that point to ultimate concerns, these immanent practices driven by contemporary institutions socialize clinicians to believe as if these concerns are chief. While few clinicians likely consider these worthy of their chief affections,[25] on the functional level, they have become the de facto ultimate concern for affiliates of secular medical institutions. In sum, this process amounts to a socialization of clinicians within immanence.

Professional Aspects of Socialization

Understanding the socialization of immanence among medical professionals requires addressing that guild of medical professionals called physicians.[26,ix] The rise of physician authority in the United States is due in large measure to the fact that medical practitioners consciously presented themselves to the American public throughout the twentieth century as engaged in a scientific enterprise.[26] Aligning medicine with science, however, was not the sole reason for the emergence of the profession of medicine during the nineteenth century in the United States. Sociologist Jonathan Imber discusses evidence that physicians were allied and morally commissioned by Protestant clergy during the nineteenth century.[27] He argues that Protestant clergy empowered the medical profession with a moral and spiritual vocation, resulting in a deeply held public trust of physicians.[27 [pp. 3–21]] This trust was not grounded only in scientific competence, but also in the moral character and spiritual credibility of doctors who were encouraged to align their medical duties according to explicit Protestant understandings.

Imber's thesis is that a confluence of factors eventually led to the current waning of trust in the profession among the American public. First, a history of "organizational realities" has transformed trust in physicians, as physicians have become an autonomous guild, leading eventually to high salaries and then a fully corporatized profession.[27 [p. 175]] These structural realities eroded public trust in physicians. Imber's analysis is quite complex, for he also argues that the profession's changing relationship with clergy, especially beginning in the final years of the nineteenth century, led clergy to "reframe the expectations" of physicians according to reason and science rather than faith.[27] [p. 72] During this period, there was further equivocation in grounding the profession within Christian ideals. Instead, the moral authority of the profession began to draw its authority from internal regulation, thus further asserting its own professional autonomy from explicit Christian truth claims.[27] [p. 94]

Imber argues that present-day public trust in the profession has declined in part because there are no highly esteemed cultural authorities, like clergy in the nineteenth century, authorizing it as a profession of high honor and moral character. Thus, the profession currently depends on scientific credentials for the profession's prestige. More importantly, Imber's thesis suggests that physicians have undergone a gradual process of developing a sense of professional autonomy disconnected from traditional religion and spirituality. As shown in Chapter 9, medicine was received by religious people based on specific theological values including medicine as a divine gift, the interconnection of body and soul, and the unique privilege of seeing the divine in the patient's presence. These ideas carried forward into the profession during the nineteenth century as religious communities sanctioned medicine and physicians to be performing holy work.

Thus, the profession has become especially secular to the degree that physicians' competencies, guild associations, and personal identities are self-consciously independent from particular religious and theological beliefs and motives. It is in this sense that the medical profession has become secular; it has moved forward by rejecting these beliefs in its institutional and professional guilds. In other words, secular medicine is not merely silent toward religion, its professional status has specifically *rejected* and *abandoned* theological endorsement. This absence socializes physicians to conceptualize their own professional identity and competencies as being disconnected from traditional spirituality and its religious communities. Yet, as this chapter has attempted to highlight, the absence of traditional spirituality and religion has not yielded a medical profession void of spirituality itself. In the place of traditional spiritual understandings is an immanent form of spirituality that socializes medical professionals into a theological belief system, governed by immanence. What does that belief system comprise?

Philosophical Accounts

Medical professionals are socialized into a moral system of immanence. Few have been more critical of this bioethical immanence than H. Tristram Engelhardt Jr., who has provocatively described and offered a critical account of medicine with a particular focus on secular bioethics.[x] Central to Engelhardt's thesis is that any attempt to do bioethics based on secular assumptions leads to a thin consensus between moral strangers.[28] Moral debate within secular medicine has led to moral differences that cannot be solved by appeal to a common rational argument. Englehardt argues that moral strangers "lack sufficient common moral premises, moral rules of evidence, and/ or moral rules of inference . . . [and lack sufficient] appeal to a mutually recognized moral authority."[28] [p. 152] He describes secular, bioethical rationality as a thoroughly immanent approach to morality in which life is lived as "if there were no transcendent God to Whom all should in humility submit."[28] [p. 138] He argues that a secular approach to medicine is a "content-full moral vision with a particular understanding of the value of autonomy or liberty . . . committed to a particular vision of autonomous self-realization."[28 [p. 140]] This secular ethos "considers suspect, if not morally deficient, moral communities that do not recognize autonomous self-determination as the keystone of moral flourishing . . . this celebration of autonomous self-determination radically brings into question traditional religious, especially ascetic pursuits. Self-fulfillment becomes fully *thisworldly*."[28 [pp. 140-141]]

Engelhardt provides five characteristics of this secular medical ethos: (1) priority to self-determination as far as it is compatible with the overall goals of financial markets; (2) the state as the mechanism to create social justice, which provides freedom from material and social constraints; (3) liberation from tradition, particularly those traditions which claim special authority; (4) freedom from traditional mores by encouraging pursuit of consensual self-satisfaction and promoting market forces that create and fulfill those needs; and (5) freedom "from transcendent or metaphysical commitments . . . setting aside transcendent and therefore democratically non-negotiable sources of obligation."[28 [pp. 142-143]] Many clinicians do not embrace these moral values within their private lives, such as a belief in self-determination, which stands in contradiction to the view that God creates moral standards and expects humans to live by them. As we have repeatedly pointed out, the tension results from the fact that clinicians are socialized to bifurcate their moral lives to follow and represent the moral beliefs of the profession when they act as medical professionals, and then within their personal lives they are free as allowed by law to follow whatever moral belief system they wish. It is usually those clinicians who do not subscribe to the moral principle of self-determination who recognize that this in itself is a content-full moral belief system, with self-determination as its first principle, and that it is being superimposed on the profession under the guise of moral neutrality. Because this moral belief system is presented as morally neutral, the profession has generally accepted this judgment, and medical trainees are deeply socialized to accept this principle without question during medical school. Debate does not seem to be allowed on this matter, and anyone who questions the principle of self-determination runs the risk of being categorized as a religious bigot, a proselytizer, or some other negative epitaph. However, if self-determination is a moral tradition rather than an adjudicator of morality, then the implication is that it forms the central creed governing a spirituality of immanence. Medical professionals inculcate and abide by this moral creed or otherwise risk losing their professional status.

Engelhardt's description of secular medicine is further augmented by Charles Taylor's analysis of what he terms "the secular age."[21] Taylor suggests that a secular age refers to "a move from a society where belief in God is unchallenged and indeed, unproblematic, to one in which it is understood to be one option among others, and frequently not the easiest to embrace."[21 [p. 3]] Taylor suggests that it is especially this final sense of the secular which now depicts our age: "A secular age is one in which the eclipse of all goals beyond human flourishing becomes conceivable; or better, it falls within the range of an imaginable life for masses of people."[21 [pp. 20-21]] But what is it that drives this third sense of secular according to Taylor? His answer is what he terms an "immanent frame."[21 [see chap. 15]] He defines the immanent frame as a constructed social order that reconfigures space, time, rationality, and nature all in immanent terms—a full-blown human social system aimed toward human flourishing that contains no necessary contingency on the reality of transcendence undergirding human flourishing. An immanent frame, according to Taylor, can be "spun" as either open or closed. An "open" immanent frame refers to a basic immanent system that can be punctuated by occasional moments of transcendence. There is mystery that is real and greater than the horizontal world around us and is characterized by a disposition "open to something beyond."[21 [p. 544]] A closed immanent frame may be defined as a disposition closed to the possibility that a greater reality exists beyond the natural, material world. Whether open or closed, an immanent frame structures human experience of social reality—space, time, rationality, and a metaphysical view of nature—nudging everyone toward a basic disposition of immanence.[21 [p. 555]]

Both immanent moral beliefs (emphasized by Englehardt) and immanent structures (emphasized by Taylor) together form what we are simply calling an ethos or spirituality of immanence. This ethos permeates the medical culture. There is, as noted by Taylor, an open immanent frame within the secular medical context. For example, patients remain free to employ their religious or spiritual values in the medical context, but when those values conflict with medical advice there is a general expectancy that those values should be subsumed to the aims of medicine.[29] Likewise, within medical institutions, chaplains, chapels, and religious rituals are provided as optional, complementary services, but they are also decentralized, marginalized services since they hold no integral position within medical care itself.[30,31] An open immanent frame does not eliminate patients' traditional religion but categorizes it among aesthetic preferences. Thus, when discussions arise concerning the goals of care within life-threatening illness, most clinicians acknowledge the patient's religious beliefs but then change the topic since this is not deemed pertinent to medical decisions.[32] Also consistent with this description are patterns of clinician referral to chaplaincy. These are infrequent[33-35] and often engendered only after medical options are exhausted.[34] When medicine can do no more, then there is some willingness to give traditional religion and spirituality space within the larger medical context.

Based on this philosophical perspective, the secular medical context is infused by an ethos of immanence so that the *shared social structures* of a secular medical context—time, economics, space, professional roles, and competencies—have little dependency on transcendent claims or realties. Irrespective of the physician's own interior and spiritual disposition, most clinicians, when caring for terminally ill patients, practice medicine shaped by *this-worldly*, immanent aims. While the five characteristics of a secular medical ethos described by Engelhardt would rarely be consciously acknowledged, Taylor's analysis reveals how an ethos of immanence is reinforced by institutional structures built into a secular medical context. Spiritual care barriers (see Tables 3.9 and 3.10) are individual aspects of this underlying milieu. When the barriers are seen in this larger context of immanence, then they form an omnipresent socialization of clinicians leading to *neglect or avoidance of spiritual care* despite their own positive opinions related to the appropriateness of nurses and physicians occasionally providing spiritual care (Table 3.6) and its perceived positive benefits for patients (Table 3.8).

Theological Aspects of Socialization

Finally, there is a theological level of analysis related to understanding the socialization process of clinicians as they are immersed within a secular medical context. Shuman and Volck have argued, based within a Christian framework, that theology names medicine as a "mysteriously animated social force.[36] [pp. 26,28] While many discussions related to medicine and spirituality have tended to instrumentalize religion as subservient to bodily health, Shuman and Volck argue that religion (and from their vantage point, Christianity in particular) ought to name medicine, harnessing its power to the service of God.[36] [p. 31] They describe medicine by drawing on the New Testament's terminology of principalities and powers.[xi] Whether visible or invisible, personal or impersonal, the powers are institutional forces that provide humanity with a social order making a shared human life possible.[36] [p. 32] However, based on a Christian narrative, the powers are both created by God and have fallen into rebellion against God. In their brokenness, the principalities and powers have a tendency to enslave mankind into a false worship, allowing human consciousness to elevate the powers into a "quasi-divine status."[36] [p. 33] According to Shuman and Volck, medicine occupies a "revered social position" in which society's general disposition is worship of medicine.[36] [p. 35] They argue that the current social context operates on a spiritually oriented fear and denial of death.[36] [p. 35] This unresolved social fear has seduced US society into falsely placing faith in the idol of medicine—a spiritual power that holds out the promise of safety and restoration against sickness and our own mortality. From this perspective, medical researchers and physicians are "sanctioned with the power to preserve life and vigor and to forestall or control death, [and] are understood within modern culture to represent, if not to possess, godlike power."[36] [pp. 37–38] Shuman and Volck provocatively suggest, "The project by which medicine becomes the chief mediator of the power of death is clearly in some respects a religious one, if by *religious* we mean pertaining to the particular objects of affection around which our lives revolve."[36] [p. 36] The authors conclude that the Christian community, especially church members receiving medical care, must resist the seduction of medicine's idolatry and harness the power of medicine only as it is rightly ordered under the authority of Christ.

Putting the Four Levels Together

The implications of this theological view further complicate our understanding of immanence and its socialization of medical professionals.

A historical analysis of hospital institutions, according to Risse,[24] yields a conclusion that postmodern hospitals are houses of high technology that displace traditional religion and spirituality from institutional concerns, impacting how academic medical professionals conceptualize the medical institutions in which they care for patients. From a sociological perspective, according to Imber,[27] the medical profession itself has undergone a process in which religion has been displaced, yielding a profession that conceptualizes itself as autonomous from traditional religion and spirituality, requiring no dependence on it for its professional identity and competencies. Philosophically, according to Engelhardt[28] and Taylor,[21] a positive (or non-neutral) moral belief system is embedded within underlying beliefs in ethics and decision-making, which is reinforced by large-scale social structures that disseminate immanence. Secular medicine is thus a social milieu in which *this-worldly* concerns are primary and other-worldly concerns are deemed optional, aesthetic concerns. These scholarly perspectives help to illuminate how medical professionals are socialized concerning traditional religion and spirituality in the medical context and why physicians and nurses may infrequently provide spiritual care. Theological analysis provides a complementary level of understanding concerning the secular medical context. If Shulman and Volck[36] are right, then what Taylor has philosophically termed an ethos of immanence, an immanence that is perceived as nonreligious, should be further understood as a full-blown, content-full spirituality.

Immanence Theologically Considered

What emerges from this analysis is a tentative conclusion that nurses and physicians within the secular medical context are socialized into a spirituality of immanence. As physicians are socialized into the profession of medicine, encased by postmodern hospitals of high technology, permeated by beliefs and structures of immanence, *a clinician's adopted spirituality qua clinician is centered on bodily health, cure, and physical comfort as ultimate telos or chief affection*. Medicine is centered around the physical and material dimensions of the patient, so that this focus emerges as its unrivaled final purpose and driving goal. Focus on the cure and comfort of the body is not intrinsically a spirituality. It becomes a spirituality in the absence of any other ultimate meaning-making system that frames the activity of medicine. In the absence of a greater or more ultimate concern, the material focus on the body is transformed into a collective love and ultimate concern.[xii]

In those contexts where medicine has been partnered with traditional religious purposes expressed, for example, in the Abrahamic traditions, then the practice of medicine is only a second-order concern, framed by a larger meaning-making system. In such cases, medicine itself is an activity that expresses the values of a spiritual worldview that seeks to care for and love the sick. When medicine is positively partnered with religious perspectives, then medicine is by default denying its focus and activities as ultimate. Yet, in the absence of a religious meaning-making system in the form of partnership, there is silence as to medicine's relationship to ultimacy. Because medicine often deals within a context of human finitude, fears, and deepest questions and holds out a potential for restoration, medicine's silence as to what is ultimate is all that is necessary for society to grant divine-like status to it. Medicine is so powerful in the human imagination that it must consciously seek to deny its own ultimacy lest patients look to it as the source of their own ultimate hope. In partnership with traditional religions, this denial was intrinsic since medicine related itself to another sphere that claimed its relationship to ultimacy. But medicine's jettisoning of traditional religion and its silence about what is ultimate creates a near irresistible enticement to elevate itself to a consecrated, religious-like status. It becomes the mediator, not of eternal life, but of a salvation of immanence. It is this immanence that enables institutions to make boasts such as "First. Best. Always." and "The World is Waiting." It also encourages patients to hand themselves over in "total and unconditional trust."

Those within the Abrahamic traditions immediately see that this is language about God. It is one of the clues that more is going on than meets the eye.

A spirituality of immanence is centered on bodily health, cure, and physical comfort as the chief *telos,* ultimate aim, chief affection. We suggest that this becomes medicine's inevitable direction when it is no longer in partnership with traditional religious structures. The severing of the analogical relationship between medicine and religion as discussed in Chapter 11—that mirroring of themes, structures, and practices, with one sphere focusing on the material and the other focusing on the immaterial—has repositioned medicine from a secondary good serving infinite ends and committed to the ultimate end of serving transcendence, to a social sphere of action that is its own ultimate *telos.* By rejecting this partnership and separating the material and immaterial, medicine's activities around the human body, previously practiced as secondary and finite, have become its chief and ultimate end.

Thus, with surprising irony, contemporary medicine continues to hold to a spirituality, with its collective efforts centered on bodily health, cure, and comfort as its chief love. While few could have conceivably intended this result, the analogical or sacramental relationship of medicine and religion, the invisible realities to which they point, the god-like adulation sometimes expressed by patients, and the hubris surrounding many of medicine's institutions, suggests that medicine comes too close to looking and acting like traditional religions. Gestures of neutrality within medicine hidden behind limited definitions of spirituality and religion do not undo the obvious linkages that become clear when we view medicine through a theological lens aided by functional understandings of religion. Failure to partner with traditional religions elevates immanence to the level of spirituality.

Conclusion

Contemporary secular medicine and spirituality have only an appearance of separation. There is an existing separation, but it is between secular medicine and Western spiritualities including Judaism, Christianity, and Islam. After recognizing that spirituality and religion are broad constructs identifiable in what is "ultimate concern" or "chief love," then the very framework of "separation" is exposed as an apologetic for a spirituality of immanence. This spirituality governs today's contemporary medicine, and it does so under a guise that it is neither spiritual or religious. The principle claim of immanence is that it can divide the material and immaterial spheres, and, through this division, the material realm is nonspiritual. In contrast, our argument in Part II has marshalled evidence that contemporary medicine looks, acts, and functions in a religious-like fashion. When life and death are on the line, spirituality and religion are inevitably close behind, so that constructed divisions between material and immaterial are implausible. Discussions about spirituality, religion, and medicine that embrace the language of "separation" between medicine and spirituality as an appropriate description of contemporary reality already concede the argument in principle. In contrast, the theological perspective offered here in Part II argues that medicine in its contemporary secular institutions and professions is both intrinsically spiritual in its ultimate concerns and loves and also infused with a veiled, quasi-religious zeitgeist embedded in its structures. Clinicians are deeply socialized into immanence, and it leads them to unconsciously avoid or neglect their patients' spiritual needs—a majority of Americans who express these needs in terms of traditional religion.

As we turn now to Part III of our argument, we begin by offering four reasons why medicine should reevaluate its partnership with a spirituality of immanence and reconsider how a conscious partnership with the world's religions is possible in light of pluralism.

Notes

i. In Sloan's defense, he merely adopts the definitions that are employed by the research that he critiques in his book. If they do not define religion, then why should that burden fall on him? Nevertheless, in part I of *Blind Faith*,[2] Sloan engages in a historical review of medicine and religion, and in part III, the book explores ethical dimensions of medicine and religion. In both sections, it is a fallacy to discuss a proper relationship between medicine and religion without also properly defining religion and defending that definition. Sloan is not only critiquing empirical research on religion, spirituality, and health; he is also defending the status quo, which also assumes specific definitions related to spirituality and religion. A book-length project pertaining to religion that fails to define and defend the conceptual nature of its key topic has a fatal flaw, not merely an oversight.

ii. It is nearly but not entirely a foregone conclusion because, even if we assume substantive definitions of religion, a thick analysis of how medicine is used in our culture suggests that at a minimum some religious-like dynamic appears to be taking place. Substantive definitions tend to blind interpretations in this direction, but not always so. Thus, even if some readers might conclude that these phenomena are not formally or technically a religion because they prefer a substantive definition, an informal and nontechnical approach to the subject suggests "religious-like" phenomenon.

iii. One way to illustrate this issue of definition is by noting the growing acceptance of complementary and alternative medicine within NIH research funding and in medical practice. Practices such as yoga and the relaxation response have become widely accepted within medicine and actively promoted in major teaching hospitals across the United States. These practices have become acceptable in a secular context because they are presented in purely secular terms, independent from theological underpinnings or religious community associations. Nevertheless, religious scholars have continued to show how these practices have embedded laden religious theories about the nature of the divine, suffering, or salvation, which remain hidden but nevertheless formative. While empirical research may focus on biological and physiological cause-and-effect relationships, which hold importance to a certain degree, the impact of these practices holds latent theological beliefs that theologically form those who practice them. While it does appear possible to suppress the tradition-rich stories and communities that produced yoga or mindfulness meditation, the underlying theological assumptions remain embedded.

For example, undergirding mindfulness meditation is a focus on human breath and being nonjudgmental. This intense focus on the moment suggested by this practice highlights a presupposition of what is most important and central. Likewise, emphasis within mindfulness meditations on nonjudgmental dismissal of thoughts suggests an underlying morality. By way of contrast, in the Abrahamic traditions, the mind is called to focus especially in worship of God, not on the breath as in Buddhism. The Abrahamic traditions also place weight upon a moral code that demands a judgment against injustice and hatred of neighbor (while rejecting a censorious spirit). In other words, only certain religions emphasize the practice of being nonjudgmental, primarily because within Buddhism there is a belief that the material reality that we live and suffer within is in fact ultimately an illusion. To be nonjudgmental is a form of actively living into acceptance that our lives are illusory. However, Western religions have seldom produced such spiritual practices because they believe in a material world that is real (not illusory). They also receive a moral code that judges human motives and actions based on a belief of real evil that inflicts pain on the innocent. Thus, implicit within practices of yoga and mindfulness meditation are latent theologies about cosmic realities. Attempts to characterize these in purely secular and nondoctrinal terms misses the embedded theological presuppositions driving the practice. It is akin to receiving the Christian Eucharist, but, rather than seeing the bread as a sign of Jesus' body, it is secularized and equated with simply having a heart of thanksgiving and gratitude for life (as *Eucharist* means "thanksgiving"), which is perhaps beneficial to one's health. While conceptualizing the Christian practice of Eucharist in nonreligious terms seems irresponsible and should be outright rejected, some Eastern spiritual practices are being accepted in secular medicine because of a problematic substantive definition for religion. Functional approaches to religion that focus on the utility of a practice aimed toward ultimate concern expose these as fraught distinctions. Eastern religious practices such as yoga or mindfulness meditation should not be framed as nonreligious and offered to patients or clinicians, while Western religious practices are overtly denied entrance. Preference for substantive definitions for religion has created these problematic distinctions

iv. The social structures of contemporary medicine appear neutral regarding human authority since they are grounded in human autonomy. Upholding human autonomy appears neutral toward religion since it upholds the individual's authority to be the final word. It appears highly congruent with religious and nonreligious choices since, in this perspective, religion is primarily a private decision. This approach presupposes, however, a substantive definition for religion, and autonomy is an applied principle only on the individual level. What is unfortunately not often considered or recognized in this view concerns the functional dimension of religion pertaining to authority and its related collective prerogative for individual autonomy. While the individual is left to decide, it is the preceding *collective agreement* that authorizes the individual. So while neutrality holds as it pertains to an individual patient's right to decide, neutrality does not exist within the underlying level of the social structure. There is a specific and constructive decision within the underlying collective that sanctions individual human authority. It is the level of the social structure itself that is biased toward individualism and individual authority. While this is not unique to contemporary medicine, these dynamics take a particular form in medicine.

This is an example of one of the ironies of the liberal tradition, where there is corporate authorization to preference an individual's right of choice and interpretation. When using a substantive definition of religion, autonomy appears as a neutral principle. But, upon employing a functional understanding of religion, it draws attention not to the individual but to the preceding collective authorization. On what grounds does the collective authorize the individual? What are the underlying assumptions that justify this claim? A creed advocating for individual choice and rights places final authority on the individual. It leaves behind the rationalities and meanings that may inform a person's choice as being inherently secondary. The fact that the reasons for a choice are deemed secondary implies that adequate justification is grounded in the individual herself, not in the rationalities or arguments justifying a choice. Thus, delegated authority rests on the individual, but it is still the collective that legitimates that authority. What this implies is that a real but hidden authority lies, not in the individual, but within the collective authority that has granted individuals a power to choose. How is this authorization different from divine authority, where the individual is expected to comply with God's will? On a functional level, social sanction of the individual is akin to divine authority, and thus, from a functional approach to religion, patient autonomy is similar to a *religious-like* creedal position. This is hardly a relativistic or neutral position, but it rather functions like divine authority that sanctions individual choice.

v. Christian Smith recently makes a case for a substantive definition oriented around "superhuman." He dismisses functional approaches such as "ultimate concern" since "many religions are concerned in part—and some are almost wholly concerned—with this-worldly, even mundane issues, like fertile crops and healing sickness, not ultimate things like eternity or "the meaning of life" (Smith, *Religion*, 24). This dismissal, however, misses that these items among certain groups function as ultimate. His definition assumes that ephemeral aims or temporary material things cannot be the object of ultimate concern or chief affection. Contrastingly, we are suggesting that, on their face, such things hold the potential to have an elevated role. Smith's dismissal of so-called ephemeral aims that are *not* associated with the superhuman ignores and miscategorizes religious-like phenomenon that we have been exploring in secular medicine.

vi. See http://www.nyp.org, accessed March 13, 2017.

vii. We want to be clear that we highly respect Dr. Richard Sloan as a scientist and as a critic of the spirituality and health movement. His own critical work has been vital in pushing researchers in the field of spirituality and health to be methodologically rigorous in its approach. In our argument, Dr. Sloan's book, *Blind Faith*,[2] represents the majority view within medicine concerning the nature of religion and medicine. Our intention is not to pick on Dr. Sloan himself. Instead, we are criticizing the majority perspective that he conveniently represents in his important book.

viii. As a historian, Risse warns that generalizations that he offers in his concluding chapter easily overgeneralize the complexity of every individual hospital. Risse offers case studies that point to general shifts that may or may not specifically apply to any one case.

ix. Medical hospitals and medical physicians have been in a symbiotic relationship but also hold distinct developments. For the relationships among physicians, hospitals, and the US medical system see Starr.[26]

x. Our account is not focused on bioethics narrowly considered, but on the underlying belief system that is often made overtly clear within bioethical accounts. Outside of the field of bioethics, underlying beliefs usually lay under the surface and are seldom mentioned or directly defended. It is usually only when there are strong disagreements (e.g., abortion) that these most basic belief considerations become clear.

xi. Shuman and Volk rely on theologian Walter Wink's view related to the principalities and powers. The powers were created by God, fallen, and will be redeemed. Wink tended to be ambivalent when describing if the powers were personal or impersonal agents. He said, "These powers are both heavenly and earthly, divine and human, spiritual and political, invisible and structural . . . (they) possess an outer, physical, manifestation and an inner . . . corporate culture or collective personality" (W. Wink. *Engaging the powers: discernment and resistance in a world of domination*. Minneapolis, MN: Fortress Press; 1992: 3). Whatever exactly the powers are in Wink's view, they intertwine invisible and spiritual dimensions with visible, material, and human characteristics. This can create expressions of hostility against persons who are institutionalized and deeply entrenched within social structures.

xii. Of course, one of the ironies of this conclusion is that it leads to classifying a material focus on the body as a spirituality. How can a material focus be "spiritual?" Here, we are encountering the limits of language since the connotation of spirituality is typically associated with what is invisible and nonmaterial. Nevertheless, such popular understandings fail to take account of how traditional Western spiritualties imbue the human body and the whole material sphere with spiritual meaning. Religions make claims over the material realm, including human bodies. Dichotomies that divide "material" and "immaterial" are constructed and superimposed on human reality and deny many religious claims that the material and immaterial are enmeshed and inseparable. The secular view claims that the material and immaterial can function separately, without doing violence or compromising either sphere. But this view of reality that leads to compartmentalization is an *unprovable claim* about the nature of the human. The secular claim—that the material and immaterial can be divided and done so without detriment to either—is itself a metaphysical assertion and one that is accepted by faith since it cannot be validated on empirical grounds. In these ways it functions like other clearly identified spiritual worldviews. So, while it appears like an oxymoron to consider the secular view focused on immanent material body as a "spirituality," we suggest that this is the most consistent and fair-minded approach.

References

1. D. P. Sulmasy. Ethos, mythos, and thanatos: spirituality and ethics at the end of life. *J Pain Symptom Manage.* 2013;46(3):447–451.
2. Richard P. Sloan. *Blind faith: the unholy alliance of religion and medicine.* 1st ed. New York: St. Martin's Press; 2006.
3. William T. Cavanaugh. *The myth of religious violence: secular ideology and the roots of modern conflict.* Oxford/New York: Oxford University Press; 2009.
4. Robert Neelly Bellah. *Habits of the heart: individualism and commitment in American life.* Berkeley: University of California Press; 1985.
5. William T. Cavanaugh. The invention of the religious-secular distinction. In: Barbieri WA, ed. *At the limits of the secular: reflections on faith and public life.* Grand Rapids, MI: William B. Eerdmans Publishing; 2014:105–128.
6. Dietrich Bonhoeffer, Eberhard Bethge. *Letters and papers from prison.* New York: Simon & Schuster; 1997.
7. Tomoko Masuzawa. *The invention of world religions, or, how European universalism was preserved in the language of pluralism.* Chicago: University of Chicago Press; 2005.
8. Daniel Dubuisson. *The western construction of religion: myths, knowledge, and ideology.* Baltimore: Johns Hopkins University Press; 2003.
9. Derek R. Peterson, Walhof Darren R. *The invention of religion: rethinking belief in politics and history.* New Brunswick, NJ: Rutgers University Press; 2002.
10. Jonathan Z. Smith. Religion, religions, religious. In: M. C. Taylor, ed. *Critical terms for religious studies.* Chicago: University of Chicago Press; 1998:269–284.
11. Candy Gunther Brown. *The healing gods: complementary and alternative medicine in Christian America.* New York: Oxford University Press; 2013.
12. John Rawls. *A theory of justice.* Original ed. Cambridge, MA: Belknap Press; 2005.
13. J. D. Yoon, Daley B. M., Curlin F. A. The association between a sense of calling and physician well-being: a national study of primary care physicians and psychiatrists. *Acad Psychiatry.* 2017;41(2):167–173.
14. J. D. Yoon, Hunt N. B., Ravella K. C., Jun C. S., Curlin F. A. Physician burnout and the calling to care for the dying. *Am J Hosp Palliat Care.* 2016:1049909116661817.
15. J. D. Yoon, Shin J. H., Nian A. L., Curlin F. A. Religion, sense of calling, and the practice of medicine: findings from a national survey of primary care physicians and psychiatrists. *South Med J.* 2015;108(3):189–195.
16. Daniel P. Sulmasy. *The healer's calling: a spirituality for physicians and other health care professionals.* New York: Paulist Press; 1997.
17. MJ Balboni. Everyday religion in hospitals. *Society.* 2015;52(5):413–417.
18. R. J. Lawrence. The witches' brew of spirituality and medicine. *Ann Behav Med.* 2002;24(1):74–76.
19. R. P. Sloan, Bagiella E., Powell T. Religion, spirituality, and medicine. *Lancet.* 1999;353 (9153):664–667.
20. Paul Tillich. *Dynamics of faith.* New York: Harper; 1958.
21. Charles Taylor. *A secular age.* Cambridge, MA: Belknap Press of Harvard University Press; 2007.
22. Gary B. Ferngren. *Medicine and religion: a historical introduction.* Baltimore: Johns Hopkins University Press; 2014.
23. Arthur Kleinman. *What really matters: living a moral life amidst uncertainty and danger.* New York: Oxford University Press,; 2006.
24. Guenter B. Risse. *Mending bodies, saving souls: a history of hospitals.* New York: Oxford University Press; 1999.
25. F. A. Curlin, Lantos J. D., Roach C. J., Sellergren S. A., Chin M. H. Religious characteristics of US physicians: a national survey. *J Gen Intern Med.* 2005;20(7):629–634.
26. Paul Starr. *The social transformation of American medicine.* New York: Basic Books; 1982.
27. Jonathan B. Imber. *Trusting doctors: the decline of moral authority in American medicine.* Princeton, NJ: Princeton University Press; 2008.

28. H. Tristram Engelhardt. *The foundations of Christian bioethics*. Lisse, Netherlands; Exton, PA: Swets & Zeitlinger Publishers; 2000.

29. F. A. Curlin. Commentary: A case for studying the relationship between religion and the practice of medicine. *Acad Med*. 2008;83(12):1118–1120.

30. R. de Vries, Berlinger N., Cadge W. Lost in translation: the chaplain's role in health care. *Hastings Cent Rep*. 2008;38(6):23–27.

31. Wendy Cadge. *Paging God: religion in the halls of medicine*. Chicago; London: University of Chicago Press; 2012.

32. N. C. Ernecoff, Curlin F. A., Buddadhumaruk P., White D. B. Health care professionals' responses to religious or spiritual statements by surrogate decision makers during goals-of-care discussions. *JAMA Intern Med*. 2015;175(10):1662–1669.

33. T. A. Balboni, Vanderwerker L. C., Block S. D., Paulk M. E., Lathan C. S., Peteet J. R., Prigerson H. G. Religiousness and spiritual support among advanced cancer patients and associations with end-of-life treatment preferences and quality of life. *J Clin Oncol*. 2007;25(5):555–560.

34. P. J. Choi, Curlin F. A., Cox C. E. "The patient is dying, please call the chaplain": the activities of chaplains in one medical center's intensive care units. *J Pain Symptom Manage*. 2015;50(4):501–506.

35. L. C. Vanderwerker, Flannelly K. J., Galek K., Harding S. R., Handzo G. F., Oettinger M., Bauman J. P. What do chaplains really do? III. Referrals in the New York Chaplaincy Study. *J Health Care Chaplain*. 2008;14(1):57–73.

36. Joel James Shuman, Volck Brian. *Reclaiming the body: Christians and the faithful use of modern medicine*. Grand Rapids, MI: Brazos Press; 2006.

PART III

RESTORING HOSPITALITY
TO MEDICINE

13

Why Medicine Should Resist Immanence

Introduction

If we are correct that medicine is informed by a spirituality of immanence, defined as a fundamental centering on bodily health, cure, and physical comfort as chief affection or ultimate concern, then should this spirituality be resisted or modified? Here, we argue that this spirituality that presently dominates medicine should be contested and altered for four reasons. First, this spirituality is incongruent with the beliefs of most American patients and their experience of life-threatening illness. Second, a spirituality of immanence fails the test of religious pluralism, an essential characteristic of medicine in the twenty-first century. Third, this spirituality enables and encourages impersonal social forces, including bureaucracy, market forces, and the technological imperative, to affect how medicine is conceived, practiced, and experienced. Finally, immanence is creating a professional socialization with negative clinician outcomes, such as burnout. In this chapter, we briefly discuss the first two reasons since Chapter 2 details patient experience of spirituality and illness, and Chapter 15 engages the issue of pluralism. Instead, this chapter focuses on the impact of immanence in creating conditions for impersonal medicine and its subsequent impact on clinician socialization.

Problem 1: Immanence Fails to Reflect Patients' Illness Experience

As demonstrated in Chapter 2, illness is a spiritual event that invokes deep questions about life. As patients seek meaning to understand, cope with, and navigate serious illness, many find solace and strength through traditional religious beliefs, relationships, and practices. Patients turn to clinicians and the medical system primarily for physical help, hoping for cure, and settling for other levels of support such as management of chronic conditions, quality of life, and alleviation of pain. Nevertheless, as patients turn to healthcare for help, they do so within their existential and relational expectations.[1,2] They are human persons, not machines or body parts.[i] Rather, illness is entwined with particular persons and individual narratives.

A spirituality of immanence, with its focus on the body, creates and nurtures a larger spiritual system that is incongruent with the spirituality embraced by many patients. Whereas a majority of patients interpret their illness in terms of specific religious beliefs and among a network of religious relationships and practices, a spirituality of immanence produces social structures that undermine patients' religious experiences. Because of the accepted narrative that the secular is neutral, it can be difficult to see how this spirituality is not patient-centered.

One way to see this is by illustrating it with an example. Imagine a Catholic patient, Mr. C., who enters a hospital named Saint Mary's Hospital, with its main building shaped in the form of a cross. While sitting in the lobby, Mr. C. sees a prominent Bible displayed in the main hospital lobby. An older nun, dressed in her religious habit, walks past as she talks with two physicians in their white coats. In such a place (we describe one of the contemporary hospitals at the Mayo Clinic in Rochester, Minnesota), our fictitious patient's religious faith is stimulated, potentially strengthened, and supported. Such a scene indicates to Mr. C. that he has not entered into a sphere that is merely about his body and disease, but one that is concerned with his whole person, even its immaterial dimension. At the same time, we also recognize that such a scene would not necessarily be welcoming for members of non-Christian religions; we will further discuss the complexities of a truly pluralistic medical setting in Chapter 15.

Now imagine the same patient entering another hospital named General Hospital. As Mr. C. waits in a main lobby, several physicians walk past but there are no recognizable religious symbols or religious persons to be seen. There is art work on the walls that display fashion drawings of women in gowns, a Warhol Campbell's Souper dress, and The Beatles with Ali.[ii] Elevator-style hotel music plays quietly in the background, and an electronic advertisement is displayed on a flat panel TV saying that "our sole mission is to defeat cancer, especially yours." In this scene, the patient is immersed in the material sphere, focused on the body, with some signaling of other immanent aspects of life. But what is central to a majority of US patients, including Mr. C., is conspicuously absent throughout the hospital ethos. There is no mention of anything besides this temporary life. His illness and the fear it invokes because it is life-threatening and may likely lead to his death can find little real comfort in ephemeral artwork or promises of victory in his "war on cancer." While Mr. C. turns to his Catholic faith for strength and solace, the hospital itself offers little public support for his spirituality.

In mainstream understanding, St. Mary's creates a religious context, whereas General Hospital is neutral; that is, being neither for nor against spirituality or religion. It is thought that if General Hospital were against religion, then the patient might encounter some subtle or overt hostility toward his faith, perhaps in the form of proselytism.[iii] By excluding traditional religion from the public aspects of the medical context, the secular view argues that it remains neutral toward it. However, there are three problems with this view.

First, it depends on a substantive understanding of spirituality and religion, rather than a functional definition that we extensively argued for in Chapter 8 and Chapter 12. The absence of traditional spiritual symbols in a hospital does not negate the possibility of ultimate concerns or chief loves in full operation. A spirituality of immanence, with its focus on *this-worldly* affairs, including its particular focus on healing the body, is spiritual because the way it functions. Having publicly removed all other traditional religious forms of ultimacy, immanence itself becomes what is ultimate. Recognition of ultimacy is the human impulse within the illness context. A secular hospital excludes traditional spirituality and religion from its public face, but it is not excluding a spirituality of immanence, which functions in similar ways as traditional spiritualities (as described in Chapters 10–12).

Second, the popular cultural understanding holds religion to be private, but this also is a myth based on substantive definitions for spirituality and religion. As suggested in Chapter 8, religion becomes embodied within the collective social and relational structures that reflect and reinforce a particular spirituality. Because the medical context is imbued with life-and-death realities, it means that ultimate concerns function at the heart of illness and throughout the medical context. While traditional religious expressions are consciously excluded in the General Hospital example, other forms of religious ultimacy replace them. In such a context as the hospital, exclusion of functional religion is impossible. Functional spirituality expresses itself throughout a hospital setting so that, whatever is included, even those things that are ephemeral and seemingly innocuous, have the ability to take on symbolic meanings. Thus, a spirituality of immanence, which looks dissimilar from the world's religions in substance, creates its own set of beliefs, practices, relationships, and symbols. Though traditional religious expressions are privatized, hospital spaces and cooperative practices continue to reflect and reinforce a collective form of spirituality centered around immanent, bodily concerns. This so-called privatization of religion and secularization theses more generally are in fact a sociological fiction that describes the exclusion of traditional religious forms from the public sphere, yet includes a functional spirituality advancing immanence. A setting like the hospital always reflects and reinforces functional spiritual and religious views that impact the patient's experience of their illness. So while Mr. C. can choose to turn to his own Catholic spirituality for support during his cancer, this is a private and individual choice. Advocates of religious privatization believe that General Hospital is being neutral toward his faith. But the secular view overlooks how the entire ethos of the hospital reflects an entirely different set of values that operate in a disguised conflict with Mr. C.'s faith commitments. While he can still center his own spirituality around the Catholic faith, he must choose this direction while simultaneously resisting a hospital ethos advocating a culture and environment championing immanence.

Third, there is deep incongruence in the United States between patient-reported levels and kinds of religiousness and spirituality in contrast to a spirituality of immanence. This raises a most basic question: Who does a spirituality of immanence serve? As shown in Chapter 2, even in the metro area of Boston, a majority of cancer patients (79%) identified with the Christian religion. Yet the secular hospitals that serve these patients offer little visible indications of acknowledgment of their experience. More than half of patients describe themselves as spiritual and religious (Table 2.1), more than half indicate that religious beliefs play a major role in coping with illness (Table 2.3), most deal with spiritual concerns in their illness (Table 2.4), and a large majority of patients turn specifically to a Christian understanding of God for connection, love, and strength within their cancer (Tables 2.2 and 2.3). Despite these large majorities, the secular hospital and medical context has been largely stripped of signs or symbols that might uphold patients' faith. This incongruity is an empirical fact, and no matter what one's personal views are concerning religion per se, patient-centered approaches should factor in the actual patients receiving care as they face life-threatening illness.

Yet because a spirituality of immanence governs the public dimensions of clinical care and hospital institutions, the incongruity is not one of deliberate neglect and avoidance of patients' particular views and experiences. Rather, patients of particular world religions—both Abrahamic and others—who carry their own faith into the medical setting are confronted by an alien spirituality within the larger medical ethos that paradoxically denies its own spiritual and religious nature. In contrast, only approximately 25% of our patient sample indicated that they were nonreligious and nonspiritual in their experiences (Table 4.2), and only 7% specified no spiritual concerns of any kind (Table 2.5). In terms of proportionality (see Table 2.3), broadly speaking, the largest patient group are those who are religious and spiritual (53%) and who predominantly identify with Christianity. Then there are those who are neither religious nor spiritual (25%), and finally those who are spiritual, not religious (19%) (see Tables 4.1 and 4.2). Surely, we expect that these percentages will change over time, and there are also currently widespread geographic differences in the United States when comparing Boston and New York[3] to Houston[4] or North Carolina.[5] Yet, as we look across the United States, the spirituality of immanence that dominates medical culture currently represents at best only one-quarter of patients. This results in a failure to reflect patients' actual spiritual experiences and viewpoints and raises the issue of pluralism as a second problem related to immanence.

Problem 2: Immanence Fails the Test of Pluralism

If medicine is controlled by an ethos of immanence, which is functionally spiritual, then it raises a second major problem in regards to issues around political pluralism. Yale theologian Miroslav Volf suggests that political pluralism refers to a philosophy "according to which freedom of conscience is guaranteed to all people, irrespective of their faith or lack of it, and they all have equal voice in running the affairs of common public life."[6 [p. 141]] Within the American hospital, which increasingly reflects trends toward globalization, a principled form of pluralism must reject both extreme positions that either exclude religion from secular hospitals or inundate the hospital domain with a single religion or ideology.[6 [p. 131]]

A spirituality of immanence dominates most hospitals and holds a religious-like monopoly over the public domain of medicine. Of course, traditional religion can be found throughout the hospital among individuals, from patients to clinicians to hospital staff,[7] but this religion is privatized, having no collective institutionalization. The focus of concern is not that patients from varied religious traditions are prohibited from practicing their faith within their encounter of medicine. Religious patients of all stripes, from Catholic, Muslim, Wiccan, and Jehovah Witnesses—to name a few—are freely permitted to practice their faith. The issue is not private practice, but the larger collective, shared, public framework of medicine embedded within its institutional and professional forms. If this underlying framework is also based on a spirituality of immanence, upholding the physical body as ultimate concern and chief affection, then the principles that underlie pluralism are in violation. This spirituality of immanence is imposed upon all who enter the courts of medicine, through mostly invisible structures that deeply socialize patients and clinicians alike to interiorize particular beliefs, values, and practices. This spirituality is not enacted through sermons or worship services but is advanced within the underlying structures of medical time, hospital space, a materialistic epistemology, interpreted meanings of disease and cure, and certain valued commitments and deep motivations, some clearly embraced and others purposely ignored. The underlying medical structures in the United States are simply not value-neutral, impartial, or areligious. They instead form a hegemony around medicine's collective structures, and this hegemony shapes the beliefs and practices of patients and clinicians in ways that are more powerful than privatized religion.

Part of the way that immanence holds its spiritual monopoly over medicine is through its prohibitions concerning proselytism.[iv] Injunctions against religious proselytism[8] focus especially on threats to the patient–clinician relationship, with special concern for the clinician advocating for traditional religious perspectives. Critics rightly point out the need to uphold trust within this relationship and, at a minimum, require patient consent in all spiritual interactions.[v] Yet what should be especially troubling is that within discussions that minimize or hold back uninvited religious ideas or discussions, there is a failure to equally acknowledge how a spirituality of immanence is also imposed on patients without consent. The issue is that a spirituality of immanence operates under the category of being nonspiritual and nonreligious, and it is therefore exempt from concerns of proselytism. If we have had any success in the argument described in Part II, however, immanence is a full-blown spiritual system, with its actual nature concealed within conceptually problematic definitions that have been accepted and perpetuated within Western culture. While traditional world-religions (e.g., Christianity or Judaism) readily recognize and admit the religious nature of their sources of ultimate concern and chief affection, immanence monopolizes medicine's professions and institutions by feigning neutrality. This pushes out other religious traditions while holding on to power without admitting its own religious-like affections.

Hence, this current medical framework fails the test of pluralism. Immanence is not neutral but instead is functionally very closely akin to other world religions. If medicine is going to reflect patients' actual experiences and worldviews, then this necessitates reconceptualizing immanence for what it really is in function: a spirituality of ultimacy with religious-like structures. This demands that the hegemony of immanence over America's medical professions and institutions be broken and for truly pluralistic structures to be reformed in partnership with what patients consider ultimate. While this claim is wide-reaching in potential implications, some will simply reassert the old claims that immanence is areligious. Here again, readers must honestly weigh our claims from Part II, evaluating issues of power, freedom, consent, and equitable ways to share in a good society. Pluralism demands that immanence be reconsidered, and, in Chapter 15, we will make a case for how pluralism can move forward in twenty-first-century American medicine.

Problem 3: Immanence Empowers
Impersonal Medicine

A third reason that a spirituality of immanence should be reconsidered is that it likely is a major contributor toward our death-denying culture, our willingness to accept a hyper-focus on the body to the deficit of the whole person, the empowerment of impersonal social forces across medicine, and the socialization of clinicians to neglect or avoid the spiritual needs of their patients. Consider the interrelationship between a spirituality of immanence and the socialization of clinicians depicted as a five-tiered "layered-cake" in Figure 13.1.

The figure illustrates multiple threads of the book's argument. The underlying values of immanence that are centered on bodily health, cure, and comfort as chief love, form the bottommost foundation (layer 1) that is infused among the other factors including underlying beliefs, social and relational directions, and an array of institutions that are necessary for clinician socialization. In layer two, plausibility structures (discussed in Chapters 6 and Chapter 7) form our cultural presuppositions that lead to a shared social imagination. In contemporary American culture, this forms a conceptual reality in terms of a litany of dualisms oriented around immanence and transcendence. From within this dualistic structure, an immanent society justifies separation of medicine and religion. This then makes plausible a psychological repression of death. Extending from this commitment to a spirituality of immanence, hospital institutions and professional guilds absorb as their primary telos the goal to cure over the energy necessary for caregiving.

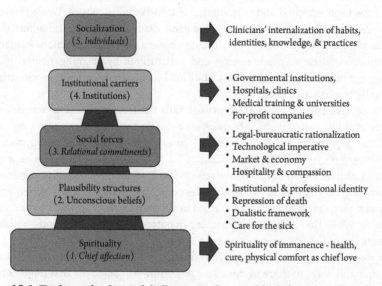

Figure 13.1 The layered-cake model, illustrating how visible dimensions of medical socialization and institutions are supported by underlying social forces, beliefs, and, ultimately, a collectively embraced spirituality or chief affection.

Layer Three: Social Forces

Out of plausibility structures develop an array of social forces (layer 3). These are institutional commitments that guide how complex relationships operate within a democratic, capitalistic society.[2] With a spirituality of immanence, impersonal legal and bureaucratic forces are central to the social system. This unleashes what Weber described as *zweckrational* or technocratic, rational social action in relation to usually utilitarian goals. These are at the same time "relational" since they oversee how human organizations relate to one another, yet they are also in their essence *impersonal forces* since they are oriented around the legal-bureaucratic, scientific-technological, and capitalistic economy. The dynamism behind these relational commitments is impersonal in the sense that their focus is on the arrangement of human affairs aimed toward production, efficiency, and material exchange—all of which presuppose indirect human relationships. A century ago, Weber described the interlocking of these three social forces (bureaucracy-market-technology) to be characterized "without regard for persons."[2 [p. 215]] The rational logic of these social forces depends on a capitalistic economy governed by maximum efficiency, calculable rules of output, specialization, and its freedom as a system from personal touch or decision-making bound within communal relationships. Weber says that these social forces develop "the more perfectly the more the bureaucracy is 'dehumanized,' the more completely it succeeds in eliminating from official business love, hatred, and all purely personal, irrational, and emotional elements which escape calculation. This is the specific nature of bureaucracy and it is appraised as its special virtue."[2 [p. 216]]

The nature of impersonal social forces caused Weber to famously describe these social forces as an iron cage since they depersonalize decision-making so that persons are secondary to the goals of the larger social system.[9 [p. 181]] Impersonal bureaucratic forces cause medical clinicians to function like replaceable cogs within the healthcare machine. Unfortunately, patients are increasingly not shielded from depersonalizing forces. One dynamic of rational and calculable bureaucratic efficiency is that it always aims toward greater compliance toward its ideal type of economic, organizational, and technical resourcefulness and competence. Efficiency generates organizational compliance toward nonpersonal ends. This results in health organizations that continuously seek higher productivity and effectiveness in every aspect of the organization. Over time, this leads to organizational measures that, by default, increase impersonal aspects of medicine aimed around cure, cost-effectiveness, and technological proficiency. As organizations more proficiently comply with increasing impersonal markers of efficiency and calculable outcomes, patients will perceive their treatment as reflecting these less personal aims. Healthcare interactions will be less between persons, and patients will feel more like an identification number (bureaucracy), a body part (technology), or a dollar sign (market economy) within their medical interactions. An impersonal medical system aimed to maximize efficiency, cure, and profit requires these impersonal measures to be increasingly acted upon by institutions and medical professionals to achieve larger social goals. Such forces indelibly imagine individual persons in terms of material ends rather than precisely as human persons. Impersonal social forces energize the importance of specialization and a division of labor, with both as necessary consequences in efficiently achieving the desired outcome of bodily health, cure, and physical comfort as the *telos* of medical care.

The aims of an efficient, technologically driven, and bureaucratic system lies in tension with a fourth social force identified as "hospitality and compassion." While Americans desire a cost- and technology-effective system, most patients desire *personal care* from caregivers who also deeply desire to provide authentic human compassion. It is only at the next level, however, that we see how these social forces play out within particular organizations such as hospitals or professional guilds.

Layer Four: Institutional Carriers

On the fourth level of the layered cake are particular institutions related to or directly engaged in medicine and health. These include government agencies, hospitals, professional guilds, for-profit companies, and university training centers that systematize themselves according to level-three social forces. By fitting into the larger relational system, organizations gain social status and are beneficiaries of economic exchange. In order for particular organizations to function and survive, especially with governmental influence playing an increasingly central role in credentialing and monetary power over the larger system, individual institutions must organize themselves according to each of the lower levels of social forces (layer 3), beliefs (layer 2), and chief values (layer 1) of the larger system. It is through this system of layering that a spirituality of immanence is absorbed by nearly every institution if organizational leaders want their institution to survive.[vi] Each layer in Figure 13.1 relies upon and assumes the layer below. It is in this manner that social participation on the organizational level absorbs a spirituality of immanence, which infiltrates every layer above it, penetrating most organizational structures, including their mission statement and choice of trustees, hiring practices, internal organizational structure, allocation of resources, and architectural designs and renovations. Every health organization or professional guild that resists immanence, in either its identification as chief love (layer 1) or the beliefs (layer 2) and social forces (layer 3) that immanence produces, directly jeopardizes that organization's ability to survive. Alternatively, every health organization that maximizes its commitment to immanence and its assumptions has greatest potential to succeed.

Each of these social forces is activated and carried forward by particular organizations that discipline their role and function within the larger healthcare matrix. Organizational structures are constructed by several local factors operative in healthcare institutions, such as origin and ethos, the composition of its trustees and leaders, its identified purpose and mission, and by the types of people selected to work within the organization. Some organizations are oriented around only certain social forces, whereas others are interconnected with some or all four social forces (see Figure 13.2). For example, the Joint Commission is an organization that is focused on the legal-bureaucratic aspects of healthcare, and it aims to certify and accredit healthcare institutions. Other organizations may be principally oriented toward one social force (such as health insurance companies, which are centered around the market), but then they may also engage a variety of financial decisions based on science-technological or legal-bureaucratic factors. Medical training organizations such as medical schools

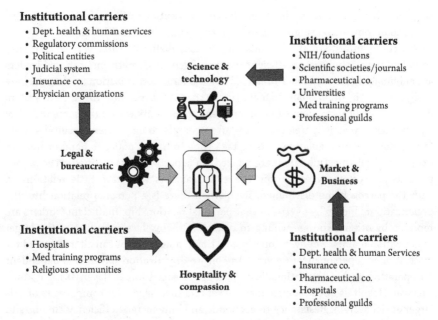

Institutional carriers
- Dept. health & human services
- Regulatory commissions
- Political entities
- Judicial system
- Insurance co.
- Physician organizations

Institutional carriers
- NIH/foundations
- Scientific societies/journals
- Pharmaceutical co.
- Universities
- Med training programs
- Professional guilds

Science & technology

Legal & bureaucratic

Market & Business

Institutional carriers
- Hospitals
- Med training programs
- Religious communities

Hospitality & compassion

Institutional carriers
- Dept. health & human Services
- Insurance co.
- Pharmaceutical co.
- Hospitals
- Professional guilds

Figure 13.2 In contrast to the proliferation of health-related organizations, which carry the aims of powerful social forces (the market, science, and bureaucracy), few health organizations are primarily or solely committed to hospitality and compassion of patients.

are primarily oriented around science-technology but are also secondarily concerned about hospitality and compassion. Perhaps the most complex organizational models are academic medical hospitals, which are simultaneously oriented by all four social forces.

Weber's analysis suggests that organizations that thrive within this bureaucratic health system increasingly conform to certain ideal characteristics.[2 [esp. pp. 196–198]] Labor is divided in order to maximize competency in a particular area and in order to increase total output. All roles and actions are highly regulated using written codes and rules that are understood by all in the organization. Similar to the military, medical organizations uphold a clear hierarchy of authority so that every worker is accountable to his or her assignment, thus minimizing chaotic actions on either the lower or upper levels of the organizations. Every worker must demonstrate competency and qualifications, and they are rewarded for their actions based on measured outcomes. The organizational structure requires a commitment to detachment regarding individual persons or personal relationships. Organizational hiring, for example, is not based on *who* you know but *what* you know as an expert and your ability to execute a particular action. Efficient organizations are committed to principles that depersonalize and disfavor relationships. Thus, ownership and workers are normally kept separate. Workers do not own production, which could compromise production, and ownership remains separated from its workers to minimize nonrational, emotion-based decisions. Within large health organizations, the most efficient institutions will conform to this ideal type and become increasingly successful in achieving their intended aims.

A well-organized system depends on depersonalizing its caregivers so that they complete their actions in an efficient manner. Even charismatic institutional leaders are sublimated (a term Weber preferred) by the larger organization so that they are easily replaced by other qualified managers as cogs of the machine. An efficient system disciplines medical caregivers to primarily engage patients within the same technical and calculable means. Caregivers who fail to comply to an efficient medical system (e.g., a doctor who regularly wants to take time to hold a patient's hand or hold an extended family meeting) are marginalized, an action which is justified on economic grounds and often forced by upper-level bureaucrats who have little relationship with the person being disciplined. Even when there is a personal relationship, the organizational hierarchy overrules that personal relationship. Inefficient workers are replaced by others who are willing to discipline themselves according to the larger organizational aims. Not even top organizational management can alter the need for institutional depersonalization since the entire organization (layer 4) is dependent on operating within the rationalization of these social forces (layer 3) for its own survival. Hospitals and academic medical centers themselves are components of this larger social system. Resistance to economic and bureaucratic efficiency amounts to organizational suicide. In fact, Weber concluded that once bureaucratic apparatuses are absorbed by organizations in relationship to each other, they result in a type of power relationship that is "practically unshatterable."[2 [p. 228]] The social psychology of bureaucratic organizations, held in place by market forces, results in disciplining those who might attempt to slow, change, or somehow threaten the machine-like structure. Even top-level chief executives will be resisted and undermined by lower level deep bureaucrats if those executives were to threaten the internal organizational structure or overall success of the organization. Thus, these organizations are constantly geared toward efficiency, resisting internal threats, and grounded in a common interest in seeing that "the mechanism continues its functions and that the societally exercised authority carries on."[2 [p. 229]]

Institutional Carriers of Hospitality and Compassion

In Figure 13.1, we included *"care* of the sick" as a core plausibility structure (layer 2) and "hospitality and compassion" as an ongoing social force (layer 3). These are social beliefs and relational energies that have a connection to immanence. Clearly, care and compassion remain bedrock commitments within American society and do not necessarily rely on overt religious rationales to reach these conclusions.

Although care of the sick in terms of compassion, care, and hospitality continues to hold a persuasive position within American society, we see a *breakdown on the institutional level in the transfer of these ideals within healthcare organizations*. As Figure 13.2 depicts, the number of institutional carriers of hospitality and compassion are limited to those organizations that are closest to patient care. Medical trainees in medical schools, nursing schools, and related clerkship programs (e.g., medical residency) form one cluster of organizations that carry on the social force of hospitality and compassion. Hospitals and smaller clinics form the nexus of the second type of organization where hospitality and compassion are cultivated and embodied toward the suffering sick. There can be little doubt that these organizations continue to desire to nurture caregivers who are caring and provide deep compassion to the sick. But there are also ongoing signs that the social forces of hospitality and compassion are eroding, not necessarily as ideals, but in some organizational practices and within the patient–clinician relationship. Signs of this erosion include less overall time for patient–clinician visits, lateraling of patient experiences to nonclinicians, increasing technological interactions, and worrisome burnout rates among clinicians. The overall evidence suggests that while the social force of hospitality and compassion remains an important ideal, it is not subsequently being sustained or nurtured on the ground by health organizations.

There are at least two contributing factors explaining why health organizations struggle to nurture and sustain the social force of hospitality and compassion within patient care.

The first is that it is unlikely that any single organization can maintain balance between the personal and impersonal aspects of caring for the sick when that organization's life depends on the financial market. There is an undeniable conflict of interest between, on the one hand, hospitality and compassion, which at its core is a personal and costly human love, and, on the other hand, the three impersonal social forces of legal-bureaucracy, scientific-technology, and a market economy. The former is organized around relating human persons, whereas the latter forces of modernity are organized by principles of depersonalization. We should hope that these competing forces might balance one another in a suitable cooperative. Patients need to be dealt with in tenderness and human love, but, at the same time, the bills need to be paid. When it comes to the care of those facing life-threatening illness, there should obviously be a merger of loving kindness, science, business, and organizational management. Care of the sick must uphold all four of these dimensions for the sake of human care, sustainability, and medical effectiveness. The contemporary evidence suggests, however, that if a single organization is expected to espouse and maintain both the personal dimensions of care as well as impersonal social forces, the gravitational pull draws organizations away from human-centered care and toward bureaucracy, science, and the market. This is the necessary direction for organizations that are interwoven and dependent on market forces. Human care and compassion is secondary to the organization's basic economic survival. Additionally, patients are socialized into passivity by the sick role,[10] which results in depersonalization being strongly resistant to market correction since patients are socialized to be passive in their need for help, neither demanding nor exercising commercial shrewdness.[vii] These factors further compromise the ability of hospitals to defend an ethos of institutional hospitality or for medical and nursing schools to form trainees to be self-consciously committed to compassion. While there are many *individuals* who are committed to the highest levels of human care, compassion, and hospitality, our point is that *institutionally*, particular organizations within the American system will be unable to stop depersonalization within the logic of their organizations because bureaucratic, technological, and economic rationalizations are too robust. Within any healthcare organization, impersonal rational forces will generally take precedence over personal ones if an organizational choice becomes necessary. These choices are increasingly necessary for health organizations.[11,12]

A second, closely related contributing factor explaining why health organizations struggle to nurture and sustain the social force of hospitality and compassion within patient care is that there is now a palpable structural absence of traditional religious organizations, such as Christian churches, Jewish synagogues, and clergy[13,14] [p. 199] influencing and supporting America's health organizations.[viii] While a spirituality of immanence cannot be directly impugned for causing impersonal social forces to expand, *we hypothesize that it is a spirituality of immanence that nonetheless creates the conditions for depersonalizing forces to expand within medicine.*

How does this work? Immanence (layer 1) and its dualistic plausibility structures and repression of death (layer 2) create the necessary conditions for impersonal forces to govern by first creating a belief system (layer 2) that requires a formal separation between health organizations and particular religious communities (layer 4). Once local religious organizations have little voice in health organizations, the check-and-balance system between impersonal and personal social forces becomes lopsided. A key organizational advocate for hospitality and compassion is substantially silenced. In the absence of traditional religious communities and the formal and informal support of health organizations by religious leaders, there is a structural breakdown among networks of local persons to mobilize and hold impersonal forces in check. There are few organizations committed to championing compassion or upholding transcendent meaning that corrects death-denial tendencies. In the absence of communities committed to spiritual transcendence, there are few, if any, institutional carriers resisting or placing into balance a death-denying culture. With the structural absence of traditional spiritualities that emphasize transcendence, a fear of death becomes formidable, and the imperative to trust in science and technology becomes irresistible. Impersonal social forces expand in the absence of organizations wholly committed to the personal aspects of caregiving.

Local religious communities hold tremendous capacity for hospitality and compassion toward the sick. As a reminder of that potential, many hospitals in the United States were spearheaded by networks of religious communities that had the imagination, desire, and will to care for the sick by establishing and initially sustaining organizations with caregiving aims.[15-17] While few local religious communities have the resources to oversee contemporary health organizations—with some exceptions including the Roman Catholic Church and the Adventist Health System—many do have the ability to partner with health organizations including hospitals, medical clinics, and medical school training centers. These local faith communities entail an evident cultural resource that is substantially large, consisting of approximately 350,000 clergy and congregations in America.[18] Just as importantly, local faith communities reside outside the bureaucratic and economic system, which means that they potentially hold a unique prophetic voice to rein in impersonal social forces, uphold transcendent meaning when facing death, and advance hospitality and compassion among the seriously ill. Immanence has partially prevented local religious organizations from serving the larger good in these ways. If there were one likely organization (level 4) that could resist large-scale rationalization (layer 3) and disenchantment in American medicine, that single type of organization is ironically the one that has been systematically impeded from direct involvement by immanence (layer 1) and dualistic plausibility structures that privatize religion and deny death (layer 2).

In considering our hypothesis, an important counterpoint is that many criticize the eroding effects of impersonal social forces but without appeal to traditional monotheistic or Eastern religions. The material body and its suffering are constant reminders that, in the words of philosopher Martha Nussbaum, "one's own weakness and vulnerability is a necessary condition for pity; without this, we will have an arrogant harshness."[19] [p. 34] Thus, there remains an underlying perception, apart from appeals to traditional religion, that there is an important cultural responsibility to care for the sick and to do justice for the poor. Surely religion remains in American society one of the major institutional catalysts calling for human compassion. Nevertheless, philosophers from Rawls[20] to Nussbaum[21] have shown that justice and compassion have robust theoretical defenses without dependence on rationales offered by traditional religion. Political philosophers have displayed somewhat convincing arguments that prudential self-interest apart from religious rationales leads to altruistic conclusions demanding social responses of compassion and justice, especially for the less fortunate and the sick. So, on these grounds, it would appear that the impersonal social forces can be critiqued and resisted without recourse to particular religious organizations, especially religious traditions like Christianity or Judaism that have been most influential in the United States.

Nonetheless, philosophical arguments, no matter how thoughtfully articulated, do not subsequently generate local communities of tightly woven networks that have the will to resist rationalization, provide transcendent meaning considering the fear of death, or the energy to sustain human compassion. While philosophical arguments reach conclusions comparable to those of traditional religions concerning a social responsibility to act and care for the sick, evidence also suggests that local religious communities develop uniquely moral intuitions and types of relationships necessary for compassionate responses.[22] In a nationwide longitudinal study, Putnam and Campbell found that after adjusting for various demographic factors including religious belief, it was a person's direct connection with his or her religious institutions that accounted for donating more time, money, and engagement in civic organizations, as well as other measures of altruism.[22] [see ch. 13] They concluded that religious institutions create social capital through direct networks and friendships, which in turn leads to multiple expressions of neighborly kindness. While we should recognize how philosophical arguments justify the importance of care and compassion without appeal to traditional religions, our concern is that these abstract and rational conclusions do not appear to lead to the creation of on-the-ground organizations or grassroots networks of persons mobilized toward action. In other words, the idea does not itself lead to social action. Putnam and Campbell concluded from their study that organizational networks are critical to altruistic action. While Nussbaum and like-minded philosophers helpfully show how human reason independent of traditional religion yields recognition of compassion and justice, what is missing from this perspective is an acknowledgment that philosophical conclusions are less likely to galvanize people into local networks nor are they as likely to generate sustained, organized action.

Contrastingly, traditional religions provide a particularly powerful kind of social cohesion that may uniquely enable these local communities to offer transcendent meaning against the fear of death and respond to philanthropic needs over the long term. Many traditional religious groups in the United States idealize (though imperfectly practice) the importance of welcoming diversity in socioeconomic backgrounds, mobilizing groups toward actions of service, and praying for those who have fallen ill. But, just as importantly, most traditional religious communities do not regularly assemble primarily for reasons of philanthropy, altruism, or social action such as caregiving. Philanthropy is an outcome rather than the primary purpose for meeting and relating. This means that traditional religious communities have intense interest in sustaining their relationships over extended periods of time precisely because their primary purpose is the worship of God, as in the Abrahamic traditions. Because of this enduring and transcendent purpose, many traditional religious groups erect strong infrastructures of internal organization, purchase property, and have clear procedures for transferring leadership to the next generation. By contrast, far fewer civic organizations have the will to perpetuate themselves with this level of intense human capital, if for no other reason than they understand their own organization's mission as temporary. Few things beside traditional religions motivate people to sacrifice the necessary investment of time, talents, or treasure over an extended period and with enormous personal effort. So, while Putnam and Campbell may potentially be correct that involvement in local organizations, not traditional religions per se, explains the increase in philanthropy, it is also clear that social capital and deep bonds of local human networks are distinctively created and sustained by traditional religious communities. Many abstractly and rationally concur that care and compassion are important beliefs, that denying death is irrational, and that impersonal social forces should be resisted. However, traditional religious communities are unlike other voluntary associations because their transcendent purpose regularly brings people together, deepens social capital, and produces communities motivated to spread their transcendent meaning that overcomes fear while offering hospitality and compassion.

These factors lead us to a tentative conclusion that the unique dynamics provided by traditional religious communities may be the only existing type of organization in the United States that has capacity to directly challenge depersonalization within medicine. Religion has the imaginative resources to resist and reorder the powers of bureaucracy, capitalism, and technology so that each takes its dutiful order in service to the patient who is the true focal point. What other institutional carrier exists that can resist bureaucracy by articulating that the patient is a person, not a number? What social force other than traditional religious communities can network people to shape the market and declare that money is *not* the bottom line within healthcare? Where else do we hear calls to transcendent meaning and courage in the face of death that still recognize science and technology as important but not ultimate? To be clear, we recognize that those who do not describe themselves as religious share in our criticism of depersonalized forces harming patient care. We suggest that the evidence indicates, however, that it is primarily the social networks created by traditional religious communities that possess the unique capacity to partner with medicine, resist the impersonal direction of certain bureaucratic social forces, and bring a needed balance among conflicting impulses.

Resistance of impersonal social forces requires an equally powerful network of people who are well organized and bound to institutional structures. Traditional religious communities have this wherewithal, but they are separated from most health organizations. A key breakdown in the layered cake (Figure 13.1) is the systematic failure to transfer the accepted social force of compassionate care for the sick (layer 3) among institutional carriers (layer 4). Health organizations cannot be realistically expected to balance personal and impersonal forces because of an inherent conflict of interest related to their dependence on market forces. Thus, traditional religious communities are the most likely and perhaps only existing institutional carriers of hospitality and compassion for the sick. Yet the plausibility structures have divided traditional spirituality from medicine. As an unintended consequence, a spirituality of immanence enables these conditions that block traditional religious institutions from exerting correction and balance upon impersonal social forces. This then leads any final hopes of hospitality and compassion to be upheld by individual professional caregivers, the top-most layer in Figure 13.1. Yet the marks of immanence can also be seen among individual clinicians who appear powerless to resist the direction that the medical system has taken. We turn to this next.

Problem 4: Immanence Harms Clinicians

A final reason that a spirituality of immanence should be challenged is that it may be an underappreciated contributor within the socialization process that results in negative clinician well-being (e.g., burnout). Immanence leads to conditions that disconnect medical trainees and professionals from spiritual and religious resources that provide meaning, a transcendent calling, resilience in the face of suffering, and positive coping in light of an impersonal health system.[23,24]

Clinician well-being—defined as having both positive (e.g., life-balance, personal satisfaction) and negative dimensions (e.g., burnout, mental health issues, substance abuse)[25]—has been shown to be associated with physician empathy[26] and patient adherence to treatment and actions in managing chronic diseases.[27] Conversely, physician burnout is associated with clinician- and patient-assessed adverse outcomes including medical errors, lower patient satisfaction, and higher mortality ratios of hospitalized patients.[28-33] Research has consistently identified a correlation between the rigors of medical training and increased clinician cynicism and lack of humanitarianism.[34-36] Nearly half of clinicians in the United States show some symptoms of depersonalization and exhaustion.[37-44] These processes are associated with thoughts of leaving medicine,[45] mental health issues, substance abuse,[46] and suicidal ideation.[47-51] Clinician burnout is also linked to physicians reducing their work hours and leaving the profession. It is also projected to become a significant contributor to a future physician shortage in the United States.[52-54] There are clear links between burnout and external system factors that have made health organizations increasingly difficult places to work.[55-57] Organizations that are perceived to be more profit-centered rather than patient-centered are associated with clinician burnout.[55] Leading physician expert Tait Shanafelt from the Mayo Clinic has identified at least six system-level contributing factors including excessive workload, increasing clerical burden, loss of flexibility and control over work environment, difficulty in integrating work and personal life, loss of meaning in work, and organizational objectives that conflict with the altruistic values of the profession.[53] Trends point to a downward spiral of clinician well-being linked to the impersonal social forces that have been on the rise throughout medicine.

How can traditional spirituality and religious communities make any difference for clinicians? Many clinical trainees enter medicine with a great deal of humanitarian idealism and deep internal desires to compassionately care for the sick.[23] Clinical training in hospitals and the medical wards acts as a "secondary socialization"[58 (pp. 138-139)] in which clinicians internalize, through habitualization, the necessary institutional practices, knowledge, and viewpoints that make clinicians spontaneously act with little reflection as clinicians. This process is necessary to form physicians and nurses,[59] but some elements of this training lead to a socialization that undermine professional ideals.[60] This is often referred to as the "hidden curriculum," which is the process of formation, largely based in apprenticeship, that instills behaviors, attitudes, and values among trainees in tension with the ideals of the medical profession.[42,60-64] On an individual level, a few preliminary studies have shown a cross-sectional association between increased clinician spirituality and lower levels of burnout.[65,66] In addition, several national surveys of medical students and physicians have shown strong links between a clinician's sense of calling and spirituality, religious affiliation, and religious service attendance.[67] These studies have also reported strong associations between a clinician's sense of calling and lower burnout, higher career satisfaction, greater energy in caring for the dying, and ongoing commitment to clinical practice.[24,41,55] This is initial evidence that clinicians who are well-formed or engaged in their spiritual and religious traditions have some individual ability to be protected from the corrosive effects of depersonalization encountered in the hidden curriculum and to maintain a sense of meaning, purpose, and calling during the rigors of training.

While the rupture in medical training between idealized and actual socialization justifies calls for greater professionalism, including clarification of standards and means of assessment,[68-70] it is not likely that medical education or professional codes of conduct can reverse the toxic elements encountered within this socialization. Internal social structures in medicine include poor behavior modeling that devalues and objectifies patients and rigid hierarchal relationships that limit correction of abuses of power. But these internal processes that harm clinicians' care for patients and their own well-being are reinforced by more formidable currents that lie beneath the surface. Clinicians have long been exposed to "corporate socialization" where they are inculcated to approach medical care "the way the plan or the company has them done."[11 [p. 448]] Institutional carriers and their social structures are forming clinical practice around market considerations, its growing legal-bureaucratization, and the technological-scientific imperative that strives against death.[71] In other words, the hidden curriculum, experienced in layer 5 of Figure 13.1, is generated by deeper systemic structures that lie beneath individual socialization. Medical training or alternative socialization processes that are individually based can partially and locally resist, but hardly correct, the underlying systemic problems.

Clinician socialization is part of a more complex social process that includes institutions, social forces, and plausibility structures and is ultimately informed by an underlying spirituality. As Figure 13.1 illustrates, clinician socialization is built and depends on a groundswell of underlying commitments, beliefs, and social organizations. Individual socialization occurs within human relationships embedded in multiple institutions. These institutions are "carriers" of deeper values, identities, commitments, and beliefs, which create a composite web of relationships that enable individual socialization to seep into one's consciousness. Socialization of medical trainees is built on the underlying levels of the layered-cake (Figure 13.1). Thus, the so-called hidden curriculum and its unwanted outcomes, such as clinician burnout, are prone to resist change unless measures are taken to fundamentally address these underlying systemic issues within the layered cake model.

This is where the role of religious organizations (and the underlying spirituality that they hold to) may be a key means to counter the impersonal dimensions of medicine that have led to poor clinician well-being. Impersonal social forces create contexts that depersonalize clinicians and place many in unsustainable career trajectories, and this in turn creates adverse clinician outcomes that are unwanted for patients, harmful to clinicians, and ironically create new inefficiencies for the medical system to solve. In attempting to solve this problem, from where will a powerful enough solution be found? In our view, it is unlikely to expect solutions arising from the very same social forces that created the problem originally and continue to drive it. The drive toward a rational and efficient system turns clinicians into the cogs of a larger, impersonal system. Will the same rational and efficient concerns governed by economic motivations be able to recover the human aspects of care and humanity of caregiving? It is difficult to imagine that such a reversal will take place from within the existing social system since whenever economics is the ultimate decision-maker in a capitalistic medical economy, we should generally expect the expansion of depersonalization, not its shrinkage.[2] The counter of these forces is not more bureaucratic, economic, or technical solutions. The respiriting of clinicians will depend on a different kind of rationality that is based first and foremost within a spirit of human care and compassion. A different kind of socialization of clinicians is needed. It is hard to imagine that this will arise from any other location than the spiritual traditions and organizations that have largely carried Western medicine forward over the past two millennia.[14]

Here again, we suggest that the issue is partially caused by the removal of traditional spirituality and religious communities from the training and sustaining of caregivers. As discussed in Chapter 5, one of the primary resources for caregivers that sustains them and provides intrinsic motivation to care is a particular spiritual identity and calling.[24,41,55,67] The separation of medicine and religion cuts off clinicians from the chance to draw strength and find resilience through resources and relationships embedded in spiritual traditions. In recognition of these issues, one promising approach suggested by Kinghorn and others is to ground the ideals and virtues of medical practice within communities which can form clinicians to internalize the virtues necessary in caring for the ill.[62,63,72] This view recognizes the socialization process and, consequently, requires creation of equally powerful social structures that enable internalization of virtuous habits and caregiving practices. Since deep structures are not easily altered, some have called for local and incremental approaches that include partners operating inside[73] and outside of medicine who foster virtues and pass on to trainees the heart of medicine.[64] While we agree with those who highlight the importance of spirituality as a critical resource within medical training,[73-77] the issue is that seeing spirituality as a resource within patient care fails to diagnose the real problem and stops short of what religious communities have to offer. Rather,

Kinghorn et al.[62] suggest several reasons that spiritual and religious communities may serve as viable partners in forming medical professionals in light of the hidden curriculum. Moral and spiritual communities aim to form members in accord with values such as compassion and upholding the personhood of patients. Spiritual and religious communities are often less influenced than medicine by hierarchal structures or the market economy's demands for efficiency. Many spiritual communities not only uphold values that are consistent with professional ideals such as compassion but additionally provide practices that socialize members into habits of virtue that generate compassion. Finally, most spiritual communities uphold robust understandings of suffering and dying, including ways that transcendent meaning overcomes the fear of death.[78,79] This can enable clinicians to serve patients within a framework of meaning and action as they encounter serious illness and the suffering that comes with it.[23]

Religious traditions and their local communities may be the one entity that has both a perspective and organizational capacity to call into account the social powers beholden to economic motivations and the denial of our dying. Throughout the medical literature, there are discussions and interventions aimed at modifying the socialization process of clinicians so that they are more compassionate, resistant to the hidden curriculum, or have better coping strategies. These approaches essentially locate blame in medical education and training and offer solutions on the individual level. This largely misses how the "train" of medicine hastens in the opposite direction of the outcomes desired by most individual clinicians (Figure 13.3).

Change must be primarily focused on the structures of medicine. Responses to medicine's direction are unlikely to change its course if we rely on more of the same dynamics that have propelled medicine and our society in the direction of impersonal medicine. Blaming individual clinicians fails to recognize how most clinicians desire to provide personal and compassionate care. The problem and its solution lies in underlying structures that are linked all the way down to our base beliefs (level 2) and

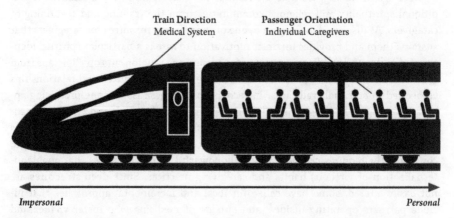

Figure 13.3 The direction of the "train" of the healthcare system, transporting compassionate clinicians oriented toward patient-centered care, but rapidly moving toward impersonal patient medicine. Thanks to Grace Pearson, graphic designer, for creating this figure.

deepest loves (level 1). Some form of "crash" is our eventual outcome unless we collectively deal with our social idolatry of medicine: centering its chief affections around immanence, the problematic beliefs oriented by dualism and a cultural fear of death, and the impersonal forces overtaking medicine. Religious organizations are far from perfect, but they uphold critical values that medicine desperately needs. No matter how much money, regulation, intellectual energy, and scientific prowess we pour into healthcare, it is not capable of giving the salvation that we desire. For this we must look elsewhere.

Conclusion

In this chapter, we have argued that a spirituality of immanence is problematic for medicine. It does not align with many patients' own spiritual and religious perspectives, and it in fact imposes on most a worldview alien to their own experience. Thus, this dynamic fails to be pluralistic as it exerts the hegemony of only one spirituality, privatizing all others. Additionally, immanence suppresses traditional religious spiritualities, unleashing impersonal forces that are directed toward ever-increasing efficiency. This creates unhealthy medical organizations that are struggling under the weight of extremely potent forces that eventually burn out an army of caring and committed nurses and physicians. Apart from the presence of traditional spiritual and religious communities that may counterbalance a system overmastered by impersonal forces, these worrisome powers will likely continue to expand.

But can religious communities be brought back into partnership with the medical system in some way that is agreeable to both religious communities and those who deeply oppose traditional religion? In Chapter 14, we consider proposals where this is considered but bound to likely fail. In Chapter 15, we propose a solution called structural pluralism.

Notes

i. Cassell illustrates how depersonalization took place in anatomical drawings. See Cassell, *The Nature of Suffering and the Goals of Medicine.*[1 (pp. 164–199)]

ii. Consider the fascinating and well-designed art display at one of Boston's premier cancer centers: http://www.dana-farber.org/About-Us/Yawkey-Center/Audio-Art-Tour/Yawkey-Center-for-Cancer-Care-Artwork.aspx Out of 47 selected pieces, not one piece displays traditional religious ideas. There are surely multiple reasons for avoiding religious themes, but it remains notable how incongruous these art pieces are in contrast to the majority of patients who walk its halls. If art is partly intended to invoke meditation and reflection, and if a majority of Boston patients find their deepest meaning in religion, then what does this absence perhaps unintentionally reveal? While including religious art would be potentially upsetting or offensive to some patients who do not share that religious viewpoint, it is also the case that the absence of religious symbols displays an equally problematic bias. Religious patients do not necessarily say they are upset (at the art that is missing), but the absence of religious symbols in this example reinforces a different spirituality—one of immanence.

iii. M. J. Balboni. A theological assessment of spiritual assessments. *Christian Bioethics.* 2013;19(3):313–331

iv. Proselytism may be defined as the act of persuasion from one person to another aimed to alter the person's spiritual commitments of ultimate concern and commitment to another spiritual commitment of ultimacy.

v. The doctrine of informed consent exists to promote a patient's self-determination and the ability to make rational decisions. Within legal reasoning, informed consent specifically legislates harm caused to a person's physical body (e.g., surgery), and, for this reason, it is unlikely that most spiritual care interventions would require informed consent since spiritual care is not a bodily intervention with physical liabilities. This would further medicalize spiritual care—a process that should be vigorously resisted. However, upholding a patient's self-determination and ability to make informed decisions is a correct and necessary principle that undergirds patient spirituality. Spiritual care must be gentle, respectful, without self-aggrandizement, and concerned to ensure that a patient does not feel manipulated, coerced, or threatened—especially in relationship to their medical care received from the clinician. Consequently, proactive spiritual care provided by clinicians must always be accompanied by a patient's consent. This is the best understanding of "patient-centered" spiritual care. It is not that the content of spiritual care necessarily conforms to the patient's presuppositions or worldview, but that the patient consents to receiving spiritual care according to the tradition to which the clinician is bound. This means that there is an appropriate and inappropriate form of proselytism. The pivotal distinction focuses on a patient voluntarily permitting the clinician to offer spiritual care and understanding that the spiritual care received will be provided according to the clinician's spiritual tradition. Inappropriate proselytism refers to the promotion of a particular religious faith without patient consent or voluntary agreement to engage in spiritual conversation with an understanding of the clinician's framework. As a word of caution, however, the issues of consent, power dynamics, and spirituality have not been carefully studied. Future research is needed to more clearly define the issue of consent as it pertains to religion in the patient–clinician relationship. How consent is defined and obtained in relation to spirituality and religion needs further investigation.

vi. In one interesting case study, Roman Catholic hospitals, though originally committed to a very different spirituality oriented by their Christian beliefs, by many accounts partly reflect a spirituality of immanence in their American institutions. This is not by conscious choice, but more likely because of the intermediary acceptance of those social forces and then the plausibility structures that justify those forces. While some Roman Catholic hospitals continue to seek their unique Christian identity as institutions, it is nearly impossible to keep immanence from holding a louder voice within the institution because of the larger social system that itself is based on immanence.

vii. One may believe that market forces would correct this outcome if it were truly important. Patients and family caregivers will object to depersonalization and be drawn to person-centered institutions. This market view fails to acknowledge, however, that patients and family members are expected to conform to the sick role,[10] which includes expectations of not complaining, following the physician's orders, and being a grateful patient. These social expectations come from a period when medicine and economics were largely kept separate by the "gauze curtain" to protect the patient–physician relationship from financial concerns. This socialization still largely exists, and so it is wrongheaded to expect a market correction.

viii. For example, we performed an informal, web-based survey of board of trustee members from the four Boston-based hospitals where we conducted the Religion and Spirituality and Cancer Care study. We found one board member who was affiliated with a religious organization (less than 1% of all trustees) and no community clergy members. In contrast, the two clearest characteristics of the trustees were their affiliation with science/technology and their ability to give or raise money. Trustees have ultimate oversight over an organization, and their own backgrounds will influence what they consider most important for that organization's success.

References

1. Eric J. Cassell. *The nature of suffering and the goals of medicine.* 2nd ed. New York: Oxford University Press; 2004.
2. Max Weber, Gerth Hans Heinrich, Mills C. Wright. *From Max Weber: essays in sociology.* New York: Oxford University Press; 1946.
3. A. B. Astrow, Wexler A., Texeira K., He M. K., Sulmasy D. P. Is failure to meet spiritual needs associated with cancer patients' perceptions of quality of care and their satisfaction with care? *J Clin Oncol.* 2007;25(36):5753–5757.
4. M. O. Delgado-Guay, Hui D., Parsons H. A., Govan K., De la Cruz M., Thorney S., Bruera E. Spirituality, religiosity, and spiritual pain in advanced cancer patients. *J Pain Symptom Manage.* 2011;41(6):986–994.
5. H. G. Koenig. Religious attitudes and practices of hospitalized medically ill older adults. *Int J Geriatr Psychiatry.* 1998;13(4):213–224.
6. Miroslav Volf. *Flourishing: why we need religion in a globalized world.* New Haven, CT: Yale University Press; 2016.
7. MJ Balboni. Everyday religion in hospitals. *Society.* 2015;52(5):413–417.
8. C. Puchalski, Ferrell B., Virani R., Otis-Green S., Baird P., Bull J., Chochinov H., Handzo G., Nelson-Becker H., Prince-Paul M., Pugliese K., Sulmasy D. Improving the quality of spiritual care as a dimension of palliative care: the report of the Consensus Conference. *J Palliat Med.* 2009;12(10):885–904.
9. Max Weber. *The Protestant Ethic and the spirit of capitalism.* New York: Scribner; 1976.
10. Talcott Parsons. *The social system.* Glencoe, IL: Free Press; 1951.
11. Paul Starr. *The social transformation of American medicine.* New York: Basic Books; 1982.
12. Rosemary Stevens. *In sickness and in wealth: American hospitals in the twentieth century.* Baltimore: Johns Hopkins University Press; 1999.
13. Jonathan B. Imber. *Trusting doctors: the decline of moral authority in American medicine.* Princeton, NJ: Princeton University Press; 2008.
14. Gary B. Ferngren. *Medicine and religion: a historical introduction.* Baltimore: Johns Hopkins University Press; 2014.
15. Charles E. Rosenberg. *The care of strangers: the rise of America's hospital system.* New York: Basic Books; 1987.
16. Guenter B. Risse. *Mending bodies, saving souls: a history of hospitals.* New York: Oxford University Press; 1999.
17. G. B. Risse, Balboni M. J. Shifting hospital-hospice boundaries: historical perspectives on the institutional care of the dying. *Am J Hosp Palliat Care.* 2013;30(4):325–330.
18. M. J. Balboni, Sullivan A., Enzinger A. C., Smith P. T., Mitchell C., Peteet J. R., Tulsky J. A., VanderWeele T., Balboni T. A. US clergy religious values and relationships to end-of-life discussions and care. *J Pain Symptom Manage.* 2017;53(6):999–1009.
19. Martha Nussbaum. Compassion: the basic social emotion. *Social Philosophy and Policy.* 1996;13(1):27–58.
20. John Rawls. *A theory of justice.* Original ed. Cambridge, MA: Belknap Press; 2005.
21. Martha Craven Nussbaum. *Upheavals of thought: the intelligence of emotions.* Cambridge/New York: Cambridge University Press; 2001.
22. Robert D. Putnam, Campbell David E. *American grace: how religion divides and unites us.* 1st ed. New York: Simon & Schuster; 2010.
23. M. J. Balboni, Bandini J., Mitchell C., Epstein-Peterson Z. D., Amobi A., Cahill J., Enzinger A. C., Peteet J., Balboni T. Religion, spirituality, and the hidden curriculum: medical student and faculty reflections. *J Pain Symptom Manage.* 2015;50(4):507–515.
24. J. D. Yoon, Daley B. M., Curlin F. A. The association between a sense of calling and physician well-being: a national study of primary care physicians and psychiatrists. *Acad Psychiatry.* 2017;41(2):167–173.

25. T. D. Shanafelt, Sloan J. A., Habermann T. M. The well-being of physicians. *Am J Med.* 2003;114(6):513–519.

26. T. D. Shanafelt, West C., Zhao X., Novotny P., Kolars J., Habermann T., Sloan J. Relationship between increased personal well-being and enhanced empathy among internal medicine residents. *J Gen Intern Med.* 2005;20(7):559–564.

27. M. R. DiMatteo, Sherbourne C. D., Hays R. D., Ordway L., Kravitz R. L., McGlynn E. A., Kaplan S., Rogers W. H. Physicians' characteristics influence patients' adherence to medical treatment: results from the Medical Outcomes Study. *Health Psychol.* 1993;12(2):93–102.

28. T. D. Shanafelt, Bradley K. A., Wipf J. E., Back A. L. Burnout and self-reported patient care in an internal medicine residency program. *Ann Intern Med.* 2002;136(5):358–367.

29. J. E. Wallace, Lemaire J. B., Ghali W. A. Physician wellness: a missing quality indicator. *Lancet.* 2009;14(9702):1714–1721.

30. J. R. Halbesleben, Rathert C. Linking physician burnout and patient outcomes: exploring the dyadic relationship between physicians and patients. *Health Care Manage Rev.* 2008;33(1):29–39.

31. N. Ratanawongsa, Roter D., Beach M. C., Laird S. L., Larson S. M., Carson K. A., Cooper L. A. Physician burnout and patient-physician communication during primary care encounters. *J Gen Intern Med.* 2008;23(10):1581–1588.

32. C. P. West, Shanafelt T. D., Kolars J. C. Quality of life, burnout, educational debt, and medical knowledge among internal medicine residents. *JAMA.* 2011;306(9):952–960.

33. T. D. Shanafelt, Balch C. M., Bechamps G., Russell T., Dyrbye L., Satele D., Collicott P., Novotny P. J., Sloan J., Freischlag J. Burnout and medical errors among American surgeons. *Ann Surg.* 2010;251(6):995–1000.

34. L. D. Eron. Effect of medical education on medical students' attitudes. *J Med Educ.* 1955;30(10):559–566.

35. A. G. Rezler. Attitude changes during medical school: a review of the literature. *J Med Educ.* 1974;49(11):1023–1030.

36. R. Christie, Merton R. K. Procedures for the sociological study of the values climate of medical schools. *J Med Educ.* 1958;33(10 Part 2):125–153.

37. L. Gundersen. Physician burnout. *Ann Intern Med.* 2001;135(2):145–148.

38. G. Deckard, Meterko M., Field D. Physician burnout: an examination of personal, professional, and organizational relationships. *Medical Care.* 1994;32(7):745–754.

39. M. Linzer, Visser M. R., Oort F. J., Smets E. M., McMurray J. E., de Haes H. C. Predicting and preventing physician burnout: results from the United States and the Netherlands. *Am J Med.* 2001;111(2):170–175.

40. S. S. Chopra, Sotile W. M., Sotile M. O. Physician burnout. *JAMA.* 2004;291(5):633.

41. H. J. Tak, Curlin F. A., Yoon J. D. Association of Intrinsic Motivating Factors and Markers of Physician Well-Being: a national physician survey. *J Gen Intern Med.* 2017;32(7):739–746.

42. M. Hojat, Vergare M. J., Maxwell K., Brainard G., Herrine S. K., Isenberg G. A., Veloski J., Gonnella J. S. The devil is in the third year: a longitudinal study of erosion of empathy in medical school. *Acad Med.* 2009;84(9):1182–1191.

43. L. M. Bellini, Shea J. A. Mood change and empathy decline persist during three years of internal medicine training. *Acad Med.* 2005;80(2):164–167.

44. L. N. Dyrbye, Thomas M. R., Huntington J. L., Lawson K. L., Novotny P. J., Sloan J. A., Shanafelt T. D. Personal life events and medical student burnout: a multicenter study. *Acad Med.* 2006;81(4):374–384.

45. L. N. Dyrbye, Thomas M. R., Power D. V., Durning S., Moutier C., Massie F. S., Jr., Harper W., Eacker A., Szydlo D. W., Sloan J. A., Shanafelt T. D. Burnout and serious thoughts of dropping out of medical school: a multi-institutional study. *Acad Med.* 2010;85(1):94–102.

46. M. R. Oreskovich, Shanafelt T., Dyrbye L. N., Tan L., Sotile W., Satele D., West C. P., Sloan J., Boone S. The prevalence of substance use disorders in American physicians. *Am J Addict.* 2015;24(1):30–38.

47. L. N. Dyrbye, Thomas M. R., Massie F. S., Power D. V., Eacker A., Harper W., Durning S., Moutier C., Szydlo D. W., Novotny P. J., Sloan J. A., Shanafelt T. D. Burnout and suicidal ideation among US medical students. *Ann Intern Med.* 2008;149(5):334–341.
48. T. L. Schwenk, Davis L., Wimsatt L. A. Depression, stigma, and suicidal ideation in medical students. *JAMA.* 2010;304(11):1181–1190.
49. J. L. Givens, Tjia J. Depressed medical students' use of mental health services and barriers to use. *Acad Med.* 2002;77(9):918–921.
50. L. N. Dyrbye, Thomas M. R., Shanafelt T. D. Systematic review of depression, anxiety, and other indicators of psychological distress among US and Canadian medical students. *Acad Med.* 2006;81(4):354–373.
51. R. Tyssen, Vaglum P., Gronvold N. T., Ekeberg O. Suicidal ideation among medical students and young physicians: a nationwide and prospective study of prevalence and predictors. *J Affect Disord.* 2001;64(1):69–79.
52. K. L. Harrison, Dzeng E., Ritchie C. S., Shanafelt T. D., Kamal A. H., Bull J. H., Tilburt J. C., Swetz K. M. Addressing palliative care clinician burnout in organizations: a workforce necessity, an ethical imperative. *J Pain Symptom Manage.* 2017;53(6):1091–1096.
53. T. D. Shanafelt, Noseworthy J. H. Executive leadership and physician well-being: nine organizational strategies to promote engagement and reduce burnout. *Mayo Clin Proc.* 2017;92(1):129–146.
54. S. J. Swensen, Shanafelt T. An organizational framework to reduce professional burnout and bring back joy in practice. *Jt Comm J Qual Patient Saf.* 2017;43(6):308–313.
55. J. D. Yoon, Hunt N. B., Ravella K. C., Jun C. S., Curlin F. A. Physician burnout and the calling to care for the dying. *Am J Hosp Palliat Care.* 2016:1049909116661817.
56. T. D. Shanafelt, Hasan O., Dyrbye L. N., Sinsky C., Satele D., Sloan J., West C. P. Changes in burnout and satisfaction with work-life balance in physicians and the general US working population between 2011 and 2014. *Mayo Clin Proc.* 2015;90(12):1600–1613.
57. T. D. Shanafelt, Dyrbye L. N., West C. P. Addressing physician burnout: the way forward. *JAMA.* 2017;317(9):901–902.
58. Peter L. Berger, Luckmann Thomas. *The social construction of reality: a treatise in the sociology of knowledge.* 1st ed. Garden City, NY: Doubleday; 1966.
59. H. Lempp, Seale C. The hidden curriculum in undergraduate medical education: qualitative study of medical students' perceptions of teaching. *BMJ.* 2004;329(7469):770–773.
60. F. W. Hafferty, Franks R. The hidden curriculum, ethics teaching, and the structure of medical education. *Acad Med.* 1994;69(11):861–871.
61. F. W. Hafferty. Beyond curriculum reform: confronting medicine's hidden curriculum. *Acad Med.* 1998;73(4):403–407.
62. W. A. Kinghorn, McEvoy M. D., Michel A., Balboni M. Professionalism in modern medicine: does the emperor have any clothes? *Acad Med.* 2007;82(1):40–45.
63. T. P. Daaleman, Kinghorn W. A., Newton W. P., Meador K. G. Rethinking professionalism in medical education through formation. *Family Med.* 2011;43(5):325–329.
64. Jack Coulehan. Today's professionalism: engaging the mind but not the heart. *Acad Med.* 2005;80:892–898.
65. R. T. Ho, Sing C. Y., Fong T. C., Au-Yeung F. S., Law K. Y., Lee L. F., Ng S. M. Underlying spirituality and mental health: the role of burnout. *J Occup Health.* 2016;58(1):66–71.
66. E. Salmoirago-Blotcher, Fitchett G., Leung K., Volturo G., Boudreaux E., Crawford S., Ockene I., Curlin F. An exploration of the role of religion/spirituality in the promotion of physicians' wellbeing in emergency medicine. *Prev Med Rep.* 2016;3:189–195.
67. J. D. Yoon, Shin J. H., Nian A. L., Curlin F. A. Religion, sense of calling, and the practice of medicine: findings from a national survey of primary care physicians and psychiatrists. *South Med J.* 2015;108(3):189–195.
68. Abim Foundation. ACP-ASIM Foundation. European Federation of Internal Medicine. Medical professionalism in the new millennium: a physician charter. *Ann Intern Med.* 2002; 136(3):243–246.

69. Project Medical Professionalism. Medical professionalism in the new millennium: a physicians' charter. *Lancet*. 2002;359(9305):520–522.

70. R. M. Epstein, Hundert E. M. Defining and assessing professional competence. *JAMA*. 2002;287(2):226–235.

71. E. J. Emanuel, Fuchs V. R. The perfect storm of overutilization. *JAMA*. 2008;299(23): 2789–2791.

72. R. M. Antiel, Kinghorn W. A., Reed D. A., Hafferty F. W. Professionalism: etiquette or habitus? *Mayo Clin Proc*. 2013;88(7):651–652.

73. C. M. Puchalski, Blatt B., Kogan M., Butler A. Spirituality and health: the development of a field. *Acad Med*. 2014;89(1):10–16.

74. Christina M. Puchalski. *A time for listening and caring: spirituality and the care of the chronically ill and dying*. Oxford; New York: Oxford University Press; 2006.

75. H. G. Koenig, Hooten E. G., Lindsay-Calkins E., Meador K. G. Spirituality in medical school curricula: findings from a national survey. *Int J Psychiatry Med*. 2010;40(4):391–398.

76. G. Lucchetti, de Oliveira L. R., Koenig H. G., Leite J. R., Lucchetti A. L., for the SBRAME Collaborators. Medical students, spirituality and religiosity--results from the multicenter study SBRAME. *BMC Med Educ*. 2013;13:162.

77. T. P. Guck, Kavan M. G. Medical student beliefs: spirituality's relationship to health and place in the medical school curriculum. *Med Teach*. 2006;28(8):702–707.

78. Joan Halifax. *Being with dying: cultivating compassion and fearlessness in the presence of death*. 1st ed. Boston: Shambhala; 2008.

79. John R. Peteet, D'Ambra Michael N. *The soul of medicine: spiritual perspectives and clinical practice*. Baltimore: Johns Hopkins University Press; 2011.

14

Problematic Rapprochement Strategies

Introduction

The current separation of medicine, spirituality, and religion is not inevitable, as if science conquered superstition, nor is it necessarily irreparable. There have been multiple attempts to reengage the relationship between medicine and religion, such as in the 1960s, when the American Medical Association created a working group with clergy,[1] and in recent decades, when the spirituality and health movement has generated enormous literature, scholarship, and activities such as academic conferences and workshops,[2 [pp. 1-3]] medical school courses,[3] and increasingly sophisticated curricula in physician competencies.[4 [pp. 420-421]] Changing attitudes toward spirituality and religion within medicine have been under way, with one of the clearest indicators being adoption of consensus standards within the field of palliative care[5,6] and by increasing recognition of the significance of religion and spirituality by the Joint Commission,[7] which oversees and certifies hospitals in the United States.

While increasing openness to spirituality and religion appears to exist in medical culture, a spirituality of immanence described in Part II creates counterforces that shape medicine's rapprochement to spirituality and religion in a manner that is less than true partnership. This chapter explores how future partnership may be envisioned between medicine, spirituality, and religion. Here, we identify three primary constituencies involved in the relationship between medicine and spirituality and three primary issues that remain obstacles to a larger synthesis. A better way forward involves all interested parties both making compromises and receiving gains. In the next chapter, we will offer a tentative but constructive proposal called "structural pluralism." This approach holds potential to make rapprochement possible by undoing the forces of a spirituality of immanence and providing a benefit where all constituents receive important gains.

Three Constituencies

Rapprochement refers to theoretically informed strategies aimed toward the resumption of harmonious relations between separated parties. When considering the broken relationship existing between medicine and traditional world religions, there are three main constituencies with partially conflicting interests in this area. For simplicity, we will classify these three groups as "skeptics," "spiritual generalists," and "religious particularists" (see Table 14.1).[i]

We refer to *skeptics* as those who are primarily aligned with the current separation of medicine and religion. They are concerned with protecting medicine's social position, growing its institutions and knowledge, and advancing medical care in its nexus with science and market forces. While this group has been generally unconvinced of rapprochement, it generally grants in principle that the relationship should be considered using empirical means of description and often under a utilitarian assumption that spirituality may have merit within medicine's foci if it serves the ends of physical health, cure, and bodily comfort. When religion is incorporated into patient care, skeptics uphold a clear division of labor between clergy and hospital chaplains on the one hand and clinicians on the other. Clinicians should focus on the body and clergy on the soul. While skeptics object to religion in medicine, many are also deeply concerned that medicine is drifting into dehumanized care.[8 [pp. 53–59]] Skeptics have not found a solution to growing dehumanization.

Spiritual generalists consist of a broad coalition of constituents who stress the universal aspects of spirituality, usually downplaying religious traditions. This group is especially concerned with broadening the scope of medical care beyond a reductionistic lens in order to include the whole person. Their protest is against biomedicine's gaze on the mechanisms of disease and its focus on the body to the detriment of other aspects of humanity (illustrated by Picasso's *Science and Charity*). Members

Table 14.1 **Issues obstructing rapprochement between medicine, spirituality, and religion**

Spirituality should be:	Skeptics	Spiritual Generalists	Religious Particularists
Instrumental, empirically informed use for health	√	√	
1 Versus			
Intrinsically relevant regardless of benefits or outcomes		√	√
Generically constituted grounded in basic humanity		√	
2 Versus			
Tradition-constituted by communities, beliefs, and narratives	√		√
Division-of-labor, professionalized spiritual credentials	√	√	√
3 Versus			
General privilege and responsibility, semi-permeable roles			√

in this group include some who are traditionally religious privately but who prefer to emphasize commonalities, not what is distinctive, among religious traditions. Some in this group hold to a theology of religious pluralism, a conviction that "all world religions are roughly equally true, provide equally valid access to the divine, foster human flourishing equally well, and are equally effective means for reaching the hoped-for everlasting life.[9 [p. 140]] The group also includes those who consider themselves "spiritual not religious" and those who stress complementary and alternative therapies such as mindfulness meditation and yoga in addition to biomedical therapies. The group's primary rapprochement strategies have focused on generic spirituality, deemphasizing religion per se, and highlighting a division of labor which advances board-certified hospital chaplains as an emerging medical profession. Chaplains are especially needed to advance spiritual care and should do so by employing empirical studies.

A third constituency, *religious particularists*, refers to those who are self-consciously aligned with traditional religious communities including Christian denominations (70.6% of the US population) and other world religions (5.9% of US population).[10] Religious particularists are sensitive to honor the beliefs and practices that are unique to their spiritual tradition. Many who hold to this perspective believe that their faith is the true faith, under an authority relevant to all peoples, and that it is the right path for everyone to follow irrespective of age, culture, or religious identification.[9 [pp. 138–139]] While presumably most do not necessarily denigrate other traditions or seek to exclude them from the public square,[9] stress is laid on faithfulness in every sphere of life. They also may have particular theological understandings in how their faith tradition shapes health and the care of the sick. A primary concern among those in this group is faithfulness to their tradition in the receipt or the delivery of medicine. Most religious particularists do not assume that all religions can be distilled down to the same underlying human experience or underlying divine mystery. There are real differences between religious groups, and these differences should be recognized and, at a minimum, accommodated within the structures of medical care. In addition, some religious traditions emphasize a hierarchy within their tradition that elevates priestly responsibilities. Sacerdotal traditions exemplified in pre–Vatican II Roman Catholicism may at times emphasize a division-of-labor approach to spiritual care. By contrast, some Protestant traditions, which historically have elevated the role of the laity in priestly functions, would resist a division of labor and prefer a democratic sharing of spiritual care across professional roles.

Whereas all three groups desire patient-centered care, there are a number of issues that make rapprochement between competing visions difficult. Each group is confronted with multiple obstacles, illustrated in Table 14.1. Each constituent group responds to these choices differently, creating partial alliances and profound disagreements. These differences result in a lack of consensus that obstructs synthesis among medicine, spirituality, and religion. It would also appear that these differences enable a spirituality of immanence to dominate and, ironically, disable an alliance strong enough to resist and redirect social forces speeding toward an impersonal medicine (Figure 13.3).

There are at least three critical issues that create alliances and disagreement among the constituencies as illustrated in Table 14.1. This table suggests competing ways that these issues have been formulated and which position is preferred by skeptics, spiritual generalists, and religious particularists, respectively. This chapter unfolds each issue and provides an argument for our viewpoint. A fourth key issue pertains to the structures of pluralism in medicine. Chapter 15 will focus on ways to engage pluralism within American medicine.

Issue 1: Instrumental Uses Versus Intrinsic Value

The first matter that divides constituents concerns the question of whether spirituality and religion are relevant to medicine because of their instrumental role in impacting physical health or because of their intrinsic value irrespective of health benefits and impact on outcomes. Accordingly, most discussions tether this concern with the use of empirical research in examination of spiritual and religious phenomenon.

An instrumental approach to religion understands religion's purpose as a means or instrument to a nonreligious end, rather than the internal ends identified by religion itself. There are multiple examples of those who put forward arguments that appear to instrumentalize and subordinate the use of religion for the purposes of health,[11–14] and this view has many critics.[15–18 [pp. 161–185]] Within a mental health perspective, for example, there can be a tendency to emphasize the purpose of spirituality and religion in service of psychological adjustment and coping.[19,20] In this account, what is important is the individual patient's internal sense of quality of life, happiness (to the extent that it is possible), and coping with disease and dying. These psychological aims are the goal, and spirituality and religion are the means to the end. From this vantage point, the actual claims of a particular meaning-making system such as that found, for example, in Islam, Judaism, or Hinduism, are secondary and its truth claims are not in view. They are "true" to the extent that they assist a patient in making meaning, but they cannot be validated in their actual substantive claims.

In responding to this reduction of spirituality and religion into psychological processes, bioethicist Jeffrey Bishop has passionately argued against this misuse of religion because it serves medicine's finite aims of physical and social control, inculcating it within a metaphysic of efficient causation.[15,17] Mental health professionals may employ religion because of its capacity to facilitate coping within illness but not based on its own claims or merits. This use of religion for medical and health ends, as Bishop has argued, is culturally insensitive because it distorts religion for purposes aside from most religions' own intrinsic ends. Based on the thought of Foucault, Bishop argues that the use of religion in medicine is part of a larger biopolitics, so that religions' effects on either health or coping in illness and dying become tools of the state, designed to efficiently control bodies and populations.[17] [p. 251] These warnings against utilitarian uses of religion for medicine are cogent and correspond to this book's thesis in regards to the hegemony of medicine's spirituality of immanence.[ii] Immanence seeks to control all other spiritual traditions by bringing them under its power and instrumentalizing them for the goals of physical health, cure, or comfort as ultimate concern.

A related question concerns whether examining spirituality and religion using empirical research may constitute an example of instrumentalization. Critics argue that research of spirituality and religion is problematic because it slips from describing what is important for a patient into an advocacy of spirituality and religion, which is "a speciously utilitarian reduction of that way of life to a series of isolated techniques.[16 [p. 26]] Similarly, Bishop takes to task the construct of religious coping as being a reductionist use of religion for merely psychological purposes in illness.[iii]

While these criticisms hold general weight, we also are concerned that opponents recognize and uphold that empirical research includes at least two legitimate purposes that are theologically consistent with the internal claims of many religious traditions.

First, empirical research plays an important role in describing the role and impact that religion holds in medicine. While secular medicine dismisses the importance of spirituality and religion in patient experience, empirical research has repeatedly demonstrated how this dismissal is biased and does not reflect the experiences or viewpoints of patients or their medical caregivers (as described in Chapter 2). Likewise, in regards to Jeffrey Bishop's argument against the reductionism of religious coping assessments, Pargament himself strongly warned against collapsing religion into psychological coping. Early on in his seminal work on religious coping, Pargament counseled, "[I] admit from the start that the psychology of religion and coping cannot provide a full accounting of religious life. There is more to religion and life than coping with stress."[20 [p. 14]] Studying the impact of religion on coping or other outcomes is not intrinsically a reductionist practice but can be done while retaining interpretative perspectives that uphold the intrinsic value of religion. Critical realist approaches to phenomena emphasize how reality is stratified into multiple levels of significance. This view resists reductionist explanations that claim to give a complete accounting of a phenomena, when in fact that account is meaningful on only one level of reality. Thus, when Pargament discusses religion using the lens of psychological coping, this should not be understood to mean that religion is merely a coping mechanism. The psychological dimension is only one level of several that are needed to move toward a comprehensive understanding of religious phenomena. In other words, it is not the act of empirical research that is instrumental, but how studies are designed and interpreted within their larger context of meaning.[iv]

Second, as the field of spirituality and health further develops, there is increasing clarity that empirical research has the potential to serve the very religious communities that it analyzes. VanderWeele suggests that as experts from religious communities are directly involved in creating assessment tools and designing the contexts of study, they have the capacity to focus research "on the particular goals and end of religious communities, taking religious variables not simply as 'exposures' but also as 'outcomes,' viewed as ends in their own right."[21 [p. 386]] Even so, prior religious criticisms of empirical research are being heeded by researchers who are developing and testing interventions that come out of and are being offered within particular theological traditions. One recent example concerns religiously integrated cognitive behavioral therapy in response to depression.[22] This form of research has the capacity to serve religious communities by developing health interventions that flow out from and advance each tradition's ultimate concerns and affections.

Spirituality, public health, and medicine need not compete with nor fail to engage one another in many instances, but they hold potential to operate within what Swinton and Mowatt describe as a "hospitable conversation" that leads to a "critical faithfulness."[23 [pp. 89-92]] On the one hand, medicine's instrumentalizing of religion fails the test of partnership and masks utilitarian ethics within a garb of neutrality. On the other hand, religion's *carte blanch* rejection of empirical modes of inquiry and statistical analysis fails the test of partnership and risks incorrectly suggesting that religion cannot learn from science or falsely suggesting that science and religion are antagonists with competing truth claims.[24]

As a way forward between instrumental and intrinsic interpretations, skeptics and spiritual generalists should abandon viewpoints that interpret religion with an instrumental framework. Such an approach privileges medicine above religion and fails to recognize how public health and medicine often assume and superimpose their own underlying spirituality of immanence. Spiritual generalists have argued that their approach is not intended to assimilate spirituality into medicine. They suggest that a realistic approach must be incremental given the general medical hostility toward religion. Therefore, some level of compromise is necessary to make small inroads toward rapprochement.[v] However, many religious particularists are loath to go along with this compromise because they believe it undermines the very nature of religion[16] and sacrifices its prophetic ability to challenge medicine's deep structures.[25 [p. 140]] If spiritual generalists and religious particularists could find an agreed-upon strategy, then these two groups together would be more difficult to resist if they both advocated for rapprochement. But, as it currently stands, this is a major point of fragmentation in the spirituality and health movement.

An additional step through this impasse is the need for religious particularists to embrace and engage in empirical research. This need not be in the form of a disciplinary biopolitics that Bishop and others warn against.[15,17,26] Rather, an embrace may come with the realization that the health sciences are a means of discovering certain levels of truth through the employment of God-gifted reason, which together work as partners with theology in advancing the kinds of health desired by religious communities. Empirical investigation encourages constructive criticism of the blind spots that particular communities can sometimes hold. Skeptics and spiritual generalists rightly champion empirical research as an important avenue toward rapprochement. Direct input in study questions, research design, development of measurements, and intervention studies will be strengthened to the degree that religious particularists participate. Failure to produce methodologically rigorous and theologically robust research should not lead to conclusions that such research holds little value, but rather that such research serves as an invitation for religious particularists to become more deeply involved in producing higher quality research. Engagement in research holds potential to enable all three constituents to work closely together. As research becomes progressively granular in its understanding of spirituality and religion, it may serve as an important way through some differences.[2 [pp. 3–6]]

Issue 2: Division of Labor Versus Semi-permeable Roles

A second rapprochement strategy is what might be described as a "division-of-labor model" to spiritual care. Within the medical literature, many agree that spiritual care is a collaborative effort, involving doctors, nurses, chaplains, and other medical caregivers.[27] Some theorize the jurisdiction of spiritual care by dividing responsibility so that chaplains and clergy handle spiritual concerns, while physicians and nurses focus on bodily matters.[27–30] Clinicians are involved by inquiring if spirituality or religion is important to the patient. If it is, then clinicians should call in a chaplain in a consultancy model. The chaplain goes beyond inquiry in spiritual diagnosis and creating a spiritual care plan.[27,31,32] This approach seeks to reassert spiritual dimensions of caring for the ill by growing and legitimizing a professional group of spiritual caregivers as specialists, employed by the healthcare system, whose primary expertise is the spiritual care of patients. As awareness of the implications of spiritual matters in medical care has grown,[2] there has been increasing momentum to professionalize spiritual care within the medical setting, with chaplains serving as the primary providers.[vi]

As a spiritual care model, the division-of-labor approach has important advantages. If clinicians regularly inquired about spiritual concerns, then spiritual care of patients would surely become more frequent in the healthcare setting. Additionally, a clearer set of roles is established by the professionalization of chaplaincy, and this could improve the frequency and quality of spiritual care. As chaplains become recognized partners in the healthcare team, they may become more integrated into the care of the critically ill.[vii] If chaplains became more widely recognized as professionals on the medical team, patient spiritual care would be integrated much earlier in the illness experience, rather than as an after-thought when medical technology reaches its limits. In becoming professionally recognized, chaplain services would be billable by the hospital to insurance companies and government agencies. Currently, spiritual care services are not recognized as a professional expertise requiring financial reimbursement. If spiritual care became reimbursable, then we would likely see a significant growth in the field of chaplaincy, and this would presumably lead to more patients receiving spiritual care from persons serving on the medical team.

Despite these advantages, Wendy Cadge's study affirmed how hospital chaplaincy struggles for legitimacy as an underfunded, optional service with low status in the hospital.[33 [pp. 105–127]] Many clinicians approach chaplains as an afterthought. For example, in a multisite national study of chaplains in the ICU, chaplains were infrequently called upon by nurses and physicians and typically only just before a patient died.[34] Well-trained providers of spiritual care are essential for the provision of caregiving in the medical context, and we affirm that hospital chaplaincy is essential not peripheral. The question we are raising is how to achieve this end? A truly integrated model of medicine and spirituality requires fluid rather than fixed professional boundaries in the collaboration and contributions from both medical providers and religious communities. So if clinicians are regularly engaged in spiritual care of patients, they will then be far more aware of its importance and be much stronger advocates for the presence of chaplains in the hospital setting. By contrast, a division-of-labor model that professionalizes chaplains as medical professionals is plagued by significant liabilities and will only further distance spiritual care from the mindset of clinicians. Such an emphasis may undermine the effort to gain chaplaincy recognition as an essential ministry.

If spiritual care of the patient and a strong chaplaincy are the primary aims, then there are four additional liabilities associated with a division-of-labor approach.

Spiritual Care Subjected to Legal-Rational Forces

A first liability is that the provision of spiritual care will become subject to empirical demonstration, and this will lead to a reshaping of pastoral care based on financial considerations. This will likely subject spiritual care to instrumental approaches to spirituality motivated primarily by cost and efficiency, rather than the intrinsic motivations suggested in the previous section.[viii] What happens to the very nature of spiritual care when it becomes commodified as a billable activity within medicine's market system? Does this cheapen the care or transform what many believe is "invaluable" into another immanent activity? Certainly, there are a number of central human activities and values in the care of the sick that should not be subjected to legal-rational measures or incentives. Compassion, for example, consists of certain human ideas, activities, and words, but it would likely harm the very nature of compassion if medicine either professionalized the activity into a guild of "compassion providers" or if it became an activity reimbursed for "compassion-based" services. Weber has clearly shown why the bureaucratic process is both highly efficient and rational, but also leads toward dehumanization that changes the worker and the very nature of the work.[35 (p. 196-244)] Like compassion, professionalizing spiritual care as an expertise will likely alter its nature.

Changes resulting from professionalization would likely affect the amount of time that chaplains are able to offer their patients. Currently, chaplains are stretched thin but they still can offer more time listening to a patient in comparison to clinicians. However, it is likely that if chaplains succeed in gaining professional status on the medical team, the ability to spend necessary time with patients will be dramatically undermined. Chaplaincy departments will be under extreme pressures to produce research results demonstrating effects on nonspiritual outcomes in order to justify ongoing reimbursement, and individual chaplains will be forced to spend significantly less time with any one patient in order to maximize efficiency and profit. While many if not most current chaplains will resent and resist changes created by the commodification of their time and its inconsistent rationalization with all traditional forms of pastoral care, bureaucratic logic and market realities will become impossible to impede.[35 (p. 228)] This will, in turn, further alter the types of people attracted into the chaplaincy profession, as modern professions with specialized knowledge do not depend on private piety or moral formation as criteria for qualification.

Chaplaincy leaders have been partly motivated to gain professionalized status within medicine's bureaucratic market system in order to gain a level of legitimacy within that system. Yet, in being legitimated by the medical system in its legal-rationalism, hospital chaplains delegitimize their present status provided by their own religious communities and ordination. A division-of-labor approach then risks transforming chaplains into servants of a spirituality of immanence, the very spirituality that obstructs traditional spiritual caregiving from religious communities. Chaplains will have little ability or incentive to stand against the bureaucratic, reductionist, and market-driven dimensions of medicine.

Marginalization of External Religious Voices

Combined with such anticipated changes to hospital chaplaincy, a second liability to the division-of-labor approach is that professionalization of chaplains will undermine the role of community clergy, religious communities, and medical professionals in offering spiritual care either as volunteers or as part of their own legitimate callings as a clinician at the bedside. If spiritual care is earmarked as a domain of expertise, then legal-rational processes will require spiritual care providers to hold a significant level of specialized training lest they be deemed unqualified to provide spiritual care. This designation will invest hospital chaplains with a higher level of control over the spiritual domain, and many potential providers including medical professionals and community clergy will lack the bureaucratically constructed medical credentials to be qualified in providing spiritual care in the hospital context.

Studies have already suggested that community clergy provide spiritual care differently compared to hospital chaplains,[36-38] and this is likely influenced by theologically driven presuppositions.[36,39] Approximately half of community clergy in the United States never receive certification in hospital chaplaincy training, partly because training offered by organizations such as the Association of Clinical Pastoral Education (CPE) is interpreted as theologically discordant from the perspectives of many theologically conservative denominations.[17,39,40] Community clergy in theologically conservative denominations, which are by far the largest religious groups in the United States, such as most Black Protestant, Hispanic Pentecostals, and White Evangelicals, will be unwilling to receive CPE credentialing, and this could conceivably prevent community clergy from providing spiritual care within hospitals.

In addition to this, medical professionals who are apt to provide spiritual care will be discouraged or conceivably reprimanded for doing so under a division-of-labor model. A clinician or hospital staff member who prays with a patient or engages in a religious conversation[41-43] will be seen by the chaplaincy community as having violated a professional boundary. But this "violation" presupposes a theological perspective on who has authority to provide spiritual care. A division-of-labor approach assumes a certain theology about who should provide spiritual care. Nevertheless, professionalizing spiritual care does not fit well with many Protestant Christian theologies or a post–Vatican II emphasis,[ix] both which stress the priestly role of the laity and the responsibility of lay persons to visit the sick. These Christian viewpoints stress how all persons in the community are afforded the privilege, honor, and responsibility to pray and care for souls, offering both a listening ear and words of spiritual comfort and direction.

Clergy are recognized in Catholic, Orthodox, and Protestant traditions as holding advanced knowledge and pastoral skills and as being formed within lives of piety. Within a larger Christian context, however, clergy equip the laity to do the work of the ministry. Nevertheless, those denominations that authorize and prepare lay persons to visit the sick contradict the inherent logic of a legal-rational healthcare system. The aim of bureaucracy is efficiency, and it executes efficiency by designating a particular domain of work for a particular professional class, which then holds exclusive rights and jurisdiction over that domain.[35 [p. 228]] In the Christian context, many clergy aim to equip the laity to be priest-like in service to others. Since under a legal-rational system, efficiency and control are the primary aims, we should then expect that a professionalized chaplaincy guild, following a division-of-labor approach, will not desire or welcome spiritual care volunteers who provide spiritual care according to their own tradition.

Reinforcement of Secular Plausibility Structures

A third liability in the division-of-labor model is that it does not correspond with how patients experience illness, but it instead corresponds with the plausibility structures that minimize the significance of spiritual care. Within the dynamics of the medical team, the model is presented as a "generalist-specialist" understanding where nurses and physicians are spiritual generalists and chaplains are spiritual specialists.[27,31,44,45] Advocates of this approach suggest that medical professionals inquire with the patient concerning religion or spirituality using a short screening tool or spiritual history-taking.[27,46,47] The primary aim in asking the patient spiritual questions is to identify if the patient should receive further spiritual engagement from a chaplain.[46]

This approach, however, does not correspond with studies discussed in Chapter 3 that demonstrate how patients' spiritual experiences of illness are intertwined with patients' medical experience and medical decision-making.[48-50] As implied previously in data from the Coping with Cancer findings,[51-53] a division-of-labor approach may lead to unrecognized and inadequately addressed spiritual gaps in the medical setting. For example, one study reported that associations between spiritual support and end-of-life medical decisions were present during spiritual care offered by the medical team but not during pastoral care services.[52] This finding likely indicates that the practice of spiritual care by nurses and doctors uniquely addresses certain dimensions of spiritual concerns, such as when spiritual and medical issues overlap. These findings suggest that spiritual care in the medical setting is not best served by a professionalized, subspecialty model but rather by an integrated, generalized, laity model. The latter is founded on the principle that bodily and spiritual matters cannot be dichotomized and hence that caregiving in the setting of illness requires attention from a diverse array of spiritual caregivers including clergy, chaplains, congregants, family members, physicians, and nurses.

Additionally, spiritual support from medical caregivers not only requires a multidisciplinary team approach, but also calls for individuals who are simultaneously comfortable in both the biomedical and spiritual dimensions of caregiving. Without a model of spiritual care that promotes the integrated involvement of both biomedical and religious communities, the contemporary medical approach dichotomizing body and soul will likely remain unchanged. Not only is an integrated, generalized model likely the only means of overcoming the chasm between medical and spiritual caregiving, it also is the most resource-rich (particularly desirable in the context of a financially strained medical system) insofar as it draws upon a multitude of skilled helpers offering necessary and complementary resources in the task of shepherding souls. In light of overwhelming spiritual concerns triggered by illness,[x] many people of different levels of spiritual care training and experience should participate in providing spiritual care to the sick according to their abilities and the level of concordance they hold with the patient.

Weakening a Prophetic Voice

A final concern regarding the division-of-labor approach is that it will further insulate medicine's institutions and structures from particular theological critiques.[54] If the work of spirituality and religion became located in or associated with a particular professional group such as hospital chaplaincy, the spirituality of immanence that currently dominates the structures and the values of medicine will be inadequately engaged. A division-of-labor approach is focused on the individual patient and clinician within a privatized form of spirituality, but it leaves the larger medical structures unexamined. Our concern is that a division-of-labor approach will safeguard medicine's spirituality of immanence rather than call its hegemony into question. A division-of-labor approach focuses on individuals rather than social structures and thus leads to an inability to critique medicine's meaning-making systems, including its legal-rational bureaucratization, commodified market-driven system, or its technological reductionism of the patient's illness experience.

A prophetic voice inspired by particular religious communities enables critique of the structures of medicine. In order to uphold and maintain spiritual voices, especially community clergy and hospital chaplains, those voices need to retain autonomy from medicine's structures, specifically, financial dependence. Holding on to a degree of independence suggests that religious communities are partners and benefactors in the care of the seriously ill and have access to patients but are not beholden to medicine's reductionist rationality, bureaucratic structures, or financial incentives. Governance is especially worrisome when clergy are financially reimbursed directly for spiritual care by a hospital or by the government. For religious communities to hold a prophetic voice in the medical system, careful thinking is needed pertaining to how clergy and chaplains structurally fit within the medical institutions that they serve. Contemporary chaplaincy funding models tie the chaplain to the hospital; we recommend a traditional chaplaincy model that allows chaplains to operate primarily as members of their faith and religious community. Under previous financial structures, congregations volunteered lay and clergy time in caring for the spiritual needs of the ill. Medical institutions should partially share in the costs related to spiritual care, but this does not suggest that chaplains work directly for a hospital or that they are directly paid by a hospital. Alternative approaches encourage reimbursement to third-party organizations, and medical institutions may partly support the spiritual services provided.[xi] It is both unwise and unrealistic to expect hospitals or the government to be principally responsible for costs related to the spiritual care of the seriously ill. There is a strong case to be made that the government has some financial self-interest in creating advantageous conditions for spiritual care to be offered to patients as long as it is voluntary and desired by the patient. The link between spiritual care and medical outcomes (discussed in Chapter 3) is sufficiently solid that there should be little doubt of these associations.[51,52,55] As long as no particular faith group is excluded from generally available resources,[56 [pp. 66-80]] there is a strong empirical case for the government to share in some costs related to spiritual care provision.

However, religious communities and community clergy have a responsibility to engage medicine and use their own financial resources toward caring for the sick. Hospitals should facilitate such a partnership by reaching out to clergy, providing education on medical issues, and working more closely with regulators so that state and federal laws (e.g., the Health Insurance Portability and Privacy Act [HIPPA]) do not hinder and obstruct volunteers such as clergy and lay people in providing spiritual care. There are approximately 5,600 hospitals in the United States, roughly 350,000 community clergy,[39] and approximately 10,000 chaplains.[33] While on average there are 1.7 chaplains for every US hospital, by contrast there are 62.5 community clergy per hospital. Thus, in meeting Joint Commission and end-of-life guidelines,[6,7] hospitals have potential access to a large, well-educated clergy network who currently provide approximately four hours per week in spiritual care to the sick and elderly.[39] Little evidence suggests that these potential partnerships are being adequately utilized.

In this account, we are *by no means* suggesting that hospital chaplains are expandable. Hospital chaplains are already ordained ministers in their own denominations and have significantly higher levels of experience and training in caring for the sick. The role of hospital chaplains should not be to professionalize their guild as a break-off group from community clergy. Instead, they should continue pastoral care as representatives of their denominations and as mediators in facilitating community clergy and lay people visiting the sick. In our view, chaplains are positioned to lead other clergy and religious communities in providing spiritual care, but they should do this first and foremost as clergy and ecclesiastical representatives, not as members of a specialized medical guild or as hospital employees.

A division-of-labor approach risks turning chaplains into handmaidens of medicine's spirituality of immanence, and this, in turn, inadvertently supports rather than speaks to a medical culture that, as Liberal Protestant theologian Stephen Pattison argues, desperately needs to hear prophetic words of truth.[54] Community clergy and chaplains who receive some financial support from their denominations or local congregations have a more influentia voice since they can speak prophetically without financial repercussion. While a division-of-labor approach will greatly clarify whose responsibility it is to provide spiritual care, it will blur who chaplains represent. In our estimation, hospital chaplains are necessary, but primarily as representatives of their religious communities, not professionally legitimatized or financially bound by the medical system.

In summary, a division-of-labor approach is an inadequate rapprochement strategy since it will widen the gap between medicine and the actual spiritual communities that currently exist in the United States. Skeptics may prefer a division of labor because it serves ultimately as a buffer between clinicians and patients' spiritual lives. Spiritual generalists promote this as a compromise with skeptics since it will increase the frequency of spiritual care but may be more palatable to skeptics. Our concern, however, is that it marginalizes community pastors, restrains clinicians from appropriately and sensitively offering spiritual care as it impacts medical decisions, and it only further emboldens a spirituality of immanence in dominating medicine's values and structures because it minimizes the voices of religious particularists.

Issue 3: Generic Versus Tradition-Constituted Spirituality

A third issue regards the nature of spirituality and religion as it relates to definitions discussed in Chapter 8. Skeptics and religious particularists recognize the historic and communal dimensions of spirituality, identifying it as a phenomenon seen in the world's religions. By contrast, spiritual generalists advocate for spirituality that exists prior to and independent of religion, emphasizing human purpose, meaning-making, and connectedness.[27] This broadens the locus of spirituality to include all people, including those who have no identification with any of the major world religions. From this perspective, all seek purpose and connectedness but not necessarily through one of the world's religions. This broadening also includes most, if not all, forms of meaning-making, in that all meanings are deemed valid, not only on legal grounds, but also morally and ontologically.

If spirituality is defined as "meaning-making," then advocates tend to deemphasize the importance of which particular meaning and instead underscore the positive presence of any meaning. One patient may find meaning in God, another in their children, and another patient may find his highest meaning in being able to watch another college football season. The content of one's meaning is relativized, whereas the general category of meaning is accentuated as it pertains to spiritual care. Within the medical system, patient meaning-making is affirmed, and the presuppositions supporting this affirmation include that meaning-making is inherently subjective, unverifiable through external or objective means, and thus unavailable for outside criticism precisely because of its subjectivity. Who are we to judge another's meaning? On what grounds can one's subjective meaning-making criticize another's?

The genius of this strategy is that allows religious people to pursue their goals within medicine, such as pursing a Higher Power, as well as allowing those with humanistic and nontheistic meaning systems to pursue their chosen ends and goals. Sociologist Wendy Cadge describes it as a "strategically vague frame."[33] [p. 195] There has been a growing segment of Americans that do not self-identify with a religion but describe themselves as "spiritual not religious"—estimated in 2012 to be 18% of the population.[57] [p. 22] Strengths of generic spirituality include that it taps into this growing movement in the United States, and it serves as a strategy in navigating issues of church and state. As medicine in its institutions and professions has become increasingly uneasy about particular religious identities or expressions, and skeptics advocate for a medicine–religion separation[58] (an extension of the separation of church and state, particularly salient after the flood of federal monies into healthcare after the establishment of Medicare in 1964[59]), spiritual generalists attempt to bypass this political and legal quagmire by arguing for a broader construct of transcendent belief.

Despite the strengths of generic spirituality there remain two critical problems that undermine this strategy for rapprochement: problems of definition and the exclusion of certain theologies.

Generic Spirituality and Definitional Problems

The first concern with generic spirituality is that it is often advocated on a definitional level without the idea of ultimacy and too often in contradistinction with religion. "If spirituality is everything that is good and positive about what is human," noted Bernard McGinn, the renowned University of Chicago scholar of mysticism, "then all it needs is a round of applause rather than cultivation and study."[60] [p. 33]

In a 2014 international consensus conference definition on spirituality, the language of ultimacy was formally incorporated into their definition: *"Spirituality is a dynamic and intrinsic aspect of humanity through which persons seek ultimate meaning, purpose, and transcendence, and experience relationship to self, family, others, community, society, nature, and the significant or sacred. Spirituality is expressed through beliefs, values, traditions, and practices.*"[61] This definition is a positive step forward within the field of spirituality and health as it narrows identification of spirituality to ultimate concern, which is an important correction to the 2009 consensus conference definition.[27,xii] Nevertheless, the 2014 consensus conference definition can be improved in two critical ways.

First, while this may seem overly particular and pedantic, definitions remain fundamental in both a research context and in conceptualizing the nature of medicine. Thus, the phrase "experience relationship to self, family, others, community, society, nature, and the significant or sacred" confuses the object of ultimacy in the definition with the means of expressing ultimacy. As it stands, the definition appears to endorse all human relationships to be spiritual (even if those relationships are not of ultimate concern). This creates the kind of ambiguity that McGinn and others have rightly complained about. A simple solution is to delete the phrase and incorporate this domain into the final sentence so that it reads: spirituality is expressed through beliefs, values, traditions, practices, and *experienced within individual and collective relationships.*

Second, an additional critical correction that is needed within the larger framework of the definition concerns the relationship of spirituality with religion. As argued in Chapter 8, spirituality (including nontheistic spirituality) always produces religious expressions, understood to be the social structures that reflect and reinforce an ultimate concern or chief love. The 2014 consensus conference does little with the concept of religion beside suggesting that spirituality is a larger concept. We suggest that conceptualizing spirituality as generically independent from and non-overlapping with religion creates confusion rather than clarity. Instead, as we argued in Chapter 8, every spirituality instinctively produces religious expressions in belief, practices, and relationships. The 2014 definition begins to recognize this as it concludes that spirituality is "expressed" through various forms. It is this external and collective expression through beliefs, practices, and relationships that brings embodiment and structure to spirituality. Thus, generic spirituality always takes on particular human beliefs, practices, and relationships, and these are functionally religious, even when in the popular perspective its own advocates say it is not a religion. Those who say they are "spiritual, not religious" intend to communicate that they are not of "that type of religion" (e.g., Christianity, Islam, etc.). Those in this category are rejecting certain religious expressions of a particular world religion, but they cannot functionally claim to lack religion themselves in their actual structures. While adopting a popular language that embraces generic spirituality and rejects religion seems prudent in our current political and cultural environment, it is conceptually flawed and bound to eventually fail as a construct.

Rather than adopting a generic spirituality, a better strategy recognizes that every spirituality is constituted by a tradition of ideas, practices, relationships, and communities passed on over time[xiii]—including those collective traditions that idealize individual pursuits of spirituality.[62] Each tradition is centered around and hands down its chief love or ultimate concern. Traditions are unique according to their chief affections and pass on their chief love through methods and practices deemed consistent with that community. Some traditions are more closely aligned than others when their chief love or ultimate concern converges on a similar object or telos. We are then able to categorize certain spiritualities in terms of continuity and discontinuity based on a variety of factors. Some helpfully refer to these patterns in terms of a family resemblance.[16 [p. 46],63] Thus, as we consider rapprochement between American medicine and spirituality, the point of focusing on definitional understandings is that *there is no single phenomenon called spirituality or religion*. Rather, there are spiritualities (objects of chief love), and there are religions (the structures supporting a chief love). As phenomena, some look more alike than others when comparing beliefs, practices, and relationships. It is akin to being sisters or close relatives. What associates each chief love or ultimate concern is the fundamental, centering role they hold in the lives of people.

The implication of these definitions is that a strategy for rapprochement requires dependence on (1) a functional understanding of spirituality and (2) engagement of a variety of tradition-constituted communities without presuming they are the same phenomenon. Thus, spiritual generalists are right to navigate toward functional understandings but underestimate how distinct each spirituality can be when compared to another. Divergent spiritualities should not be collapsed into one another as if they share the same underlying human experience. This is often the mistake of generic spirituality. Moreover, skeptics and religious particularists are correct to highlight the uniqueness and differences between spiritualities, but misstep in favoring substantive definitions rather than functional understandings of spirituality and religion. Future rapprochement needs to combine these two characteristics by incorporating a functional understanding of spirituality and religion while recognizing the uniqueness of each of the world's spiritualities.

Generic Spirituality Is Theologically Exclusive

A second objection to generic spirituality is that while it promotes itself based on its claimed inclusivity and nonjudgmental disposition, it is in actuality a particular theology obfuscated by an apologetics of neutrality. Generic spirituality claims to precede theological beliefs, narratives, and communities,[64] and this implies that it is applicable for both nonreligious patients and a religiously plural patient population. Within patient care, generic spirituality allows the patient to dictate the spiritual ideas, morals, and practices that are most important to the patient. Those who offer spiritual care (chaplains or clinicians) simply follow the patient's lead. This appears neutral, balanced, and atheological, so what is the objection?

Our concern is that there is a theology that undergirds and is coextensive with generic spirituality and its subsequent interfaith approach to spiritual assessment and care.[40] Applying the work of Bevans,[xiv] generic spirituality is characterized by seven theological claims.

1. It is marked by a theology of divine immanence, which locates the ultimate *within* rather than *outside* the world.[xv]
2. It presupposes that human nature and human culture are intrinsically good, and
3. That divine revelation is primarily immanent (located within nature and humanity) rather than primarily transcendent or located outside of nature and mankind.
4. Generic spirituality views any form of divine revelation or scripture to be conditional, not an infallible or inerrant revelation.

5. It holds to a methodological reliance on the human sciences as necessary and autonomous sources for guiding and revising theological claims.
6. It results in a practice that advocates listening to individuals and collective society for the very Word of God, which resides within each person.
7. It elevates the individual's unique and subjective spiritual experience of the divine as holding primary importance.

As evidenced by this list, though spiritual generalists claim that their view of spirituality is theologically neutral and all-encompassing, embedded underneath this claim are particular theological beliefs concerning the nature of God, the self, and the extent of salvation.[40] The theological presuppositions of generic spirituality only become clearer when compared to nonimmanent theologies.[xvi] Thus, the assertion that all spiritual meaning-making systems lead to the same positive goal is one made from within a certain theological perspective that privileges its view of God, the self, and understanding of salvation. Advocates of a generic spirituality do not appear to recognize that there is a significant portion of both US congregations[39] and the population[65] that resists the notion that every path leads up to the same spiritual mountain peak. Our point is not to argue for particularist theologies, but simply to point out that those who champion a generic spirituality adhere to certain theological tenets that result in excluding alternative theological claims.[xvii] Thus, on its own terms, a generic spirituality strategy fails to include all meaning-making systems.

Rather than solving the problem of pluralism, generic spirituality alienates the claims and practices held by particular religious communities. While generic spirituality attempts to broaden the spectrum of meaning-making to include nonreligious meaning-making systems, it introduces particular theological views that are in tension with many traditional religious values. Upon equating all meaning-making systems regardless of content, universal spirituality distances certain religious communities who are ironically the strongest partners to a future rapprochement of medicine and spirituality.

To be clear, we believe that advocates of generic spirituality should have every opportunity to engage with medicine and patients because it is an important theological position. However, it is only one theological view, and it is a position often misrepresented within the medical community as a solution to the problems of pluralism because it claims to encompass all spiritual traditions. However, it is in fact closed to other theological views, even those that are majority positions among clergy in the United States.[xviii]

The possibility of neutrality in spiritual care, while an incredibly alluring idea given the structural tensions raised by pluralism, is not achieved through this construct. If rapprochement is going to occur between medicine and spirituality, we are not convinced that this is a strategy that will achieve that end. In order to realize rapprochement, each religious tradition must be enabled to have its own engagement with medicine's beliefs and structures, lest each tradition be truncated into a form of belief or practice that is less than what it espouses. Otherwise, religion is restrained through generic spirituality by being transformed into something less than what each tradition claims. True rapprochement with medicine must include religious traditions in their fullness.

Conclusion

In this chapter, we outlined how current rapprochement strategies for medicine and spirituality are in tension with three distinct constituencies. In order to realize rapprochement, each constituency needs to compromise in a fashion that does not harm the core values of each. Skeptics need to compromise in allowing religion back into the culture of medicine in some form of real partnership. If there were a way to do this in a pluralistic fashion, skeptics would gain by having an alliance with the social force of religions, which may alone carry the capability of holding in check a market economy and bureaucratic forces unleashed. Spiritual generalists should move away from insisting that generic spirituality be accepted by all while still having a place at the table to advocate for their particular view. Distancing the movement of spirituality and health from religion provides a few short-term gains, but it is an approach that from its start cannot bring meaningful transformation to the powers of medicine. Religious particularists need to embrace a functional definition of religion, a willingness to accept an alliance with religious traditions other than their own, and the importance of empirical research of spirituality and religion. While finding common ground among these diverse groups is challenging given our current social context, new strategies are necessary for rapprochement to take place. In the next chapter, we propose an alternative strategy called *structural pluralism*. Here, we identify a way forward that could align these three constituencies and, by doing so, enable stronger resistance to social and economic forces heading toward impersonal medicine and a move toward a medical ethos that socializes clinicians to engage patients' spiritual needs within serious illness.

Notes

i. Readers may find that their own views do not completely correspond with any one constituency described here. These are ideal types, not well-formed groups. Indeed, our own position is that all three constituencies are missing important elements contained in the other positions. Thus, the point of this chapter is to argue for a new way.

ii. Shuman and Meador conclude similarly about instrumental uses of religion for health: "That is, they are advocating a *particular religion*—albeit one that is vaguely defined and nontraditional—with its own particular account of the ends of human life and its own implicit doctrine of God, humanity, and the rest of creation."[16 [p. 40]]

iii. Religious coping "is primarily concerned with the promotion of medical, psychological, and sociological intervention to assist patients in becoming or remaining functional within their society."[15 [p. 244]]

iv. Another example of this is a study associating spiritual care and costs in the last week of life (see T. Balboni et al. Support of cancer patients' spiritual needs and associations with medical care costs at the end of life. *Cancer*. 2011;117(23):5383–5391). The same data could interpret religion using instrumental or intrinsic perspectives. An instrumental view would argue that if medical teams provide spiritual care, then the cost of medicine would decrease. Spiritual care serves economic purposes. An intrinsic view argues that neglect of spiritual care leads to increased costs, which implies that when an important aspect of care is avoided, then this carries negative consequences, even within the economic realm. The first argues that clinicians should do spiritual care for the sake of lower costs. The latter argues, as this work does, that since spiritual care is intrinsic to good patient care, costs increase significantly when essential elements of care are neglected. The same data produce either interpretation. We agree with others that instrumental rationalities should be vigorously avoided because of their tendency to distort. But this does not lead to avoiding empirical research in spirituality and health.

v. For example, Rumbold concludes, "contemporary models of spiritual care must avoid assimilation to health service models even while accepting that a cost of incorporating spiritual care in healthcare is a degree of conceptual narrowing and functional application of spiritual insights" (see Bruce Rumbold, Models of spiritual care. In: Mark Cobb Christina Puchalski, Bruce Rumbold, eds. *Oxford textbook of spirituality and healthcare.* New York: Oxford; 2012: 182.).

vi. Articles advocating a professionalized healthcare chaplaincy include: Tim Ford and Tartaglia, Alexander. The development, status, and future of healthcare chaplaincy. *Southern Med J.* 2006;99: 675–79; Larry VandeCreek and Burton, Laurel. Professional chaplaincy: its role and importance in healthcare. *Journal of Pastoral Care* 2001(55):81–97. Sociological study observing professionalization tendencies includes Raymond de Vries et al. Lost in translation: the chaplain's role in health care. *Hastings Center Report* 2008;38:23–27.

vii. For purposes of our argument, this book's focus is not on specialized professional spiritual caregivers such as hospital chaplains. Advocates of the division-of-labor approach may find the absence of a focus on chaplaincy problematic, but this would be to misunderstand our argument. It is generally a noncontroversial point to believe that community clergy and hospital chaplains should be deeply involved in the spiritual care of patients. This is certainly the case. Instead, the focus of our argument is on the role of clinicians in providing spiritual care, primarily physicians and nurses, since it is they who are on the frontlines of medicine and who have the most regular interactions with patients facing serious illness. Our argument is not intended to undermine the critical role of clergy or chaplains.

viii. While we concur with efforts in doing empirical research of spirituality and religion in medicine, the motivations and the context behind the research are essential. Motivations to improve the application of pastoral care to patients so that spiritual care is both theologically sound and so that it yields spiritual transformation are excellent motives for empirical research. But the current effort for chaplaincy research appears to be motivated by a desire to establish chaplaincy as a profession and prove that spiritual care is important to medicine and healthcare. This serves as a practical illustration showing how inherent versus instrumental approaches to spirituality differ. Using research to prove the value of chaplains or their work will prove to be disastrous for spiritual care if the goal is to establish chaplaincy and receive financial reimbursement. Instead, the aim must be focused exclusively on improving the interactions among theology, pastoral care, and patient spiritual growth and transformation.

ix. See *Lumen Gentium: Dogmatic Constitution on the Church* for a post–Vatican II Catholic approach, which sees the laity within terms of a more general priestly role.

x. In one study, 85% of cancer patients reported to have had at least one religious or spiritual need. The same study reported that 53% were seeking a closer connection with God, 47% were seeking forgiveness, and 28% felt abandoned by God. See Sara A. Alcorn et al. "If God wanted me yesterday, I wouldn't be here today": religious and spiritual themes in patients' experiences of advanced cancer. *J Palliative Med.* May 2010:581–88.

xi. One example of a third-party approach is the Healthcare Chaplaincy Network located in New York City. This organization provides some administrative and staff chaplaincy services to hospitals around New York. This can be a financial model that offers financial independence of individual chaplains from the hospital institutions where they serve while still enabling for highly trained pastoral presence. This third-party model also cuts down on administrative costs for each hospital organization.

In addition, religious denominations can begin to heal the breach that exists between medicine and spirituality by providing personnel and resources in this area. For example, the Roman Catholic Archdiocese of Boston employs several priests who work as chaplains in some of Boston's largest academic hospitals. This is one example of how religious groups can take financial responsibility in providing spiritual care. In this example, these Catholic chaplains work primarily for a religious organization even as they work closely with hospital administrators.

xii. The 2009 palliative care consensus conference definition did not capture this critical qual-ification of "ultimacy," which leaves spirituality as a vague and unidentifiable concept. By contrast, while our functional understanding of spirituality in Chapter 8 is much broader than only the major world religions, ours emphasizes that spirituality is concerned with what is "chief" or "ultimate" and on which a person centers life. In contrast, it is problematic and confusing to define spirituality as human purpose, meaning-making, or connectedness without also indicating that these refer to the primary and most central purposes, meanings, or connections for a person. The object of meaning or purpose must hold an ultimate role lest spirituality have no conceptual anchor. Thus, while "ultimate concern" can refer to any object or person, thus making it broader than only the major world religions, it is also quite specific because it must be an object functioning at the very center of a person's life and qualifying it as spiritual. Proponents of generic spirituality need to include an adjective such as "ultimate," "chief," or "primary" to avoid vague and unhelpful definitions. This 2014 international defini-tion moves in the right direction.

xiii. It is helpful to recall Alsdair MacIntyre's definition of tradition: "A living tradition then is a historically extended, socially embodied argument, and an argument precisely in part about the goods which constitute that tradition."[62 [p. 222]]

xiv. Theologian Stephen Bevans suggests that there are two basic theological orientations to-ward the issue of human experience, spirituality, revelation, and context: a creation-centered and a redemption-centered perspective. The creation-centered perspective is akin to generic spirituality and oriented around what it means to be human (*anthropos*). The term *anthropos* highlights the goodness and potentiality of every person with the consequence that "theology chiefly involves attending and listening to that situation so that God's hidden presence can be manifested" (Stephen B. Bevans. Models of contextual theology. Rev. and expanded ed. Maryknoll, N.Y.: Orbis Books; 2002., p. 55). *Anthropos* also relies heavily on the social sciences that are fundamentally orientated around the study of human relationships and meaning.

xv. Grenz and Olson define divine immanence to refer to the reality that "God is present to crea-tion. . . . The divine one is active within the universe, involved with the processes of the world and of human history" (Stanley Grenz, Olson Roger E. 20th Century theology : God & the world in a transitional age. Downers Grove, Ill.: InterVarsity Press; 1992, p. 11).

xvi. A countercultural (or nonimmanent) theological model to spiritual care emphasizes (1) a the-ology marked by divine transcendence and that rationality is primarily tradition-mediated; (2) that human nature and culture are primarily sinful and broken; (3) the completeness of divine revelation; (4) a view of the human sciences, human experience, and context as sub-ordinate to a religious tradition; (5) the primary importance of the practice of repentance because of human sinfulness; and (6) the place for community in offering truth claims for the wider world.

xvii. For example, this is seen most easily when exclusivist understandings of religious salvation govern the type of spiritual care offered, even in a nonreligious hospital or clinic. In this context, worries concerning an inappropriate proselytism—promotion of a particular reli-gious faith without patient consent or agreement to engage in spiritual conversation with knowledge of the clinician's framework—are understandably disconcerting. But a theological hegemony is also present, for example, though much less conspicuous, with those who view salvation as a subjective, nonhistorical, interior reality. Pluralistic theologies of salvation equally exert a theological hegemony over the structure of spiritual care. The irony is that generic spirituality excludes exclusivist theologies within spiritual care.

xviii. Why should medical leaders care about so-called fundamentalist theologies, which are passé and include only a small portion of the population? In fact, religious data from around the world indicate that most people are religious exclusivists.[9 [p. 254, n. 257]] While in the United States approximately 29% agree that only their faith is the right way, these percentages in-crease to about half when people negatively evaluate specific religious groups. This suggests that the religious exclusivist position is far more common than often recognized. Yet even if exclusivist positions represented a small portion of the population, a culturally sensitive approach to spiritual care of patients should attempt to make space for such groups. Moreover, exclusivist positions are not a small minority but in fact comprise a majority of congregations in the United States. Pluralistic theologies, which attempt to speak for all religious groups, alienate some of the largest religious communities in the United States. Such alienation privileges one theology over another.

One example illustrating how generic spirituality excludes is by focusing on American black Christians and white Evangelicals, who make up more than 40% of the US population and comprise approximately 53% of all US clergy.[39] Despite comprising a majority of US clergy, these two groups alone constitute only 14% of hospital chaplains in the United States.[33] [p. 48] While there are multiple reasons that explain why the largest religious groups are significantly underrepresented among hospital chaplains, a likely reason is that black and white evangelical ministers are dissuaded from joining or are rejected by hospital chaplaincy because of the chaplain's professional commitment to not proselytize (VandeCreek and Burton, Professional chaplaincy). Understandably, many argue that proselytization of patients is ethically problematic because patients are vulnerable and their abilities to resist spiritual manipulation are decreased because of their illness (see Daniel P. Sulmasy. Ethical principles for spiritual care. In: Mark Cobb Christina Puchalski, Bruce Rumbold, eds. Oxford textbook of spirituality in healthcare. New York: Oxford University Press; 2012:465–470). But the alternatives are not as clear as sometimes supposed.

Clearly this is an important issue in pastoral care, even if well-intended clergy may push a patient to a spiritual place that the patient does not desire. While a nonproselytizing policy offers an important protection for patients, it has become a professional norm that is inconsistent with an approach that believes all meaning-making systems are valid. Generic spirituality explicitly invalidates certain spiritual viewpoints to create spiritual safe places for patients no matter their tradition. The irony in this position, however, is that it excludes a majority of clergy whose traditions reject pluralistic views of salvation. Setting aside debate on whether Evangelical and conservative Black ministers are wrong concerning proselytism, our point is that generic spirituality is not a neutral spiritual care policy, but is informed by certain theological beliefs that exclude ministers who believe in the centrality of spreading their good news. This challenges the notion that universal spirituality is, in practice, broader than the construct of religion. The rubric of universal spirituality appears to be broad in its claims but, in practice, it excludes religious viewpoints that do not agree with its theological pluralism.

References

1. D. T. Kim, Curlin F. A., Wolenberg K. M., Sulmasy D. P. Back to the future: The AMA and religion, 1961–1974. *Acad Med.* 2014;89(12):1603–1609.
2. Michael J. Balboni, Peteet John R. *Spirituality and religion within the culture of medicine: from evidence to practice.* New York: Oxford University Press; 2017.
3. Najmeh Jafari Marta Herschkopf, Christina Puchalski. Religion and spirituality in medical education. In: M. Balboni, Peteet J., eds. *Spirituality and religion in the culture of medicine.* New York: Oxford University Press; 2017:195–214.
4. Mark Cobb, Puchalski Christina M., Rumbold Bruce D. *Oxford textbook of spirituality in healthcare.* Oxford: Oxford University Press; 2012.
5. National Cancer Institute. *Spirituality in cancer care.* 2011; http://www.cancer.gov/cancertopics/pdq/supportivecare/spirituality/HealthProfessional/page1. Accessed August 8, 2011.
6. National Consensus Project. *NCP clinical practice guidelines for quality palliative care.* 2013; Third Edition:http://ww.nationalconsensusproject.org/guideline.pdf. Accessed March 28, 2013.
7. Joint Commission. 3.7.0.0 ed: E-dition; 2013:PC.02.02.13.

8. Richard P. Sloan. *Blind faith: the unholy alliance of religion and medicine.* 1st ed. New York: St. Martin's Press; 2006.

9. Miroslav Volf. *Flourishing: why we need religion in a globalized world.* New Haven, CT: Yale University Press; 2016.

10. Pew Research Center. *Religious landscape study.* 2015; http://www.pewforum.org/religious-landscape-study/. Accessed October 1, 2016.

11. Herbert Benson, Proctor William. *Beyond the relaxation response: how to harness the healing power of your personal beliefs.* New York: Times Books; 1984.

12. Herbert Benson, Stark Marg. *Timeless healing: the power and biology of belief.* New York: Scribner; 1996.

13. Larry Dossey. *Prayer is good medicine: how to reap the healing benefits of prayer.* 1st ed. San Francisco, CA: Harper San Francisco; 1996.

14. Dale A. Matthews, Clark Connie I. *The faith factor: proof of the healing power of prayer.* New York: Viking; 1998.

15. Jeffrey Paul Bishop. *The anticipatory corpse: medicine, power, and the care of the dying.* Notre Dame, IN: University of Notre Dame Press; 2011.

16. Joel James Shuman, Meador Keith G. *Heal thyself: spirituality, medicine, and the distortion of Christianity.* New York: Oxford University Press; 2003.

17. Jeffrey P. Bishop. Biopsychosociospiritual medicine and other political schemes. *Christian bioethics: Non-Ecumenical Studies in Medical Morality.* 2009;15(3):254–276.

18. Daniel P. Sulmasy. *The rebirth of the clinic: an introduction to spirituality in health care.* Washington, DC: Georgetown University Press; 2006.

19. Kelly M. Trevino, Pargament Kenneth I. Medicine, spirituality, religion, and psychology. In: M. Balboni, Peteet J., eds. *Spirituality and religion within the culture of medicine: from evidence to practice.* New York: Oxford University Press; 2017:233–262.

20. Kenneth I. Pargament. *The psychology of religion and coping: theory, research, practice.* New York: Guilford Press; 1997.

21. Tyler J. Vanderweele. Religion and health: a synthesis. In: M. Balboni, Peteet J., eds. *Spirituality and religion within the culture of medicine: from evidence to practice.* New York: Oxford University Press; 2017:357–401.

22. H. G. Koenig, Pearce M. J., Nelson B., Erkanli A. Effects on daily spiritual experiences of religious versus conventional cognitive behavioral therapy for depression. *J Relig Health.* 2016;55(5):1763–1777.

23. John Swinton, Mowatt Harriet. *Practical theology and qualitative research.* London: SCM; 2006.

24. Gary B. Ferngren. *Science and religion: a historical introduction.* 2nd ed. Baltimore: Johns Hopkins University Press; 2017.

25. Stephen Pattison. *The challenge of practical theology: selected essays.* London; Philadelphia: Jessica Kingsley Publishers; 2007.

26. M. Therese Lysaught. Beguiling religion: the bifurcations and biopolitics. In: J. Levin, Meador K., eds. *Healing to all their flesh.* West Conshocken, PA: Templeton Press; 2012:150–187.

27. C. Puchalski, Ferrell B., Virani R., Otis-Green S., Baird P., Bull J., Chochinov H., Handzo G., Nelson-Becker H., Prince-Paul M., Pugliese K., Sulmasy D. Improving the quality of spiritual care as a dimension of palliative care: the report of the Consensus Conference. *J Palliat Med.* 2009;12(10):885–904.

28. S. G. Post, Puchalski C. M., Larson D. B. Physicians and patient spirituality: professional boundaries, competency, and ethics. *Ann Intern Med.* 2000;132(7):578–583.

29. A. B. Astrow, Puchalski C. M., Sulmasy D. P. Religion, spirituality, and health care: social, ethical, and practical considerations. *Am J Med.* 2001;110(4):283–287.

30. B. Lo, Ruston D., Kates L. W., Arnold R. M., Cohen C. B., Faber-Langendoen K., Pantilat S. Z., Puchalski C. M., Quill T. R., Rabow M. W., Schreiber S., Sulmasy D. P., Tulsky J. A. Discussing religious and spiritual issues at the end of life: a practical guide for physicians. *JAMA.* 2002;287(6):749–754.

31. G. Handzo, Koenig H. G. Spiritual care: whose job is it anyway? *South Med J.* 2004;97(12):1242–1244.

32. Christina M. Puchalski, Ferrell Betty. *Making health care whole: integrating spirituality into health care.* West Conshohocken, PA: Templeton Press; 2010.

33. Wendy Cadge. *Paging God: religion in the halls of medicine.* Chicago; London: University of Chicago Press; 2012.

34. P. J. Choi, Curlin F. A., Cox C. E. "The patient is dying, please call the chaplain": the activities of chaplains in one medical center's intensive care units. *J Pain Symptom Manage.* 2015;50(4):501–506.

35. H. H. Gerth, C. Wright Mills. *From Max Weber: essays in sociology.* New York: Oxford University Press; 1946.

36. J. J. Sanders, Chow V., Enzinger A. C., Lam T. C., Smith P. T., Quinones R., Baccari A., Philbrick S., White-Hammond G., Peteet J., Balboni T. A., Balboni M. J. Seeking and accepting: US clergy theological and moral perspectives informing decision making at the end of life. *J Palliat Med.* 2017;20(10):1059–1067.

37. V. T. LeBaron, Cooke A., Resmini J., Garinther A., Chow V., Quinones R., Noveroske S., Baccari A., Smith P. T., Peteet J., Balboni T. A., Balboni M. J. Clergy views on a good versus a poor death: ministry to the terminally ill. *J Palliat Med.* 2015;18(12):1000–1007.

38. V. T. LeBaron, Smith P. T., Quinones R., Nibecker C., Sanders J. J., Timms R., Shields A. E., Balboni T. A., Balboni M. J. How community clergy provide spiritual care: toward a conceptual framework for clergy end-of-life education. *J Pain Symptom Manage.* 2016;51(4):673–681.

39. M. J. Balboni, Sullivan A., Enzinger A. C., Smith P. T., Mitchell C., Peteet J. R., Tulsky J. A., VanderWeele T., Balboni T. A. US clergy religious values and relationships to end-of-life discussions and care. *J Pain Symptom Manage.* 2017;53(6):999–1009.

40. M. J. Balboni. A theological assessment of spiritual assessments. *Christian Bioethics.* 2013;19(3):313–331.

41. M. J. Balboni. Everyday religion in hospitals. *Society.* 2015;52(5):413–417.

42. M. J. Balboni, Babar A., Dillinger J., Phelps A. C., George E., Block S. D., Kachnic L., Hunt J., Peteet J., Prigerson H. G., VanderWeele T. J., Balboni T. A. "It depends": viewpoints of patients, physicians, and nurses on patient-practitioner prayer in the setting of advanced cancer. *J Pain Symptom Manage.* 2011;41(5):836–847.

43. M. J. Balboni, Sullivan A., Amobi A., Phelps A. C., Gorman D. P., Zollfrank A., Peteet J. R., Prigerson H. G., Vanderweele T. J., Balboni T. A. Why is spiritual care infrequent at the end of life? Spiritual care perceptions among patients, nurses, and physicians and the role of training. *J Clin Oncol.* 2013;31(4):461–467.

44. T. Gordon, Mitchell D. A competency model for the assessment and delivery of spiritual care. *Palliat Med.* 2004;18(7):646–651.

45. G. F. Handzo. Best practices in professional pastoral care. *South Med J.* 2006;99(6):663–664.

46. G. Fitchett, Risk J. L. Screening for spiritual struggle. *J Pastoral Care Counsel.* 2009;63(1-2):4-1–12.

47. C. Puchalski, Romer A. L. Taking a spiritual history allows clinicians to understand patients more fully. *J Palliat Med.* 2000;3(1):129–137.

48. J. A. Roberts, Brown D., Elkins T., Larson D. B. Factors influencing views of patients with gynecologic cancer about end-of-life decisions. *Am J Obstet Gynecol.* 1997;176(1 Pt 1):166–172.

49. G. A. Silvestri, Knittig S., Zoller J. S., Nietert P. J. Importance of faith on medical decisions regarding cancer care. *J Clin Oncol.* 2003;21(7):1379–1382.

50. K. E. Steinhauser, Christakis N. A., Clipp E. C., McNeilly M., McIntyre L., Tulsky J. A. Factors considered important at the end of life by patients, family, physicians, and other care providers. *JAMA.* 2000;284(19):2476–2482.

51. T. A. Balboni, Balboni M., Enzinger A. C., Gallivan K., Paulk M. E., Wright A., Steinhauser K., VanderWeele T. J., Prigerson H. G. Provision of spiritual support to patients with advanced cancer by religious communities and associations with medical care at the end of life. *JAMA Intern Med.* 2013;173(12):1109–1117.

52. T. A. Balboni, Paulk M. E., Balboni M. J., Phelps A. C., Loggers E. T., Wright A. A., Block S. D., Lewis E. F., Peteet J. R., Prigerson H. G. Provision of spiritual care to patients with

advanced cancer: associations with medical care and quality of life near death. *J Clin Oncol.* 2010;28(3):445–452.

53. A. C. Phelps, Maciejewski P. K., Nilsson M., Balboni T. A., Wright A. A., Paulk M. E., Trice E., Schrag D., Peteet J. R., Block S. D., Prigerson H. G. Religious coping and use of intensive life-prolonging care near death in patients with advanced cancer. *JAMA.* 2009;301(11):1140–1147.

54. Stephen Pattison. Dumbing down the spirit. In: H. Orchard, ed. *Spirituality in health care contexts.* Philadelphia: Jessica Kingsley Publishers; 2001:33–46.

55. T. A. Balboni, Vanderwerker L. C., Block S. D., Paulk M. E., Lathan C. S., Peteet J. R., Prigerson H. G. Religiousness and spiritual support among advanced cancer patients and associations with end-of-life treatment preferences and quality of life. *J Clin Oncol.* 2007;25(5):555–560.

56. John D. Inazu. *Confident pluralism: surviving and thriving through deep difference.* Chicago; London: University of Chicago Press; 2016.

57. Pew Research Center. *"Nones" on the rise.* 2012. http://www.pewforum.org/2012/10/09/nones-on-the-rise. Accessed May 14, 2018.

58. N. Scheurich. Reconsidering spirituality and medicine. *Acad Med.* 2003;78(4):356–360.

59. G. B. Risse, Balboni M. J. Shifting hospital-hospice boundaries: historical perspective on the institutional care of the dying. *Am J Hosp Palliat Care.* 2013;30(4):325–330.

60. Bernard McGinn. The letter and the spirit: spirituality as an academic discipline. In: E. Dreyer, Burrows M. S., eds. *Minding the spirit: the study of Christian spirituality.* Baltimore: Johns Hopkins University Press; 2005:25–41.

61. C. M. Puchalski, Vitillo R., Hull S. K., Reller N. Improving the spiritual dimension of whole person care: reaching national and international consensus. *J Palliat Med.* 2014;17(6):642–656.

62. Alasdair C. MacIntyre. *After virtue: a study in moral theory.* 2nd ed. Notre Dame, IN: University of Notre Dame Press; 1984.

63. Doug Oman. Defining religion and spirituality. In: R. F. Paloutzian, Park C. L., eds. *Handbook of the psychology of religion and spirituality.* New York: Guilford Press; 2013:23–47.

64. Peter H. Van Ness. *Spirituality and the secular quest.* New York: Crossroad; 1996.

65. US Religions Landscape Survey. 2008; http://religions.pewforum.org/maps. Accessed August 1, 2011.

15

Structural Pluralism for Medicine and Religion

Introduction

We have attempted to show that a spirituality of immanence plays an important role in limiting patients' receipt of spiritual care within serious illness and in silencing traditional religions that have significant capacity to push back against impersonal social forces in medicine. Immanence has gained hegemony over these other spiritualities within medicine based in its claims of religious neutrality. Yet we have concluded that expectations that the medical profession remains neutral toward spirituality and religion[1] is itself a blind faith. It is blind to the cultural dynamics in which care for the sick, rather than being morally or spiritually neutral,[2,i] produces religious-like values and phenomena as described in Part II. Neutrality is not possible when existential questions of human finitude and mortality are at stake and when most patients actively seek to discuss such questions with their clinicians.

In this penultimate chapter, we reimagine the possibilities for partnership between traditional religious communities and medicine. Rather than accept the domination of immanence or advocate for problematic rapprochement strategies (as discussed in Chapter 14), we underscore three building blocks for a future partnership that we call *structural pluralism*. This form of pluralism upholds the tradition-dependent nature of spirituality and spiritual care, maintains that spirituality in medicine must protect religious freedom against all forms of spiritual coercion, and identifies an incremental and scientific manner in which to move from the structures of immanence to pluralism.

This chapter points to ways that American medicine and multiple religious traditions can find better synergy and agreement. There are no simple solutions, but, as we look to the decades ahead, we suggest that a new structural pluralism that honors tradition-based differences is essential for medicine to flourish in America in the twenty-first century.

From Immanence to Pluralism

If our larger argument concerning how secular medicine resembles religious-like values, structures, and goals (see Chapters 9–12) holds some merit, then future directions should move away from discussions of "rapprochement" between medicine and religion. Rapprochement assumes an existing separation. But as the dominant spirituality, immanence continues a structural exclusivism over medicine by protecting itself through a "wall of separation" that has become more recently interpreted to be intolerant of structural expressions of traditional religions.[1,3] [p. 9] Yet discussions of "separation" or "rapprochement" can be misleading because they are based on problematic understandings of religion. These definitions blind viewers from seeing the functional presence of spirituality in the form of immanence already in operation. Since immanence itself operates as a functional spirituality in the absence of traditional religion, our discourse should shift away from discussions of rapprochement and refocus on structural pluralism as the pathway forward for secular medical organizations and clinical professions.

By structural pluralism within medicine we refer to a conscious organization of coexistence and toleration within shared medical structures of different religions, moral systems, and worldviews. If employed within medicine, then "multiple spiritual and cultural traditions (e.g., Jewish, Buddhist, Secular humanist, Native American, Christian, etc.) would have equal opportunity to shape their own 'plausibility structures' and their particular practices related to patient care."[4] [p. 1594] This type of pluralism guarantees freedom of conscience and "equal voice in running the affairs of common public life."[5] [p. 141] Pluralism is not merely the fact of social difference or extending cultural sensitivity to a minority, but, as Diana Eck has argued in her Harvard-led Pluralism Project,[ii] it includes engagement of that diversity by seeking understanding through dialogue and encountering the commitments of others within relationships.[6,7] Pluralism itself is not necessarily an ideal to be celebrated,[iii] but rather a social compromise between moral strangers[8] who, despite best efforts to find consensus through overlapping reason,[9] recognize the incommensurability of distinct traditions of rationality and action.[10] [p. 222],[11]

Structural pluralism seeks to avoid imposing a single good over communities of people who deeply contest the meaning, purpose, and ethics of medicine. Thus, rather than creating a wall of separation between church and state, the better ideal within liberal democracies is to morally enable varying spiritual interpretations of a particular good and to call for state impartiality toward those moral and religious views.[12] [pp. 115–116] Political pluralism has been rooted in Western religious history as it upholds the freedom of religion, the moral value of all citizens, the separation of religion and rule, and the impartiality of the state.[5] [pp. 134–135] Yale theologian Miroslav Volf has also recently shown how religious exclusivists (i.e., those believing that their religion is the only right belief system) nevertheless have been and continue to be strong proponents of political pluralism.[5] [pp. 155–160] This is based on a religious conviction that authentic spirituality comes from the depths of a person's heart, freely given, and not forced through fear of the sword.[iv] While not all religious proponents share these views concerning religious liberty, Volf describes how a great many people from all of the world's religions embrace religious freedom as a social ideal despite many fundamental differences.[5] [pp. 137–160] Against this pluralism are exclusionary viewpoints that silence other claims in what amounts to either religious or secular zeal. Rather than insist on a single view of the good imposed by one group on another, structural pluralism denies the necessity for consensus. Medicine can be simultaneously practiced by a variety of moral and spiritual traditions, and this will include significant overlap in practice but also enable deviation, with no single tradition establishing a norm for others to follow.

Certainly, religious freedom is an ideal shared by most religious and secular people in the United States, one that lays the groundwork for what legal scholar John Inazu calls "confident pluralism."[13] Inazu suggests that this form of pluralism acknowledges that, as a society, we may not come to substantive agreement over deep spiritual, religious, or moral issues, and yet, within our steadfast convictions we may provide equal and adequate toleration within our laws to those with whom we may disagree. This type of pluralism insists on a commitment to share power over social and public structures. It also protects minority views so that dissent is not eclipsed by coercive acts of the majority. Rather, each tradition aspires toward humility and patience even as one endures the views and practices of another tradition considered intolerable or even morally repugnant.[13]

A spirituality of immanence in medicine, however, rejects religious freedom on the structural and collective levels. Immanence locates the free exercise of religion exclusively within the private domain practiced by individuals, especially patients, but the presence of traditional religion is denied on a structural level for many of medicine's organizations, professions, or shared public spaces. Since clinicians are identified more closely with their secular professions, it is argued that in their roles as clinicians, their religious beliefs, moral positions, identities, and spiritual practices should be publicly muted and should remain private.[1,3] This is a structural exclusivism whereby hospitals and clinical professions are "highly partial to one ideology . . . employ[ing] coercive mechanisms to exclude others from participating in public life."[5 [p. 140]] From the secular viewpoint, an exclusion of traditional religion appears impartial and neutral. It is considered neutral because it applies to all the world's religions. However, we have attempted to show in this volume that this position is based on faulty conceptions of the nature of religion (Chapter 8). It also ignores how immanence is religious-like in its view of values (Chapter 9), understanding of personhood (Chapter 10), the analogical structures of medicine (Chapter 11), and its all-too-common willingness to receive reverential, worship-like esteem (Chapter 12). Thus, the structures of American medicine have not been impartial concerning spirituality. Rather, they have marginalized traditional Abrahamic religions and other faiths through problematic claims of structural neutrality, with the result that immanence now holds an exclusive monopoly over social structures both within medicine and throughout society. As American medicine's structures have become increasingly stripped of traditional Jewish, Catholic, and Protestant religious influences over the past two centuries,[14] their absence created a spiritual vacuum filled by immanence. But, rather than achieving impartiality, we now hold to a healthcare system that looks much like the world religions in function, even ironically adopting exclusionary and fundamentalist stances against rival positions. Privatizing spirituality and religion within the context of illness, healing, and dying is not possible.

The current healthcare situation, therefore, calls for new efforts to reimagine our understanding of the relationships among spirituality, religion, and medicine. Reconsideration of this relationship is not merely a tertiary or aesthetic interest, but lies near the heart of what ails medicine in the United States. As described in Chapter 13, pleas to rehumanize medicine will likely fall short without wide support and partnership from the world's religions and, in particular, Catholics, Protestants, and Jews in the United States. The social powers swirling around economics, technology, and bureaucracy are now so daunting that only equally formidable spiritualities, particularly those gathered within strong local communities,[15] hold much chance of countering and realigning impersonal and dehumanizing trends within medicine.

We also understand concerns about spiritual coercion and proselytism. What does structural pluralism imply in regards to proselytism? It views all forms of spiritual engagement that impinges on human freedom or uses external means of coercion or pressure to engender a spiritual conversion as morally intolerable. For example, it would be ethically wrong for a patient to feel threatened by a clinician to "get religion" lest the patient not receive medical attention. It would also be problematic if a patient consented to spiritual care in order to gain some medical advantage or additional privileges with his or her physician. Either negative or positive motivations infringe on the human freedom that spirituality inherently requires, undermining the intrinsic motivations of chief love and ultimate concern that are consistent with spirituality. Spiritual engagement cannot be linked to any strings of external benefit or loss since these extrinsic incentives infringe upon the intrinsic motivations required of spirituality as *ultimate* concern and *chief* love.

The best solution to this issue is "following the patient's lead,"[16 [p. 1640]] which does not eliminate the possibility of mistakes in spiritual care provision[v] but stresses the importance of listening to the patient rather than having a preset agenda. This may then lead to circumstances that involve spiritual discussions across religious traditions (e.g., a Jewish clinician talking to a Christian patient), or prayer led by the clinician, or the clinician initiating a spiritual question or discussion. "Following the patient's lead" means that that clinician must ask about and listen to the patient's faith background before assuming or suggesting any particular kinds of engagement. Prohibitions concerning proselytism are generally correct but also in need of careful nuance depending on what the patient needs and desires. Some discussions fail to recognize spiritual care in terms of a spectrum and balance notions of physician power with a patient's desire for spiritual growth.[17 [p. 467–468]]

Of course, there are also many clinicians who do not have the personal capacity to engage spiritual and religious concerns raised by a patient, and here, too, clinicians must enter into such circumstances without compulsion.[18] Some clinicians may hold strong negative feelings toward some spiritual or moral viewpoints,[18] and it is important that these feelings be accounted for so that these do not interfere with the patient–clinician relationship. For example, a clinician may hold negative feelings toward all traditional religions, making conversations with her patient challenging or emotionally difficult. In such cases, the clinician should involve clergy in the spiritual care of the patient and, when medical decisions are involved, include other medical colleagues who are more comfortable in guiding patients in how their decisions are informed by their faith. Another example is when the patient and clinician hold strongly different religious views. Conversing across religious difference can sometimes be taxing, but, in other instances, it may greatly encourage the patient, even across religious traditions. Following the patient's lead remains the critical principle that should guide clinicians in cases of both spiritual concordance and discordance.

While consensus standards call for medical professionals to inquire about spirituality and religion and refer to others for help,[19] this should not be interpreted to limit engagement when a clinician has greater comfort or knowledge of a particular spiritual tradition or when there is an established level of trust in the relationship that allows for cross-religious engagement. Following the patient's lead is based not in synthetic rules, but in wisdom, respect, and candor.[20] Spiritual inquiry and referral by the clinician is the minimum standard within life-threatening illness. It is not a boundary violation for clinicians to engage spiritually with their patients when the patient desires or expresses need and when consent is freely provided. A boundary violation takes place when spiritual care has not included the patient's voluntary agreement and consent.

Given these protections, how might medicine transition from its current stance of privatization of traditional religion toward its incorporation within the structures of healthcare? Is such a project conceivable? In reimagining the relationship between secular medicine and traditional religion,[vi] future partnership will be marked by three parameters for pluralism to operate. The following is a brief description of each factor.

Tradition-Dependent Spirituality

The first aspect of future partnership is that each spiritual tradition must be permitted to express itself within its own natural, thick way of life, without truncation or reduction.

Communities unsurprisingly form over time around deeply shared loves, many of which are centered on a transcendent object (e.g., God), and other communities are centered on some other perceived *summum bonum*. These communities form traditions of beliefs, practices, and social structures that are intended to facilitate and sustain their chief affection as they are handed down over time to generations that follow. While such communal traditions are not static, as they are influenced by many contingencies, the longest lasting communities appear to survive because of some combination of the intensity of human love, the intensity of encounter with the object of chief affection, and the ability of communities to overcome theoretical and practical difficulties related to their chief love.[10] It is important to understand that these creeds, practices, and experiences develop into thick traditions, carried on by what MacIntyre calls particular living communities,[10,vii] which hold an intermediate position between the individual and the universal.

In light of the thick communal and tradition-dependent nature of spirituality, advocates of pluralism—or, as we termed this ideology in the previous chapter, spiritual generalists—have tended to perpetuate a few misdirections as they discuss engagement of spirituality and medicine. They often promote a form of spirituality that is generic, dehistoricized, and ultimately private. While certainly some spiritualities have a propensity to be individualistic and private, the Abrahamic traditions tend to be totalizing, since they embrace claims that encompass all life, both public and private. Collapsing all the religions into one system disrespects their actual claims and undermines the unitive goal of coexistence.

Consequently, partnership between medicine and spirituality upholds and honors the uniqueness of each spiritual tradition. Between the individual and universal are these thick communal traditions that have wisdom for the practice of medicine and shelter for patients facing serious illness. Thus, a critical parameter to a future pluralism includes protection and acknowledgment of the particularity of each spiritual tradition in its theology, practices, chosen assumptions, and modes for spiritual care. Privatization or generic spirituality does not amount to partnership. Medicine will need to accept each spiritual tradition in its fullness to move toward partnership.

Noncompulsory, Voluntary Arrangements

The second aspect of a pluralistic partnership is that patients and clinicians hold freedom to participate and identify with the spiritual tradition of their choosing, without coercion.

An important counterweight to tradition-specific spirituality is that spirituality and religious affiliation need to be freely and voluntarily chosen by patients and clinicians. Freedom of religious choice and safeguarding against coercive influences is essential for partnership between medicine and spirituality. There is overwhelming consensus on this point both in the medical literature and among most religious thinkers.[19] Few argue that it is part of the common good for a sick person to be confronted by a foreign spiritual tradition that is unforeseen and unwanted while receiving medical care. Patients and clinicians (see Chapters 2–5) suggest that spiritual interactions between patients and clinicians are highly positive experiences on the condition that they are exchanged within a growing clinical relationship and emphasize patients freely sharing their spiritual identities, struggles, and questions in response to a clinician's questions.[21] Spirituality and religion carry multiple benefits for medicine when entered into with relational sensitivity and mutual consent. Spirituality should not be forced, and care is necessary to avoid even subtle pressure.

One of the implications of structural pluralism is that it beneficially changes social expectations concerning spirituality and patient consent by removing certain subtle pressures. Clinicians are characterized as neutral toward spirituality within a secular model, but an abundance of counterevidence suggests that moral and spiritual views remain operative among clinicians in patient care, and a spirituality of immanence shapes physician conduct.[2,22,viii] Advocacy of clinician neutrality is not only fictitious and impossible, it also threatens the informed consent process. Patient decision-making is deeply influenced by clinicians' prudential judgments and their spoken and unspoken values. Since bifurcating personal values from professional ones is not truly possible, structural pluralism openly draws attention to each caregiver's moral and spiritual tradition. Thus, when a patient faces a challenging moral or spiritual question related to decision-making (e.g., physician assisted-suicide or considering life-sustaining treatment because of a belief in a miracle), patients' informed consent is better safeguarded when their medical advisors openly disclose their moral and spiritual worldviews. Though this is not a license for physicians to provide medical counsel that solely fulfills their own spiritual needs rather than their patients' needs, the power gap between patients and clinicians is significantly lessened if the clinician's underlying moral and spiritual identity is openly acknowledged. Medical advice, with its potential moral implications, or spiritual care, with its implicit theologies, no longer rests solely on perceived neutral scientific evidence or unbiased values. Patients can more clearly judge a clinician's ethical counsel or spiritual care since clinicians have identified with a particular spiritual tradition with openness and candor.[20] Structural pluralism improves the consent process since it unearths hidden values through up-front disclosure, allowing patients to weigh their clinician's suggestions based within the patient's freely chosen values.

Additionally, structural pluralism creates an equitable sharing in the power structures of medicine concerning ethical issues where moral presuppositions vary significantly and agreement is unlikely. Some have concluded that moral perspectives need to be further eliminated from American clinicians so that they reflect neutrality in their roles as professionals.[23] Yet this advocacy is another example of immanence, upholding its rigid bifurcations and exerting power over alternative moral and spir-itual traditions. In contrast, a pluralistic power structure does not require medical professionals to uniformly practice certain procedures or uphold only certain pre-ferred moral views, but offers multiple spiritual traditions flexibility in how they promote health according to those values that are internally consistent with each tradition's legacy of spiritual care of the sick.[24 [pp. 214-215]] Most worrisomely, without a generous pluralism toward those with whom we disagree, healthcare will remain a major battleground for culture wars. Too much is at stake when moral uniformity is the norm for the medical profession. New medical structures are clearly possible that deescalate our moral disagreements, but this calls for both traditional religious voices to defend the freedom of "unbelievers" to practice moral views they find disagree-able and for secular humanists to protect the varied spiritual positions of religious professionals and institutions. Structural pluralism is consequently a call to share and make room for one another within the social powers of medicine despite incommen-surable difference.

Our general argument should not be construed to suggest that the Abrahamic traditions, particularly Christianity, as the dominant religion in the United States, should get free rein or exert power over patients. We are not arguing for the diminishment of one power (a spirituality of immanence) to reestablish some other spiritual power (Christianity, Judaism, or any world religion). We are not merely arguing for the freedom to constructively engage religion privately within medi-cine, but rather claim that American medicine has become gripped by a religious-like phenomenon that we have called a spirituality of immanence. Our argument is not against patients or clinicians who freely opt to follow the beliefs associated with a spirituality of immanence. Our challenge is not against immanence itself but against its domination and exclusionary power over medicine's structures. In its stead are needed new pluralistic structures across medicine that share power and emphasize freedom between our varied spiritual traditions, from the spirituality of immanence to all the world religions.

But what about a spiritual tradition that insists on proselytizing patients, believing that this is for the person's spiritual good, regardless of whether the patient desires it?[17 [p. 467]] Any viewpoint that insists on using medicine as a pretext for pushing reli-gion on a patient, against the patient's consent, stands in violation as a subversive force to structural pluralism. It is an action against the freedom of religion and should be on its face rejected. For a pluralistic society to flourish, every spiritual tradition must at a minimum affirm the freedom of choice in regard to spirituality and religion.

Likewise, each tradition must "embrace the principle of reciprocity. Whatever rights and privileges they want to claim for themselves, they must grant the same to all others."[5] [p. 192] In regards to medicine, spiritual care can only be offered in response to a patient's desire and free request. Imposing one's belief system in contradistinction to the patient's free request takes wrongful advantage of both the larger pluralistic system and the particular patient. Thus, structural pluralism by necessity must insist on certain basic limits that threaten the freedom and liberty of individuals as well as the prospering of each larger spiritual tradition. One obvious limit to religious freedom is the exclusion of coercive acts of violence or threats of violence against another tradition. For a pluralistic system to operate, all spiritual traditions must reject acts of physical violence or spiritual coercion. Each tradition must also refuse political violence against every other tradition.

There is overwhelming consensus that a non-religious medical context should not be a sphere that fosters unwanted religious conversation or spiritual coercion.[17,19,25] The point is that patients should not be coerced, spiritually manipulated, or subtly threatened in regards to spiritual matters in the medical context. Patients who enter a religiously-affiliated medical institution (e.g., Adventist Health) should reasonably expect that care provided from within that hospital will be shaped by particular religious viewpoints. But within what we today call "secular" hospitals, medicine should be a spiritually safe place for patients. Since many patients desire spiritual encouragement, proper apprehension about spiritual coercion should not result in medicine silencing its clinicians or creating a "spiritual-free zone." Such a result does not create neutral ground, but merely authorizes a spirituality of immanence. Instead, all interactions pertaining to spirituality or religion should be *freely desired* and entered into by the patient and the clinician's free will and consent.[ix] The most fundamental guide concerning spiritual and religious interactions between patients and clinicians must be based on mutual desire and consent to freely participate in spiritual conversation or discussion. Upholding a patient's self-determination and ability to make informed decisions is a correct and necessary principle that undergirds patient spirituality. All forms of spiritual care must be tender, respectful, without self-aggrandizement, and concerned to ensure that both the patient and clinician are not manipulated, coerced, or threatened—thus, enabling the choice to engage in a spiritual interaction or discussion. Spiritual care when offered by clinicians must always be accompanied by mutual consent and agreement. In terms of spirituality, this is the best meaning to the concept of "patient-centered" spiritual care.

Excursus: Concerning the Ethics of Spiritual Care and Proselytism

What does structural pluralism imply in regards to proselytism? It demands that any form of spiritual engagement that impinges on human freedom or uses external means of coercion or pressure to engender a spiritual conversion is morally intolerable. For example, it would be ethically wrong for a patient to feel threatened by a clinician to "get religion" lest the patient not receive medical attention. It would also be problematic if a patient consented to spiritual care to gain some medical advantage or additional privileges with his or her physician. Either negative or positive motivations infringe on human freedom that spirituality inherently requires, undermining the intrinsic motivations of chief love and ultimate concern that are consistent with spirituality. Spiritual engagement cannot be linked to any strings of external benefit or loss since these extrinsic incentives infringe upon the intrinsic motivations required of spirituality as *ultimate* concern and *chief* love.

Concerns that clinicians risk infringing on patient freedom in this area have led to prohibitions that are envisioned to eliminate spiritual coercion and protect patient freedom. These prohibitions have included that clinicians may ask about spirituality and religion but not directly engage it; should avoid cross-religious or interfaith discussions; should not actively lead in practices like prayer; and should insist that the patient, not the clinician, initiate all spiritual interactions. While these prohibitions are well motivated, it is less clear that they ensure patient freedom and may at times undermine it. This issue became clearer to us during the Religion and Spirituality and Cancer Care (RSCC) study, where we noticed that many patients welcomed spiritual interaction with their clinician but then stated that they would never directly ask for spiritual engagement from a nurse or physician. At the same time, clinicians are socialized to neglect spirituality and religion, perhaps since they worry about crossing a perceived professional boundary or perhaps because they are waiting for the patient to bring up the topic. These dynamics foster a huge gap in spiritual care, where the elephant in the room remains sidestepped out of crossed signals and worry of professional reprisal and is further aided by plausibility structures that invite separation (discussed in Chapters 6–7).

The greatest level of consensus among clinicians is "to follow the patient's lead."[16] [p. 1640] "Following the patient's lead" means that that clinician must ask and listen about the patient's faith background before assuming or suggesting any particular kind or level of engagement. Approaching patients in this manner requires, as one study found, an "intuitive, heuristic, case-by-case" approach to spiritual assessment and engagement.[26] [p. 20] This disposition does not guarantee miscues or mistakes, but it is primarily relational compared to stringent policies that cannot account for the particularities of each patient or their peculiar spiritual questions, desires, or needs. Following a patient's lead does not mean that the clinician should wait for the patient to initiate since many patients indicate that they will never make such a request. Clinicians need to rely on their intuitions and be alert to subtle patient cues,[26] and they also need professional permission to pursue spiritual inquiry and engagement when the patient and particular circumstances are weighed. This may then lead to circumstances that involve spiritual discussions across religious traditions (such as our earlier example of a Jewish clinician talking to a Christian patient), or to prayer led by the clinician, or to the clinician initiating a spiritual question or discussion. While consensus standards call for medical professionals to inquire about spirituality and religion and refer to others for help,[19] this should not be interpreted to limit greater engagement when a clinician has greater comfort or knowledge of a particular spiritual tradition or when there is an established level of trust in the relationship that allows for cross-religious engagement. Some patients need and desire a level of spiritual interaction from their clinician, and, in circumstances where clinicians can provide that interaction, it should be welcomed by professional standards, not discouraged by dire warnings.

Clinicians should consider important relational conditions that signal when it is appropriate to ask a spiritual follow-up question, weigh patient–clinician prayer, or engage a patient's spiritual needs. These conditions include the patient's level of vulnerability (e.g., age, mental status, etc.), the length and quality of the clinical relationship, prior history of spiritually related conversations, spiritual concordance between the patient and clinician, and the degree to which a patient freely expresses desire and consent to receive spiritual care from the particular clinician. Each of these are important conditional factors that hold a role in discerning the extent and depth appropriate in the clinical encounter, including engagement over a patient's desire to commit or recommit to a spiritual tradition of his or her choosing. Whenever spiritual care is delivered by the clinician with motivations of personal guilt, with signs of manipulative tactics, or without a patient's freely expressed desire to engage over spiritual issues, then spiritual care, including proselytism, are unethical. However, discussions that equate proselytism directly and without qualification to spiritual coercion are more problematic because they fail to recognize spiritual care in terms of a spectrum, underestimate how illness can be a spiritually illuminating time of clarification and transformation, and misunderstand the nature of clinician power (see note for details[x]).[17] [pp. 467–468] Discussions of proselytism also assume physician neutrality, and thus a move toward structural pluralism would alter the relational dynamics between patients and clinicians because it strengthens patient consent in a process that openly discloses a clinician's spiritual tradition. Thus, conditions within the relationship as well as larger cultural assumptions affect how to consider ethical actions related to spiritual care, including the question of proselytism. Following the patient's lead remains the highest standard for clinical practice, pursued within a matrix of relationship conditions.

Nevertheless, there are also some clinicians who do not have the personal capacity or comfort to engage spiritual and religious concerns raised by a particular patient, and here, too, clinicians must enter into such circumstances without compulsion.[19] Some clinicians may hold strong negative feelings toward some spiritual or moral viewpoints, and it is important that these feelings be accounted for so that these do not interfere with the patient–clinician relationship. Though following the patient's lead remains the critical principle that should guide clinicians in cases of both spiritual concordance and discordance, these interactions are ultimately relational, conditional, and based in the exercise of practical wisdom. Thus, clinician spirituality should also be protected so that they, too, are not placed into a coercive position that transgresses conscience or spiritual comfort. The consensus recommendations call for clinicians to inquire about patient spirituality and then refer to chaplains and clergy.[19] This approach attempts to balance patients' needs as well as protect clinician freedom. Neither patients nor clinicians should be coerced to spiritually engage in ways that transgress their own tradition-specific beliefs or undermine the voluntary nature of spiritual interactions at every level.

Incremental, Structural Change

The third aspect of a future pluralistic partnership is that each spiritual tradition creates its own visible social structures within medicine, which are incrementally developed and publicly accessible through scientific evaluation and understanding.

Upon safeguarding freedom to participate in the spirituality of one's own choosing, genuine partnership will uphold new ways for each spiritual tradition to claim a stake in medicine's plausibility structures, social forces, and processes of socialization. This parameter modifies traditional spiritualities from the private realm to the public. There are two principle reasons for inclusion of structural pluralism in medicine. On a practical level, spiritual care provided by clinicians to patients with life-threatening illness will remain rare without an open public endorsement of traditional spiritualities. There is a strong link between religious privatization and clinicians' willingness to ask their patients about spiritual matters. Spiritual care is infrequent partly because of these structural barriers.[27] Additionally, on a theological and political level, we live in a society that has taken pains to avoid establishing a state-sponsored civil religion. Secular approaches of religious disestablishment have sought to construct neutral public spaces where religious symbols, practices, and rationalities are absent since it is argued that these doctrines and practices do not meet basic standards of freedom and equality among a diverse public of many religions or those who claim none.[9] As we have previously argued, however, secular neutrality is a political position that poorly applies to the context of medicine and serious illness, which are thoroughly intertwined with existential questions and spiritual experiences connected to suffering, fear, and hope. While the plausibility for a sacred–secular division (see Table 7.1) may be suitable in other sectors of American society, it is misapplied to the field of healthcare.

While it is difficult to imagine alternative approaches to our spiritual differences, it is vital to remember that our society has been in constant flux on this issue since the beginning of the American experiment. In her analysis of historical engagements of religious difference, Diana Eck has described distinct episodes of American approaches including exclusivism, assimilation, and pluralism.[6 [pp. 48–77]] In parts of the nineteenth and earlier twentieth centuries, religious minorities encountered deep resistance from a dominant Protestant culture that viewed religious and cultural differences with hostility. Other religions were resisted.[28–30,xi] In the latter half of the twentieth century, assimilation into the "melting pot" eclipsed sheer discrimination. In this approach, religious and cultural differences were generally suppressed by the majority perspective. Religious minorities were welcome, but in exchange for their acceptance they had to become standardized members of society, accepting its assumptions, blending into its ethos, and privatizing those religious convictions not already well-accepted by the mainstream. Within the assimilation model, there has been more recently a greater appreciation for multiculturalism and growing expectations that medical institutions and professions become culturally aware and sensitive to patient needs. Cultural sensitivity is an important and more recent development but operates in terms of an accommodation for patients who express distinct religious and cultural needs outside the dominant ethos of immanence. Yet structural pluralism recognizes that "accommodation" is hardly a partnership. Thus, even the briefest sketch of the American experiment clarifies that pluralism has been a social enterprise with many twists and turns, with the future story remaining unwritten. Purported battle lines drawn separating a secular immanence and religious transcendence are not fixed but can be—and, we argue, should be—innovatively reimagined beyond the sacred–secular division.

What new structures might facilitate authentic partnership is difficult to foresee. Reimagining structural dimensions connected to spirituality should be approached experimentally and, thus, incrementally. As an ally to a future cluster of projects, the scientific method provides a reasonably strong pathway for hypothesis testing, careful measurement, and consensus building between scientific and religious communities in identifying exposure variables and outcomes of greatest interest.[31] As VanderWeele has rightly argued, partnership between medicine and traditional religion will in itself benefit through intense research.[31 [p. 388]] Researching future social structures that facilitate spirituality is not de facto a utilitarian project, at least not when each spiritual tradition is part of the process and shaping its goals. Nor is our proposal about "slipping in religion" under the guise of science or genuflecting to almighty science but instead a genuine partnership, *pace* Gould,[32] between magisterial modes of inquiry that overlap and constructively influence the other. By approaching these questions experimentally, with diverse financial partnership, in shared collection of data, and then in rigorous academic debate around best interpretations, this could emerge as an exemplary process where medical and varied spiritual communities partner under the umbrella of pluralism, with shared control over cultural and structural elements.[xii] This process is the very best chance of breaking the hegemony of immanence as it maintains freedom of and from religion. Structural pluralism decreases the likelihood of ideological disputes and political posturing between traditions with greater opportunity to enjoy equal and proportionally distributed access to power structures.

Creating and testing new medical structures that provide visible opportunity for spiritual traditions to take expression in life-threatening illness are not impossible to imagine. Here, we will provide three brief examples of how structural pluralism might move forward.

Patient–Clinician Religious Concordance

One possible direction of structural pluralism is that it would explore the benefits of systems that facilitated and intentionally created spiritual care encounters of shared beliefs between patients and clinicians. Imagine a spiritual patient who could request her medical care to be offered by a clinician of a concordant faith. This concept is less amendable to operationalize in certain specialty circumstances such as in the intensive care unit or within the emergency department. Yet it does fit within primary care, outpatient clinics, obstetrics, psychiatry, some inpatient hospital circumstances, and palliative and hospice care. For example, we could imagine a primary care practice that facilitates spiritual practices of yoga and mindfulness meditation for patients desiring this component to be part of their regular care. Or imagine an Islamic family medical practice that is sensitive to Islamic sexual ethics for adolescents. Inpatient palliative care units might have specific rooms for patients tailored to different religious faiths such as Catholic or Hindu, and these patients might receive care from nurses and physicians who share the patient's tradition.

Providing patients opportunities to be cared for by clinicians of similar spirituality holds some precedent and carries potential benefits. A growing body of research exists suggesting that patients and physicians who hold identity concordance in areas such as race, sex, and age are positively associated with patients' trust, satisfaction, use of medical services, and involvement in medical decisions.[33-39] Concordance is also associated with patients' identification with physician communication styles.[40] However, concordance is multifactorial and involves both visible (e.g., age, gender, race, and language) and invisible characteristics (e.g., beliefs, attitudes, values, preferences, and role orientations).[33] Given the role that spiritual traditions play in shaping beliefs and values, patient–physician spiritual concordance may likewise influence the patient–physician relationship, though studies have not yet examined this effect of spirituality on the clinical bond.

From the structural pluralism perspective, patients could opt into receiving care from a clinician or team of clinicians who share a certain spiritual identity. Within an inpatient setting, for example, certain patient hospital rooms might use tradition-specific symbols. The patient's experience of time or the daily routine might be reordered according to daily prayers drawn from the patient's tradition. Clinicians who share faith with the patient could be matched with that patient, and, if desired, patient–clinician interactions might naturally include a shared spiritual practice such as prayer,[21] a sacred reading, or deeper conversation over a clinically relevant issue that intersects with patient medical decesions.[4,41] For example, in an outpatient setting, a Roman Catholic patient experiencing major depression within his cancer care might opt to receive mental health care from a psychiatrist who shares the same tradition. Or a Pentecostal patient being treated for head and neck cancer might request a Christian oncologist because she thinks her illness is a part of God's punishment, which is why she doesn't show up for some of her treatments. Or a humanist patient, deeply committed to alternative healing through energy and reliance on crystals, worries she will be judged by physicians and would thus prefer a clinician who also shares in her metaphysical beliefs.[42,xiii] We hypothesize that patient–clinician concordance, when freely entered into by patient and clinician, would increase trust, facilitate greater communication in navigating certain issues of tension between spirituality and healthcare, effect patient satisfaction, reduce physician burnout, and lead to higher spiritual well-being. Some research also suggests that patient–clinician concordance may facilitate spiritual care that impacts medical decision-making and costs.[41,43] While structural pluralism could provide far-reaching new directions in the patient–clinician relationship, an incremental approach nestled within research would safeguard against missteps and allow cultural change to take place gradually in partnership with the benefits of the scientific method.

Structural Space

Another small step in the direction of structural pluralism concerns the design of publicly accessible religious spaces for worship and prayer, such as hospital chapels and the display of religious symbols. Hospital chapels can reinforce the secular–sacred divide if they are interpreted to mean that some space is sacred and medical space is secular. Here, traditions differ as to the purpose of chapels as they relate to the meaning of secular and sacred space. Some traditions may believe that certain spaces are especially hallowed and dedicated for spiritual purposes, whereas other spaces are ordinary and do not hold that sacred meaning. Other traditions reject a stark dichotomy in the interpretation of space, seeing all space as holding a level of sacredness. Following this latter view, some organizations placed religious symbols in public, non-chapel locations, and this signaled a sacredness to the entire sphere, including space, professionals, and patients. The point is that even in the way one interprets the meaning of a chapel space or spiritual symbol, interpretations are tradition-specific and there are no neutral positions. This includes advocates of a spirituality of immanence who assume strict demarcations between sacred and secular space. In rejecting this imposition of a space's meaning, structural pluralism recognizes that each tradition must be granted freedom to implement its own meaning of space as well as carry out its implications. When we move beyond immanence's monopoly of hospital space, pluralism's practical implications are challenging to imagine. Hospital chapels with only one tradition-specific chapel fail the test of pluralism. Likewise, hospitals that have employed multifaith and interfaith chapels fail to be tradition-specific. Not having a chapel only further ensconces the power of immanence. American hospitals have wrestled with how to provide hospital architectural spaces that signal something beyond immanence but also welcome patients and families from multiple religious traditions.[44 [p. 55–76]] There is little consensus on how to solve these differences, especially since the absence of religious symbols is the theological position of immanence.

We would propose that the way toward a solution(s) is through theological imagination and research. Little empirical research or scholarship exists[44–46] on healing spaces or spiritual symbols within a medical setting. Data do not exist concerning the frequency of chapel visits, the importance of their location within a medical center, how chapel spaces are used, or the association between the presence of chapels and potential health outcomes. Nor does research exist on patient desirability or health-related effects of religious symbols in public hospital spaces. Similarly, little is known of how a tradition-specific religious symbol, such as the *Christus Consolator* at Johns Hopkins,[47] affects patients who identify with that symbol in comparison to those who do not. Similarly, it is not clear if multifaith or interfaith chapels are used more frequently or viewed as more welcoming in comparison to tradition-specific chapels. There is also little evidence guiding chapel sizes in proportion to other public spaces in hospitals, such as cafeterias, sitting areas, art galleries, or other shared public spaces. Is patient healing promoted when chapel spaces are small and in discrete locations, or when they are large or central? Do spiritual symbols in public hospital spaces cause encouragement, offense, or indifference? Many American hospitals have provided particular religions proportionally insignificant space, whereas exponentially larger spaces are now expressly given to nonmedical, immanent, aesthetical considerations within contemporary architecture and design. Do hotel-like spaces that have abandoned tradition-specific symbols promote patient healing and wellness? The desirability and impact of these architectural practices are unknown without well-designed research.

From the perspective of structural pluralism, the design, location, and use of chapels and spiritual symbols are a helpful starting point in reimagining space. While many hospital chapel spaces are being renovated away from tradition-specific spaces into multifaith or neutral chapels,[44 [p. 73]] none of these changes is grounded in empirical studies. These changes are based on untested ideology, and this should trouble everyone. Moreover, it is highly doubtful that most religious traditions would opt to create neutral spiritual space or interfaith space since these make it difficult to express one's content-rich viewpoint in a co-shared space of only a few hundred square feet. We hypothesize that the architectural design of hospital chapel spaces matters, especially concerning their location, size, and symbolism, as well as in how well they reflect the associated religious characteristics of the visitor. We hypothesize that the degree of concordance is an important factor related to a person's ability to pursue his or her spiritual goals within that space. We also hypothesize that religious symbols, thoughtfully placed in different parts of a hospital, will be well-received and encouraging. Yet we (and everyone else) are all just guessing until well-designed and executed studies are performed in this area. Based on experimental approaches, multiple permutations of sacred spaces would examine these factors to understand and identify the characteristics of those spaces best suited to facilitate patient and family spiritual, psychological, and physical healing. Within such projects, multiple spiritual traditions, including traditional religious and humanist, would give shape to how this research is carried out and offer future design guidelines for hospital chapels as well as hospital architecture more generally.

Structural pluralism rejects the monopoly of immanence and thus calls for a public conversation that upholds the importance of tradition-specific beliefs and practices, that protects the voluntary nature of spiritual participation, and that engages publically accessible scientific evidence designed to answer questions agreed to by major spiritual traditions. The future design of healing space that is engaged by varied traditions is an area where structural pluralism can be modeled.

Professional Socialization in Medicine

A third example of where structural pluralism may yield important benefits is within medical education and professionalism. Structural pluralism invites medical educators to consider building partnerships with local clergy, hospital chaplains, and religious communities in order to formally consider the implications of spirituality and religion on the practice of medicine. Many clinicians instinctively approach medicine in this way,[48,49] but, with a few exceptions, it is rarely formally embraced within medical education itself.[50]

While immanence tends to marginalize spirituality and religion, or at a minimum circumscribe these to a small dimension of a clinician's competencies, structural pluralism recognizes this as an example of the monopoly of immanence shaping medical education. A pluralistic model, by contrast, recognizes how each tradition idealizes and aims to shape the totality of clinicians from heart, to mind, to hands. Each tradition—Humanism, Islam, Catholicism, and others—idealizes a "good physician" based within a composition of heart (spiritual and moral formation), mind (the knowledge and wisdom necessary to be a healer of persons, including but not limited to medical knowledge), and hands (especially the technical competencies and practical know-how associated with bodily care). Traditions share significant overlaps among these competencies but there are also key differences that pluralism recognizes, expressed especially around topics such as the meaning of compassion[51,52] and approaches around bioethical issues,[22,53] as well as the theological underpinnings connected to the interpretation of illness and healing.[48,xiv]

While many important labors already exist that attempt to provide spiritual support to medical trainees and professional clinicians,[25] most efforts have not yet received formal institutional endorsement and fail to receive research support necessary for change. To our knowledge, few studies have attempted to describe if and how medical students and residents receive spiritual support from religious communities, or if participation in spiritual support groups tied to medical education holds measurable effects. Structural pluralism calls for educational experiments of medical trainees who enroll into formal arrangements with thick moral and spiritual traditions,[54] facilitated by clinical mentors, clergy, and chaplains, and in partnership with local faith communities. Students could choose a variety of spiritual traditions voluntarily opted into (e.g., Buddhist, Christian, Hindu, Humanist, Jewish, Muslim) and, from within these parallel support groups, trainees would receive education in spiritual care; ethics training; shadowing opportunities; moral and spiritual direction from religiously minded clerkship directors, associated religious ministers, or group leaders; and peer-based spiritual companionship. These groups would be sponsored and recognized for credit but not mandated by a medical or nursing school, and they would provide a rich moral and spiritual environment throughout the years of medical training. There have been some small but important efforts under way experimenting with these ideas.[xv] For example, the Loyola University School of Medicine's Physician Vocation Program has been offering a four-year Ignatian spirituality directive for medical students. Loma Linda University Medical Center, a Protestant Seventh-Day Adventist institution, offers its students and residents ongoing opportunities for spiritual practice, lectures, and clerkships based on its mission of continuing "the teaching and healing ministry of Jesus Christ." The University of Chicago's Initiative on Islam and Medicine provides educational opportunities for Muslim physicians and focuses on the implications of Islam for the practice of medicine. Duke Divinity School's Theology, Medicine, and Culture Program provides a one-year course in Christian theology intended for clinicians. The Emory School of Medicine's "Emory–Tibet Partnership" offers immersion experiences and a 10-week mindfulness mediation training course based within Tibetan Buddhism. Each of these programs provides an example of how a tradition-based curriculum might find partnership within nursing and medical education. Structural pluralism proposes that larger training organizations have the capacity to provide tradition-dependent medical education tracks simultaneously throughout the training years.

These examples only begin to indicate the direction in which such training and research could develop. In terms of potential areas for spirituality and medical education to engage, consider the six domains of clinical competency identified by the Accreditation Council for Graduate Medical Education (see Box 15.1). Within a structural pluralism framework, spirituality and religion would not be a separate domain or merely an extracurricular add-on, as sometimes limited to those aspects of

---

Box 15.1 **Physician core competencies of spiritual pluralism based on the Accreditation Council for Graduate Medical Education and the American Board of Medical Specialties**[xxi]

- **Practice-based Learning and Improvement**
  Show an ability to investigate and evaluate *tradition-specific* patient care practices, appraise and assimilate scientific evidence, and improve the practice of medicine *for patients in a tradition-specific way*.
- **Patient Care and Procedural Skills**
  Provide care that is compassionate, appropriate, and effective treatment for health problems and to promote health *within a tradition-specific framework of health and well-being*.
- **Systems-based Practice**
  Demonstrate awareness of and responsibility to the larger context and systems of health care *including tradition-specific systems and practices of care delivery in a pluralistic society*. Be able to call on system resources to provide optimal care (e.g., coordinating care across sites or serving as the primary case manager when care involves multiple specialties, professions, or sites).
- **Medical Knowledge**
  Demonstrate knowledge about established and evolving biomedical, clinical, and cognate sciences and their application in *all aspects of whole person* patient care.
- **Interpersonal and Communication Skills**
  Demonstrate skills that result in effective information exchange and teaming with patients, their families and professional associates (e.g., *based within a tradition-specific framework that recognizes pluralism*, fostering a therapeutic relationship that is ethically sound, uses effective listening skills with nonverbal and verbal communication; working as both a team member and at times as a leader).
- **Professionalism**
  Demonstrate a commitment to carrying out professional responsibilities, adherence to ethical principles *within personally held spiritual traditions (religious, humanist, or otherwise)* and sensitivity to diverse patient populations *and their spiritual commitments*.

Emphasis (italicized text) is added to the AMBS listed core competencies: see http://www.abms.org/board-certification/a-trusted-credential/based-on-core-competencies/

---

a clinician's cultural sensitivity or communication skills. Instead, a pluralistic framework cuts across each of the physician competencies necessary in the care of patients.

What this box suggests is that, within the education of clinicians, there are multiple, interpenetrating constructs that lead to professional socialization. Box 15.1 does not capture the larger cultural aspects of socialization, but the aspects identified do largely reflect critical components that can be directly engaged by medical educators. Although some traditions may understandably prefer moral ("formation") rather than technical-bureaucratic language ("competencies") associated with these ideals,[xvi] the actual listed abilities are near-universally appreciated by most spiritual traditions. This argues that, as spirituality and religion is considered within medical education, research efforts should consider educational interventions in partnership with tradition-specific programs geared toward each area of clinical aptitude.

In terms of possible significance, we hypothesize that clinical trainees who participate in spiritual- and religiously based formation programs like those just mentioned would gain important internal resources for caregiving and personal well-being and strengthened fortitude in resisting aspects of the hidden curriculum. We previously described how immanence supports a groundswell of social factors that harm clinicians through burnout, loss of well-being, and "driving the heart out of medicine"[55] through corporate socialization of impersonal factors including bureaucratic, technological, and market-driven forces (discussed in Chapter 13). Among other outcomes, the so-called hidden curriculum[56] leads, among medical trainees and attending physicians, to increased levels of cynicism, emotional exhaustion, and a tendency to devalue the humanity of their patients. Structural pluralism hypothesizes that overt spiritual partnership within tradition-dependent communities will enable caregivers to retain their deepest and original motivations of compassion in the care of the sick.[50] Spirituality may also offer a protective effect that enables clinicians to identify and resist the most corrosive elements of the hidden curriculum that they encounter in clinical work.[50] Thus, medical education remains a critical way forward to implement incremental changes in partnership with trainees and religious communities. If such education allowed trainees to voluntarily opt into the tradition of their choice, there are many potential gains that can be assessed on an incremental basis through peer-reviewed research.

Resocialization and Medicine's Renewal

In Chapter 5, we noted a finding from the RSCC study indicating that receiving training in the provision of spiritual care is by far the most powerful measured predictor of whether or not nurses and physicians offer this service (discussed under hypothesis six). Medical education in spirituality and religion can be viewed instrumentally, in terms of giving our nurses and physicians skills to engage patients, help them cope, and deal with clinician burnout. This approach to spiritual care training is bound to fail because it does not address the core problems of an impersonal medicine driven by a spirituality of immanence. The better approach is to understand medical education and spirituality in terms of the overall formation of clinicians as healers[57-59] who have imbued through learning, modeling, and experience the necessary virtuous capacities to wisely engage patient spirituality and who hold professional resilience grounded in virtue rather than technique. Professional socialization conceived in this manner will be in partnership with tradition-dependent communities, rather than despite them.

Additionally, medical education, spiritual care training, and partnership with religion also suggests another possible result—a renewal of a personal and hospitable medicine. While the impersonal forces driving medicine toward increasing disenchantment appear nearly impossible to slow, let alone reverse (Figure 13.3), the implementation of structural pluralism may enable two preconditions necessary to change course against a dispirited medicine.

First, the responsibility to transform medicine from impersonal to personal rests primarily on clinicians. The forces toward impersonal medicine will almost surely not be changed by patients, government bureaucrats, business-minded executives, science researchers, or by any direct intervention of clergy or religious communities. If there is any chance for positive renewal in medicine, it will be generated and led by nurses and physicians themselves—the ones on the frontlines of illness and caregiving. Nurses and physicians by far hold the greatest level of professional prestige within society based on opinion polls illustrated in Figure 15.1.[xvii] Though the so-called "Golden Age" of medicine is over in light of cultural complaints against medicine,[60] our society still looks to its nurses and physicians with enormous respect.[xviii]

These data suggest that clinicians alone hold the best chance of renewing medicine if they take on this responsibility. They retain the greatest amount of understanding of medicine and the deepest knowledge of what is necessary in caring for the sick. Fortunately, clinicians retain a mostly unsullied reputation required to overcome these extremely powerful social forces.

A second precondition for renewal is that clinicians would need to be largely unified in resisting the social powers of the market, bureaucracy, and science, refusing to allow these concerns to dictate or undermine patient-centered care. However, for nurses and physicians to be truly unified as members of their respective professions, they would need to share in a deep moral vision that is powerful, persistent, and unwilling to stand down to hostile powers surrounding medicine. By standing together, clinicians could change the system for the sake of patients. But is such a united vision possible in our increasingly shrill, pluralistic society?

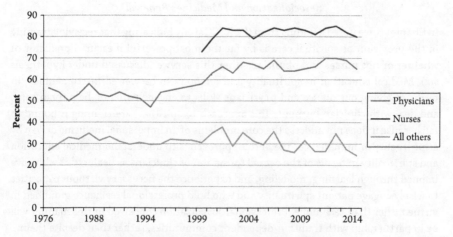

Figure 15.1 Gallup trend comparison of participants reporting as "high" to "very high" the honest and ethical standards of nurses, physicians, and the average of 14 other professions.

As one examines the largest spiritual traditions operative in American medicine,[61-63,xix] it becomes increasingly clear that these traditions hold in common certain moral ideas pertaining to the sick and their care. If clinicians were to begin to imagine the practice of medicine not merely as individuals, but from within their traditions and spiritual networks of local communities, the result would not be a cacophony of competing ideologies[5 [p. 92-93]] but heightened moral clarity and far greater unity pertaining to patient-centered care.[xx] The antinomy we are highlighting is that professional unity will not be borne by muting the traditions within medicine or stripping their richness down to a generic universal core. Instead, we are suggesting that renewing medicine's unified vision will proceed out of nurses and physicians returning to the roots of their respective spiritual traditions. Upon being formed in the abundance of wisdom, certainty of vocation, and embedded within spiritually based relational networks, clinicians will be far better grounded in a moral passion and connected to the deepest human motives in the caring for the sick. The typical narrative is that religion causes divisions or worse;[64-67] our hypothesis is that within the field of medicine and care of the sick the opposite is the case. Allow nurses and physicians to assume their identities as Buddhists, Christians, Hindus, Humanists, Jews, and Muslims, and each tributary will culminate in a powerful river that demands patient-centered care, refusing to bend to the hostility of money-focused, bureaucratic-driven, or technological-centered medicine. Structural pluralism applied to medical education provides an incremental and experimental pathway to constructively enable this approach to be put into operation.

Nurses and physicians have been mostly helpless to take on the powers that control their professional and health organizations because they ultimately lack unity due to a lack of support toward a shared moral vision. Such moral vision in the care of the sick will not come about despite spirituality and religion, but will be found in these foundations. But what is that moral vision that could unite clinicians to stand as one voice against the hostilities threatening patient care? We make that argument next.

Conclusion

A spirituality of immanence has led to the privatization of other spiritual traditions in the practice of medicine. This creates social structures where it is increasingly difficult for patients to receive spiritual care from within their own spiritual traditions. Structural pluralism goes to the root of the issue because it identifies and challenges the hegemony of immanence by imagining an alternative way to practice medicine. This form of pluralism argues for an intermediate space for communal traditions to hold structural space within the deep practices of medicine. In highlighting these tradition-dependent structures, patients are better protected because they will be more immediately conscious of the forms of spirituality that lie under the surface of medicine. Rather than feigning clinician neutrality, patients would be confronted with choices around religion in their care, and this would ultimately safeguard their self-determinative freedom and mitigate the ongoing problem of spiritual coercion advanced under immanence. Our proposal does not call for a radical or immediate cultural shift, but a gradual unfolding through scientific testing, trial, and public evaluation toward the common good. Such a path will likely enhance spiritual care for patients facing life-threatening illness without imposing religion on patients or clinicians. Structural pluralism is not itself an end, but a third way beyond the culture wars, seeking peace and spiritual flourishing for strangers despite entrenched spiritual and moral differences. However, structural pluralism alone cannot yield peace among strangers or rein in the hostile powers that threaten medicine. For this to be possible, a unified moral vision is necessary, one that is intuitively based on each tradition's own terms, able to bring clinicians together in reforming the impersonal, hostile powers menacing patient care. As we turn to the final chapter, we argue that such a unifying vision and partnership between medicine, spirituality, and religion remains possible by recovering the practice of hospitality.

Notes

i. Individual and collective actions in caring for the sick are drawn from thick moral belief systems that consist of a complex set of moral actions that privileges certain beliefs about personhood, relationships, and human love. It is contradictory to ask clinicians to be neutral toward spirituality and religion when their very actions at the bedside are inevitably drawn from underlying spiritual and religious histories and beliefs. Likewise, the analogical parallels which exist between medicine and especially the monotheistic religions, as described in Chapter 11, create a contradiction between calls to religious neutrality among clinicians and these underlying medical structures that appear religious-like.

    While a so-called secular medicine argues that it is neutral toward traditional religions, neither affirming or denying religion, the social structures themselves do not actually reflect neutrality. While we appreciate that those who defend a secular neutrality genuinely believe that contemporary medicine is neutral toward spirituality and religion, our point is that the rhetoric does not withstand scrutiny of medicine's existing values and structures. It is furthermore troublesome to imagine how the care of the sick and dying could ever be conceived in terms of neutrality in the first place, given the high stakes of illness and mortality. Thus, if neutrality were possible in regards to spirituality and religion, it does not appear to be an ideal as it may be in other contexts such as business or politics. Our conclusion, however, is that spiritual or religious neutrality is in fact not possible within a context such as medicine, and alternative models are needed.

ii. See the Harvard University Pluralism Project: http://pluralism.org/what-is-pluralism/.

iii. Religious diversity is a growing empirical fact in the United States, but it is a step too far to claim that this diversity is an ideal to be celebrated. This latter perspective is certainly the one the underlies Diana Eck's *A New Religious America*,[6] where she tends to berate religious exclusivists for claiming a divine authority that belongs within God's provenance alone (for example, see pp. 24, 383). In contrast, Volf[5] draws a conceptual distinction between religious and political exclusivism, where the former refers to one religion being more true than another and the latter refers to one religious or ideological perspective using legal means to isolate or outlaw other competing worldviews. Volf shows how many religious exclusivists are not political exclusivists. From this religious perspective, one may strongly disagree with another religion or ideological perspective, believe that the other view is morally or spiritually wrong or harmful, but then still provide political protection of that view, extending freedom of religion and equal protection under the law. This view does not celebrate religious diversity but recognizes it as an empirical reality that needs to be accommodated and permitted for a variety of prudential reasons.

iv. The writings of Roger Williams. *The bloudy tenet, of persecution, for cause of conscience* [1644]), John Milton (*Areopagetica* [1644]), and John Owen (*Indulgence and toleration considered*

[1667]) serve as classic American and English expressions that argue against the use of state coercive powers for overtly religious goals.

v. This disposition does not guarantee miscues or mistakes, but it is primarily relational compared to rule-based boundary crossings, which cannot account for the particularities of each patient and his or her peculiar spiritual questions, desires, or needs. Clinicians need to develop and rely on their intuitions and then exercise good judgment in pursuing spiritual inquiry and engagement when the patient and particular circumstances are weighed. Some patients need and desire a level of spiritual interaction from their clinician, and, in circumstances where clinicians can provide that interaction, it should be welcomed by professional standards, not discouraged.

vi. Our comments are focused on secular medical organizations and professions. While explicitly religious hospitals and clinics may also endorse some of these principles, the dynamics are different since religious healthcare is openly admitting its spiritual viewpoint, whereas secular organizations and professions explicitly deny their religious-like orientation. Patients should understand and foresee the type of organization that they are engaging premised on the importance of voluntary consent. Religious clinics and hospitals are explicit about their own spiritual identity, and this alone offers patients some protection since receipt of care from a religious clinic or hospital includes some degree of consent. Many religiously based hospitals in the United States, including Catholic and Adventist organizations, publicly acknowledge their purposes, but they also provide additional measures to avoid religious coercion.

In contrast to overt religious organizations, so-called secular health organizations do not explicitly acknowledge their underlying spirituality of immanence. Rather, there is a denial of their spiritually informed and valued-laden approaches to health and disease. The failure of secular medical organizations to acknowledge their spiritually imbued values, structures, and practices is a great threat to patient consent in regards to proselytism and religious coercion. If so-called secular organizations explicitly informed their patients of their spirituality of immanence, then there would be more parity with religious hospitals. However, current practice fails to disclose these commitments. This is why our focus in the chapter is on secular health organizations.

vii. In MacIntyre's view, a moral community "consists of any group of persons who, in the context of life together, share in practice and in theory some concept of the ends of human life and appropriate human behavior."[10 [p. 221]] Shared and sustained moral reflection and a quest for ideal human ends over time slowly develop into a moral tradition. He also defines a living tradition as "a historically extended, socially embodied argument, and an argument precisely in part about the goods which constitute that tradition."[10 [p. 222]]

viii. For example, after surveying nearly 6,000 participants in multiple representative samples of physicians, Farr Curlin and his colleagues have shown how, across a breadth of moral and spiritual issues, the degree of a clinician's religiosity is a major contributor (even after adjusting for demographic and practice characteristics) in how clinicians conceptualize moral issues and spiritual considerations and how physicians clinically engage those issues with patients. For an overview, see Farr Curlin. Religion and spirituality in medical ethics. In: Balboni and Peteet, eds. *Spirituality and religion within the culture of medicine.* New York: Oxford University Press; 2017:179–194

ix. The doctrine of informed consent exists to promote a patient's self-determination and the ability to make rational decisions. Within legal reasoning, informed consent specifically legislates harm caused to a person's physical body (e.g., surgery), and, for this reason, it is unlikely that most spiritual care interventions would require informed consent since spiritual care is not a bodily intervention with physical liabilities. This would further medicalize spiritual care—a process that should be vigorously resisted.

x. Daniel Sulmasy makes a case against "proselytizing" but does not provide a clear definition or distinction between it and spiritual care more generally.[17] "Proselytism" is a term that is often referenced in the literature as an unethical act, but it is also seldom defined. I (this note is written by Michael Balboni only) recommend moving away from this term unless it is carefully explained. Sulmasy seems to have in mind a patient converting to a religious tradition

that is held by the clinician providing spiritual care. While I agree with Sulmasy that proselytism may be coercive and an abuse of the physician's role, here I also suggest five qualifying
remarks related to the ethics of proselytism.

First, the difference between indirect spiritual care and proselytizing is in degree of engagement, not in kind. While Sulmasy appears to dichotomize between proselytism and spiritual care, they are better conceptualized on a spectrum of spiritual interactions. Even asking
a spiritually based question contains implicit norms and beliefs that can influence a patient
in a particular spiritual direction. Thus, differentiation is in degree but not in kind between
asking a spiritual question and other forms of spiritual engagement such as prayer or considering a patient's desire to newly commit or recommit to an object of love and devotion. It is
impossible to categorically separate a patient converting to a religious tradition from other
"milder" forms of spiritual expression.

Second, Sulmay's case is premised on a belief that a sick patient cannot freely offer consent to spiritual transformation or conversion if the physician is involved. But this claim
does not sufficiently weigh how illness is a clarifying experience for many patients in regards
to their life meaning and greatest love. It is often during the time of illness that patients
testify to seeing their world more intensely and clearly. In such cases, patients can offer
consent according to the principles of freedom. Patient vulnerability does not itself negate
human freedom, but in fact can better enable patients to see, consider, and evaluate their
fundamental spiritual commitments. Thus, for a clinician to participate with the patient in
this spiritual seeking and evaluation by no means suggests that the serious illness context
undermines free consent. Spiritual vulnerability and patient freedom are not themselves opposed to one another.

Third, while there is clearly a power imbalance between patients and clinicians, issues
around power must assess both the substantive issue in question and associated procedural
concerns. If one uses power to influence another to do evil, then it is an immoral use of that
power. However, if one uses human power to influence another toward good, then it satisfies
the first moral dimension of its substantive good. Upon settling this first point, procedural
issues pertaining to the use of power must be considered. Procedurally, power can be used in
partnership with a person that recognizes and allows for human freedom and dissent. Power
can also be wielded in a way that dominates another, overriding, or at least limiting that
person's freedom. There is an important moral difference between using power to influence
toward the good while maintaining respect for human freedom to choose evil or using power
to influence toward the good but dominating another through fear, retaliation, loss, or some
other alien motivation disconnected from the material end. Thus, the use of clinician power
over the patient toward a spiritual goal, which does not respect a patient's free will, should
clearly be considered unethical. Here, I agree with Sulmasy. However, a clinician may rightly
engage in the material end of spiritual care, including a range of interactions from asking
questions, to praying, to engaging questions of "conversion," *if the patient is the one who truly
desires such a material end*. This is a proper use of power in that it both serves the good and
respects human freedom, meeting both the substantive and procedural dimensions of ethics.

Fourth, Sulmasy's comparison of proselytism and sexual relations in the patient–clinician
relationship is an unfortunate comparison and misconstrues the material issue and procedural dynamics. Among the Abrahamic religious traditions, sexual relations outside of the
marriage covenant is immoral, regardless of issues of consent or power imbalance. Among
these traditions, the issue of a power imbalance may decrease blame for the person being
taken advantage and increase blame for the one who misuses power. However, what makes
sexual relations immoral is not the dynamic of power itself, but breaking one of God's com-
mandments that forbids sexual relations outside of the marital covenant (the substantive
dimension). The misuse of power by the clinician is an additional evil as the clinician used his
or her position to induce the patient toward evil actions. The presence of a power differential,
however, is not what makes an action unethical.

Fifth, these preceding considerations assume a sacred–secular division (see Chapter 7) in
which the physician is assumed to be spiritually neutral. By contrast, I have argued that the

clinician is not neutral toward spirituality and religion. Structural pluralism highlights this truth, and, within a pluralistic framework, many of these ethical concerns are removed. Structural pluralism suggests that patients need to be more directly and immediately aware of the underlying spiritual tradition that frames the clinicians' perspective. This then alters clinicians' power and allows patients to more clearly choose to participate in overt spiritual conversations.

In summary, I am not arguing that clinicians have free rein to convert their patients. Rather, clinicians should follow their patient's lead, including those patients who are actively reassessing their spiritual commitments. Clinicians will most normally be passive in this process and encourage the patient to discuss these issues with an appropriate clergy member. There may be certain circumstances and multiple conditions in which it is generally appropriate for the clinician to discuss basic questions around spiritual commitment. It depends on various factors and should not be axiomatically ruled out as I understand Sulmasy's argument to imply. The fundamental rule, as Sulmasy himself stresses in the same article, is to follow the patient's lead. This is the more important principle when weighing spiritual care interactions since it is grounded in the patient's free will and consent.

xi. For example, attitudes of exclusivism in the United States compelled Jews and Roman Catholics to create their own institutional hospitals. The dominant Protestant culture of that time was unwilling to reform the social structures to adequately fit patients' religious and cultural needs. Likewise, those who were seeking training to become physicians were actively discriminated against so that they did not receive medical and residency positions since Protestant candidates were preferred.

xii. This approach needs to be funded by diverse stakeholders including the National Institutes of Health, professional clinician agencies, a diverse set of private foundations, and by individual philanthropy. If our theological assessment of immanence is correct, then avoidance of public funding from the US government is unwarranted since even "hard science" medical research is intermeshed with some narrative of spiritual values and deep, often hidden, chief affections.

xiii. We describe and discuss several patient case examples that could be explored from a structural pluralistic perspective.[42]

xiv. In the context of serious illness, traditions vary considerably in how they envision the meaning of compassion of a good physician, a physician's ethical response at the end of life, matters of theologically related meaning of illness, or a good physician's level of engagement and responsibility toward a patient. First, the meaning and essence of compassion are debated especially between Buddhist, Humanist, and Christian perspectives. These traditions imagine compassion in distinct ways, and these differences affect how clinicians should be properly formed to exhibit compassion. Second, there are major differences in how a good physician might respond to ethical matters at the end of life including physician-assisted suicide, sedation unto consciousness, and withdrawal of life-sustaining treatments, including artificial hydration and nutrition. Third, concerning theological interpretation, traditions shape the good physician differently in how to interpret the meaning of suffering, the possibility of miracles, the degree of divine sovereignty over illness, and the role of evil and demonic spirits in illness. Fourth, traditions shape differently the level of responsibility that pertains to a good physician's response to a patient. These differences arise around the level of importance given to patient autonomy, matters surrounding a physician's conscience and conscientious refusal, and the degree to which a physician is responsible to offer directive versus indirect medical counsel. All four of these areas are grounded on a particular spiritual tradition and the ways each tradition imagines the character and response of a good physician.

xv. For more information on each program, see Loyola Chicago: https://hsd.luc.edu/bioethics/content/physicianvocationprogram/; Loma Linda: https://medical-center.lomalinda health.org/about-us; Chicago: https://pmr.uchicago.edu/iim; Duke: https://tmc.divinity. duke.edu; Emory: https://tibet.emory.edu/academic-and-cultural-programs/mind-body-sciences-summer-abroad/index.html;

xvi. The term "competency" itself may be understandably objected to by some traditions since it is language that reflects technological and bureaucratic perspectives rather than the language of virtue and formation that is preferred by major religious traditions. Competency suggests a technological skill, whereas virtue suggests a moral disposition from which skills flow.

xvii. Consider the Gallup results (Figure 15.1) to the following question about nurses and medical doctors: "Please tell me how you would rate the honest and ethical standards of people in these different fields—very high, high, average, low, or very low." Out of all professions listed, nurses and medical doctors have consistently topped the list as professionals considered to act with a high level of honesty and ethical standards. Nurses received the highest ratings among all professions. Physicians were rated only slightly lower than nurses. Even more surprising in light of the erosion of the "Golden Age of medicine," since 1976, public recognition of higher ethical standards among physicians has increased, hitting a low point of 50% in 1981 and its highest rating in 2011–2012 at 70%. Thus, Figure 15.1 demonstrates that perceptions of medicine in general are not to be equated with the most prominent persons operating within healthcare—nurses and physicians. The public continues to view nurses and physicians with a great deal of respect and trust.

Data for Figure 15.1 were gathered from online sources from Gallup: http://www.gallup.com/poll/1654/honesty-ethics-professions.aspxDataAccountants. The other professions were averaged together, including advertisers, bankers, building contractors, business executives, chiropractors, clergy, college professors, dentists, journalists, lawyers, police officers, psychiatrists, and US congressmen.

xviii. To say that we have a complaint against medicine does not entirely mean that there is a "chronic attitudinal malaise" toward it.[60] [p.2] Medicine's Golden Age seems muted but hardly lackluster. Positive opinions of nurses and physicians in particular remain impressively high, significantly greater than any other comparable profession. These findings suggest that medicine's Golden Age has not entirely come to an end in our cultural imagination.

xix. In the most recent national surveys of physicians, 51% identified with Christianity (26% Catholic, 23% Non-Evangelical Protestant, 8% Evangelical Protestant), 10% with Judaism, 10% were Muslim, and 7% Hindu.[62] Of these, we would roughly estimate that between 20% and 25% of all physicians are nominally religious but consider themselves moderately to very spiritual (based on Curlin et al.[63] and unpublished analysis from our Boston RSCC study). Although additional research is necessary to establish this, it would appear that 20–25% of physicians might *functionally* be categorized as Humanist, although we are not aware of any studies that have yet attempted to establish this directly.

Thus, the largest representative traditions among physicians (we are unaware of national surveys among nurses in this regard) would be Christian, Humanist, Jewish, Muslim, and Hindu. These five categories would likely include most nurses and physicians in the United States. The Buddhist tradition has been an active one, represented by a number of notable physician-writers and researchers. In sheer numbers, surveys suggest that they comprise less than 1.5% of physicians in the United States.[63] For spiritual traditions that have far fewer persons available in a single location, medical education approaches could, for example, take advantage of online forums for training, formation, and networking.

xx. Surely Volf is correct in his conclusion about the world religions: "Even though world religions have distinct metaphysical frameworks, readily distinguishable accounts of life worth living, and differing notions of the human predicament and of salvation, they have, as I argued earlier, structural affinities and, equally important, they share some basic principles that guide human interaction, such as the commitment to truthfulness, justice, and compassion as well as the conviction that ethical norms apply universally, to coreligionists and outsiders."[5] [pp. 92–93] There is an impressive unity and shared vision in caring for sick persons, so that healthcare provides a unique cultural opportunity to seek new religious partnerships within a structural pluralism.

xxi. This box was suggested and co-drafted with Dr. Bill Pearson, a medical educator at the Medical College of Georgia. It is used with his permission.

References

1. N. Scheurich. Reconsidering spirituality and medicine. *Acad Med*. 2003;78(4):356–360.
2. D. E. Hall, Curlin F. Can physicians' care be neutral regarding religion? *Acad Med*. 2004;79(7):677–679.
3. Richard P. Sloan. *Blind faith: the unholy alliance of religion and medicine*. 1st ed. New York: St. Martin's Press; 2006.
4. M. J. Balboni, Puchalski C. M., Peteet J. R. The relationship between medicine, spirituality and religion: three models for integration. *J Relig Health*. 2014;53(5):1586–1598.
5. Miroslav Volf. *Flourishing: why we need religion in a globalized world*. New Haven, CT: Yale University Press; 2016.
6. Diana L. Eck. *A new religious America: how a "Christian country" has now become the world's most religiously diverse nation*. 1st ed. San Francisco: Harper San Francisco; 2001.
7. Diana L. Eck. Prospects for Pluralism: voice and vision in the study of religion. *J Am Acad Relig*. 2007;75(4):743–776.
8. H. Tristram Engelhardt. *The foundations of bioethics*. New York: Oxford University Press; 1986.
9. John Rawls. *Political liberalism*. Expanded ed. New York: Columbia University Press; 2005.
10. Alasdair C. MacIntyre. *After virtue: a study in moral theory*. 2nd ed. Notre Dame, IN: University of Notre Dame Press; 1984.
11. Nicholas Wolterstorff. *Justice: rights and wrongs*. Princeton, NJ: Princeton University Press; 2008.
12. Robert Audi, Wolterstorff Nicholas. *Religion in the public square: the place of religious convictions in political debate*. Lanham, MD: Rowman & Littlefield Publishers; 1997.
13. John D. Inazu. *Confident pluralism: surviving and thriving through deep difference*. Chicago; London: University of Chicago Press; 2016.
14. Gary B. Ferngren. *Medicine and religion: a historical introduction*. Baltimore: Johns Hopkins University Press; 2014.
15. Robert D. Putnam, Campbell David E. *American grace: how religion divides and unites us*. New York: Simon & Schuster; 2010.
16. D. P. Sulmasy. Spirituality, religion, and clinical care. *Chest*. 2009;135(6):1634–1642.
17. Daniel P. Sulmasy. Ethical principles for spiritual care. In: Mark Cobb, Pulchski C., Rumbold B., eds. *Oxford textbook of spirituality in healthcare*. New York: Oxford University Press; 2012:465–470.
18. A. C. Phelps, Lauderdale K. E., Alcorn S., Dillinger J., Balboni M. T., Van Wert M., Vanderweele T. J., Balboni T. A. Addressing spirituality within the care of patients at the end of life: perspectives of patients with advanced cancer, oncologists, and oncology nurses. *J Clin Oncol*. 2012;30(20):2538–2544.
19. C. Puchalski, Ferrell B., Virani R., Otis-Green S., Baird P., Bull J., Chochinov H., Handzo G., Nelson-Becker H., Prince-Paul M., Pugliese K., Sulmasy D. Improving the quality of spiritual care as a dimension of palliative care: the report of the Consensus Conference. *J Palliat Med*. 2009;12(10):885–904.
20. F. A. Curlin, Hall D. E. Strangers or friends? A proposal for a new spirituality-in-medicine ethic. *J Gen Intern Med*. 2005;20(4):370–374.
21. M. J. Balboni, Babar A., Dillinger J., Phelps A. C., George E., Block S. D., Kachnic L., Hunt J., Peteet J., Prigerson H. G., VanderWeele T. J., Balboni T. A. "It depends": viewpoints of patients, physicians, and nurses on patient-practitioner prayer in the setting of advanced cancer. *J Pain Symptom Manage*. 2011;41(5):836–847.
22. Farr Curlin. Religion and spirituality in medical ethics. In: M. Balboni, Peteet J., eds. *Spirituality and religion within the culture of medicine*. New York: Oxford University Press; 2017:179–194.
23. R. Y. Stahl, Emanuel E. J. Physicians, not conscripts—conscientious objection in health care. *N Engl J Med*. 2017;376(14):1380–1385.

24. M. J. Balboni, et al. Ethical considerations and implications for professionalism. In: John Peteet, D'Ambra Michael, eds. *The soul of medicine: spirituality and world view in clinical practice.* Baltimore: John Hopkins University Press; 2011:200–224.

25. Christina M. Puchalski, Ferrell Betty. *Making health care whole: integrating spirituality into health care.* West Conshohocken, PA: Templeton Press; 2010.

26. F. A. Curlin, Roach C. J. By intuitions differently formed: how physicians assess and respond to spiritual issues in the clinical encounter. *Am J Bioeth.* 2007;7(7):19–20.

27. M. J. Balboni, Sullivan A., Enzinger A. C., Epstein-Peterson Z. D., Tseng Y. D., Mitchell C., Niska J., Zollfrank A., VanderWeele T. J., Balboni T. A. Nurse and physician barriers to spiritual care provision at the end of life. *J Pain Symptom Manage.* 2014;48(3):400–410.

28. E. C. Halperin. The rise and fall of the American Jewish hospital. *Acad Med.* 2012;87(5):610–614.

29. Bernadette McCauley. *Who shall take care of our sick?: Roman Catholic sisters and the development of Catholic hospitals in New York City.* Baltimore: Johns Hopkins University Press; 2005.

30. J. H. Baron. The Mount Sinai Hospital--a brief history. *Mt Sinai J Med.* 2000;67(1):3–5.

31. Tyler J. Vanderweele. Religion and health: a synthesis. In: Michael Balboni, Peteet John, eds. *Spirituality and religion within the culture of medicine.* New York: Oxford University Press; 2017:357–401.

32. Stephen Jay Gould. *Rocks of ages: science and religion in the fullness of life.* 1st ed. New York: Ballantine Pub. Group; 1999.

33. L. A. Cooper, Beach M. C., Johnson R. L., Inui T. S. Delving below the surface. Understanding how race and ethnicity influence relationships in health care. *J Gen Intern Med.* 2006;21 Suppl 1:S21–27.

34. L. A. Cooper, Roter D. L., Johnson R. L., Ford D. E., Steinwachs D. M., Powe N. R. Patient-centered communication, ratings of care, and concordance of patient and physician race. *Ann Intern Med.* 2003;139(11):907–915.

35. L. Cooper-Patrick, Gallo J. J., Gonzales J. J., Vu H. T., Powe N. R., Nelson C., Ford D. E. Race, gender, and partnership in the patient-physician relationship. *JAMA.* 1999;282(6):583–589.

36. W. D. King, Wong M. D., Shapiro M. F., Landon B. E., Cunningham W. E. Does racial concordance between HIV-positive patients and their physicians affect the time to receipt of protease inhibitors? *J Gen Intern Med.* 2004;19(11):1146–1153.

37. T. A. Laveist, Nuru-Jeter A. Is doctor-patient race concordance associated with greater satisfaction with care? *J Health Soc Behav.* 2002;43(3):296–306.

38. T. A. LaVeist, Nuru-Jeter A., Jones K. E. The association of doctor-patient race concordance with health services utilization. *J Public Health Policy.* 2003;24(3-4):312–323.

39. S. Saha, Komaromy M., Koepsell T. D., Bindman A. B. Patient-physician racial concordance and the perceived quality and use of health care. *Arch Intern Med.* 1999;159(9):997–1004.

40. R. L. Street, Jr., O'Malley K. J., Cooper L. A., Haidet P. Understanding concordance in patient-physician relationships: personal and ethnic dimensions of shared identity. *Ann Fam Med.* 2008;6(3):198–205.

41. T. A. Balboni, Paulk M. E., Balboni M. J., Phelps A. C., Loggers E. T., Wright A. A., Block S. D., Lewis E. F., Peteet J. R., Prigerson H. G. Provision of spiritual care to patients with advanced cancer: associations with medical care and quality of life near death. *J Clin Oncol.* 2010;28(3):445–452.

42. Tracy A. Balboni, Michael J. Balboni. Religion and spirituality in palliative medicine. In: Michael Balboni, Peteet John, eds. *Spirituality and religion within the culture of medicine.* New York: Oxford University Press; 2017:147–164.

43. T. Balboni, Balboni M., Paulk M. E., Phelps A., Wright A., Peteet J., Block S., Lathan C., Vanderweele T., Prigerson H. Support of cancer patients' spiritual needs and associations with medical care costs at the end of life. *Cancer.* 2011;117(23):5383–5391.

44. Wendy Cadge. *Paging God: religion in the halls of medicine.* Chicago; London: University of Chicago Press; 2012.

45. John Inge. *A Christian theology of place.* Aldershot, Hampshire, England; Burlington, VT: Ashgate; 2003.

46. Philip Sheldrake. *Spaces for the sacred: place, memory, and identity.* Baltimore: Johns Hopkins University Press; 2001.

47. N. McCall. The statue of the Christus Consolator at the Johns Hopkins Hospital: its acquisition and historic origins. *Johns Hopkins Med J.* 1982;151(1):11–19.

48. John R. Peteet, D'Ambra Michael N. *The soul of medicine: spiritual perspectives and clinical practice.* Baltimore: Johns Hopkins University Press; 2011.

49. Sarah S. Schnitker Abigail M. Shepherd, G. Michael Leffel, Ross A. Oakes Mueller, Farr A. Curlin, John D. Yoon & Tyler Greenway. Developing the good physician: spirituality affects the development of virtues and moral intuitions in medical students. *J Posit Psychol.* 2017;13(2):143–154.

50. M. J. Balboni, Bandini J., Mitchell C., Epstein-Peterson Z. D., Amobi A., Cahill J., Enzinger A. C., Peteet J., Balboni T. Religion, spirituality, and the hidden curriculum: medical student and faculty reflections. *J Pain Symptom Manage.* 2015;50(4):507–515.

51. Joan Halifax. *Being with dying: cultivating compassion and fearlessness in the presence of death.* 1st ed. Boston: Shambhala; 2008.

52. Christopher P. Vogt. *Patience, compassion, hope, and the Christian art of dying well.* Lanham, MD: Rowman & Littlefield Publishers; 2004.

53. Robert M. Veatch. *Hippocratic, religious, and secular medical ethics: the points of conflict.* Washington, DC: Georgetown University Press; 2012.

54. W. A. Kinghorn, McEvoy M. D., Michel A., Balboni M. Professionalism in modern medicine: does the emperor have any clothes? *Acad Med.* 2007;82(1):40–45.

55. Jack Coulehan. Today's professionalism: engaging the mind but not the heart. *Acad Med.* 2005;80:892–898.

56. F. W. Hafferty, Franks R. The hidden curriculum, ethics teaching, and the structure of medical education. *Acad Med.* 1994;69(11):861–871.

57. R. M. Antiel, Kinghorn W. A., Reed D. A., Hafferty F. W. Professionalism: etiquette or habitus? *Mayo Clin Proc.* 2013;88(7):651–652.

58. T. P. Daaleman, Kinghorn W. A., Newton W. P., Meador K. G. Rethinking professionalism in medical education through formation. *Fam Med.* 2011;43(5):325–329.

59. W. A. Kinghorn. Medical education as moral formation: an Aristotelian account of medical professionalism. *Perspect Biol Med.* 2010;53(1):87–105.

60. Charles E. Rosenberg. *Our present complaint: American medicine, then and now.* Baltimore: Johns Hopkins University Press; 2007.

61. T. F. O'Connell, Ham S. A., Hart T. G., Curlin F. A., Yoon J. D. A national longitudinal survey of medical students' intentions to practice among the underserved. *Acad Med.* 2018;93(1):90–97.

62. C. L. Smyre, Tak H. J., Dang A. P., Curlin F. A., Yoon J. D. Physicians' opinions on engaging patients' religious and spiritual concerns: a national survey. *J Pain Symptom Manage.* 2018;55(3):897–905.

63. F. A. Curlin, Lantos J. D., Roach C. J., Sellergren S. A., Chin M. H. Religious characteristics of US physicians: a national survey. *J Gen Intern Med.* 2005;20(7):629–634.

64. Mark Juergensmeyer. *Terror in the mind of God: the global rise of religious violence.* 3rd ed. Berkeley: University of California Press; 2003.

65. Martin E. Marty, Moore Jonathan. *Politics, religion, and the common good: advancing a distinctly American conversation about religion's role in our shared life.* 1st ed. San Francisco: Jossey-Bass Publishers; 2000.

66. Charles Kimball. *When religion becomes evil.* Rev. and updated ed. New York: HarperOne; 2008.

67. Richard E. Wentz, Wentz Richard E. *Why people do bad things in the name of religion.* Macon, GA: Mercer University Press; 1993.

16

From Hostility to Hospitality

The movement from hostility to hospitality is hard and full of difficulties. Our society seems to be increasingly full of fearful, defensive, aggressive people anxiously clinging to their property and inclined to look at their surrounding world with suspicion, always expecting an enemy to suddenly appear, intrude and do harm. But still—that is our vocation: to convert the *hostis* into a *hospes*, the enemy into a guest and to create the free and fearless space where brotherhood and sisterhood can be formed and fully experienced. X[pp. 65-66]

—Priest and Theologian Henri Nouwen, 1975

Summary of Argument

This book has been centered around three questions exploring medicine, spirituality, and religion.

A. Why is spiritual care infrequently provided by clinicians in serious illness?
B. Is, and if so, how is spirituality connected to medicine's basic social structures?
C. Is partnership among medicine, spirituality, and religion possible given our secular and pluralistic milieu?

In response to these questions, the book's arguments are summarizable in five points.

1. In response to Question A, there are multiple, overlapping reasons for its infrequency, but we conclude that the greatest contributor is *the socialization that clinicians receive* through medicine's structures to neglect and avoid patients' spirituality. This socialization removes spiritual and religious considerations from acknowledged relevance of the medical realm. As found in Chapter 5, formal training in spiritual care is not considered intrinsic to clinical care. As discussed in Chapter 6, within our broader cultural beliefs, clinicians have been willing accomplices in the larger project of death denial, aligning themselves with scientific identities and technological promise and simultaneously distancing themselves from religious associations that are affiliated too closely with the reality and reminder of death. These cultural beliefs are further reinforced by the accepted plausibility that conceptualizes separation of sacred and secular (Table 7.1) as a

possible or even almost a natural outcome of the advancement of science. Within the daily grind of the hospital wards, religious issues are rarely engaged by clinicians, all but reinforcing its avoidance and neglect, especially among young clinicians training in our academic centers. The social structures bifurcate the material and immaterial realms, with the immaterial (i.e., nonmaterial reality) reinterpreted as "immaterial" (i.e., unimportant).

2. We also offered a theological engagement, in Chapters 8 through 12, describing an underlying spirituality operating within the deep structures of medicine. Here, we identified a spirituality of immanence, referring to a collective life centered on bodily health, cure, and physical comfort as chief love or ultimate concern. Of course, we do not mean to imply that this is a sinister human plot, but rather that, in the privatization of traditional religions, life centered on bodily matters becomes religious-like because a secular–sacred framework does not fit human experience within the context of medicine and illness. Serious illness raises such deep and basic questions for most people that spirituality and religion are intrinsically irremovable from medicine. Thus, the consequence of applying the secular–sacred bifurcation has led to immanence (ironically) functioning within the privatization and practical absence of traditional religion for the collective in a religious-like way. Though hardly the intention of the advocates of immanence, spiritual dynamics express themselves in contrast to Abrahamic values (Chapter 9), especially seen around beliefs of personhood (Chapter 10), institutional structures (Chapter 11), and culminating in a tendency toward clinician and organizational veneration (Chapter 12). In response to Question B, therefore, there is a collective spirituality interwoven within the practice of medicine and its deep social structures. The privatization of traditional religions did not eliminate spirituality from medicine, but instead imbued immanence itself in holding this position. Having driven out one set of religious values (Abrahamic), a spirituality of immanence took its place.

3. Upon coalescing the empirical, sociological, and theological dynamics at play within medicine, we are led to conclude that together they form a powerful impetus for the socialization of clinicians to neglect and avoid the spiritual care of seriously ill patients. What is especially surprising is that these dynamics have created a myopia among clinicians concerning how a large majority of patients experience the intersection of spirituality and illness. This is even more surprising given the association of religious rationales with varied medical outcomes (see Chapter 3) ranging from health,[1] to medical decisions,[2,3] and end-of-life costs.[4] Neglect of spiritual care is made more surprising since clinicians themselves are relatively spiritual and religious,[5] believe that spiritual care is appropriate and beneficial among adult patients facing serious illness (see also Chapter 5),[6] and desire to provide spiritual care more frequently in their practices.[7] This suggests that socialization within immanence through these varied, invisible social structures and cultural beliefs is enormously formative. This socialization holds enough power to overcome even the interior desires of many clinicians, coloring what is seen and heard among their patients. Although there have been many well-intended efforts to advocate for spiritual or religious sensitivity among clinicians, we conclude that only an

equally powerful collective social structure, currently nonexistent, is able to resist and overturn the monopolization of immanence over medicine.

4. A spirituality of immanence has inadvertently led to the increasing marginalization of certain conditions necessary for human compassion and care and has allowed impersonal social forces to increasingly overtake the care of patients with serious illness. Our hypothesis (argued in Chapter 13) is that immanence, through its privatization of traditional religions, sidelines said religions, which themselves have some wherewithal to properly order market considerations, technology, and bureaucratization in the service of patient care. While secular humanists and those in traditional religious groups share an ethic of profound human care toward the sick, it is a demographic reality that only the latter have local and national communities and organized networks which are largely not influenced by market forces. Traditional religious groups in America, including Catholic, Evangelical, Mainline Protestant, and Jewish, are mainly on the outside of the medical profession or its varied health institutions. Thus, the only organizations that have the values, sheer mass, deep networks, and uncompromised organizational identities to resist impersonal forces are those very same groups that immanence has disallowed from influencing medicine's deep structures. These same impersonal forces aimed toward rational efficiency have been taking their toll on physicians and nurses, who are worn out cogs in the impersonal machine of medicine, facing alarming levels of burnout (Chapter 13). Most who work in medicine know well that the forces of which we speak are having widespread and deleterious effects on the care of patients. Weber's icy night of instrumental rationalization imperils medicine.[8] Against these currents, social networks created by traditional religious communities uphold the importance of care and compassion and are less beholden to impersonal social power. No doubt most clinicians, as most Americans, believe that the patient should come first, yet there are no large and influential organizations, outside of traditional religions, with the imagination, will, or size to hold back the tide of impersonal social forces rising over medicine or medical practitioners. In response to Question B, therefore, immanence has marginalized traditional religion from medicine's deep structures, and this removal has enabled other forces—namely, money, technology, and bureaucratic order—to structure the practice of medicine. There is no doubt that in moderation these forces are essential to the care of patients; however, these genies have been set loose to the degree where it is often unclear if they serve the care of patients or if they exist primarily for other ends. Every major response to the problems that ail medicine seems to be oriented around more money, better technology, or greater bureaucratic control. These larger cultural forces influencing medicine are interwoven with and have everything to do with spirituality and religion.

5. In response to Question C, we provided in Chapter 15 a pathway describing a future medical–religious partnership. Inviting traditional religion back into partnership with medicine engages certain entrenched problems, including the best way to address patient spiritual care in serious illness, the problematic monopoly that a spirituality of immanence exerts over medicine, and the unchecked rise of impersonal social forces harming patients and clinicians. Partnership with traditional religion will likely have a positive and constructive effect at each of these levels.

Clearly, however, a reintroduction of traditional religion within the structures of medicine carries with it enormous challenges given our American assumptions concerning secular structures and pluralism. In response, we outlined a proposal called structural pluralism, defined as a coexistence of multiple communities within shared medical structures consisting of different religions, moral systems, and worldviews. Within structural pluralism, medicine would partner with religious and/or other moral communities (e.g., Catholic, Protestant, Hindu, Muslim, Humanist, etc.). Each community would have access to organizational and professional structures to incrementally develop its unique, tradition-dependent spiritual viewpoints and practices for the sake of serving and caring for the seriously ill who identify with each tradition. Patients and clinicians would have the opportunity to opt into receiving or providing care from within a tradition, but always free from coercion. As outlined in Chapter 15, each tradition identifies and tests the applicability of its healing aims, makes them publicly accessible through hypothesis-testing research, and then incrementally expands its practice according to patient needs and related local demographic variables. A future partnership must maintain the tradition-rich perspectives of spirituality, defend freedom and protect against coercion, and pursue its ends of health and healing in concord with scientific knowledge. If these three dimensions are creatively held together, a beneficial partnership can be imagined and is incrementally achievable.

Hostility Caused by Pluralism

Structural pluralism will face substantial resistance and skepticism from the medical establishment because it would be believed to undermine medicine's hard-won cultural authority,[9,10] risking its financial monopoly over patient care, and destabilizing its perceived unity.[11] For example, structural pluralism could lead to clinicians shaping their medical practice around subtraditions such as Atheism, Buddhism, Roman Catholicism, Evangelicalism, Judaism, Humanism, and so on.[i] Clinicians might receive supplemental training and formation from within their traditions, and this may, over time, lead to the incorporation of different healing practices. Each tradition might emphasize distinct spiritual healing practices such as mindfulness meditation, intercessory prayer, positive thinking, or anointing with oil. Yet this diversity also carries the possibility of numerous challenges and potential pitfalls. Some traditions may advocate physician-assisted suicide as a moral practice, whereas other traditional religious groups will morally oppose it.[12,ii] What if one moral or religious tradition began to disparage another tradition? What if Tradition X became outwardly critical of the healing practices of Tradition Y? Such a cacophony could risk undermining medicine's reputation as a coherent and consistent practice, harming public confidence in medicine as a practice grounded in objective evidence or weakening standards safeguarded by professional organizations.[11]

While these are legitimate worries, there are three foundational values shared among almost all spiritual traditions that outweigh the likelihood of fragmentation.

The first value is patient-centered care, which cuts across all major traditions. Medicine believes in and must continually affirm that its purpose is the healing and care of the patient. All the major traditions uphold the centrality of the patient. Structural pluralism is more likely to reinforce patient-centered care by resisting impersonal social forces.

A second overlapping value is that medicine will facilitate a positive and ongoing partnership with science and the empirical method. With few exceptions, most major spiritual traditions are supportive of and receptive to the realities of health and illness disclosed through the medical sciences.[13,14] But this does not mean that spiritual traditions recognize the empirical sciences as the sole or final arbiter of reality. Every tradition (whether called religious, humanist, or secular) is grounded in ideological beliefs about health, illness, and healing, and so should come into dialogue with the physical and social sciences as it pertains to medicine and healing. From the position of critical realism,[15–17] a spiritual tradition (e.g., Christianity, Islam) and the empirical sciences may operate on distinct strata of reality but they also overlap since both are tacitly theory-laden, holding personal dimensions of knowledge.[18,iii] Keeping this dialogical relationship in mind, structural pluralism would neither coronate nor denounce science. The practice of medicine needs to be evidence-based, but cannot be *only* based on the scientific method. In such a partnership, science holds the potential to yield new discoveries as the health sciences become more directly aware of its presuppositions, and each tradition examines external evidence that may confirm or challenge its presuppositions about healing. This holds the potential to yield new paths of human discovery and advance how a tradition interacts with the reality of health and illness. Within a system of structural pluralism, each tradition would be expected to pursue its own distinct hypotheses, but in a form of partnered triangulation, using the scientific method for cross-tradition engagement and internal criticism.[iv]

The final overlapping value that most spiritual traditions share is the practice of hospitality, which refers generally to a gracious disposition toward strangers. The activity of medicine is lived out and displayed as one of several contexts within a larger practice of hospitality. Even today this idea is still embedded in medicine's language of *hospital* and *hospice*. Every major world tradition extolls the centrality of stretching, despite human imperfection, toward a gracious kindness to strangers.[19–36]

Hospitality is a critical value in light of structural pluralism, which openly admits that our society comprises morally strange and incommensurable traditions.[v] A collective ethos of hospitality, in which conflicting traditions uphold a gracious disposition toward other spiritual communities, is the shared spirit that can hold these rival traditions together. Hospitality is not merely a truce or a cold war, but a communicative relationship cultivated within and between communities.[37] Hospitality is a prized value, shared across traditions, and it provides an alternative model that creates space for our fundamental differences without resorting to domination.

Under a structural pluralistic model, medicine has a better chance to hold together because all the major spiritual traditions, despite their uniqueness and differences, emphasize the centrality of caring for the patient, a constructive and positive relationship with medical science in health and healing, and the value of receiving strangers in a gracious hospitality. These shared values provide a foundation in sharing in the care of the sick, despite some incommensurable differences.

Hostility in the Patient–Clinician Relationship

A paradigm shift from a spirituality of immanence to structural pluralism is necessary not only because it will break the monopoly of immanence[vi] and create conditions conducive to patient spiritual care, but also because it is one of the only forces that can properly restrain bureaucratic, market, and scientific social forces from overtaking the care of the seriously ill. As argued in Chapter 13, immanence has enabled impersonal social forces to gain nearly unstoppable momentum. Our argument is not against immanence having a voice in medicine, but against its exclusive voice shaping medicine's structures. Apart from a renewed partnership with multiple traditional spiritualities in a model such as structural pluralism, it is likely that clinicians and hospitals, though they clearly desire to be directed by an ethos of personal care of patients (Figure 13.3), are powerless to counterbalance these impersonal social forces threatening care.

If we are correct in suggesting that the practice of medicine is irreducibly connected to spirituality, then this subsequently requires acknowledgment that the patient–clinician relationship is a spiritual interaction between persons. But what is the nature of this spiritual interaction? How should it be described? The ways we conceptualize the patient–clinician relationship is often subtle, embedded in unconscious metaphors and partially revealed in common nomenclature. Medical language reflects and reinforces presuppositions concerning what is ultimate, the nature of personhood, and the purpose of the interaction between patients and their caregivers. Consider the following language and the implications that it holds for patients and caregivers. .

A sick person is often referred to (but not directly addressed) by several possible terms (Table 16.1).[38,39] Although most of those who enter hospitals in illness prefer the term "patient,"[40] some object that it suggests a paternalistic medicine that enhances the passiveness of the sick role.[38,39,41 [pp. 3–4],42] However, alternative language for those who are sick is far more problematic, including market-based language ("client," "consumer," or "customer"), scientific terms ("case" or "subject"), or bureaucratic ("user"). Shared terminology around sickness reveals the underlying framework of relational meaning, reflecting not normative proposals for the patient–clinician relationship,[43] [see chapter 15] but instead the most dominant social forces shaping medicine and the clinical encounter. Hence, to call patients "customers" or clinicians "providers" frames the medical encounter as a financial exchange shaped by market forces. Money becomes the central framework of meaning and exchange. If a clinician says, "I have a case scheduled at 10 A.M.," his language suggests that he sees the patient as an object rather than a person. To call patients "users" is to orient the framework in terms of consumption that has a managerial quality ("users" often refer to a login phrase on a computer).

Terminology reflects an unconscious belief system about what it means to be sick as well as what it means to take care of those who are seriously ill. Our choice of language reflects and reinforces cultural presuppositions. There are presently four dominant relational frameworks (Table 16.1) that provide ways to see patients and clinicians. Three of these are based within objectivized or depersonalized modes of

Table 16.1 **Language and metaphor undergirding the patient–clinician relationship**

Social Force	Patient–Clinician Relationship	Associated Terminology
Science	Object–Observer Relationship	Scientist/Specialist, Case
Economics	Buyer–Seller Relationship	Provider, Customer
Bureaucracy	User–Manager Relationship	Professional, User
Hospitality	Guest–Host Relationship	Clinician, Patient

meaning. These frames of meaning draw on impersonal social forces that we have been discussing including the scientific, economic, and bureaucratic.[vii]

First, the scientific type conceptualizes clinicians primarily as objective scientists. In this meaning-making system, the sick are viewed as material "bodies" to be examined, tested, diagnosed, and cured. As suggested in Chapter 10, this is a distant gaze that objectifies the patient and clinician into an *object–observer* relationship. It is well illustrated by Picasso's *Science and Charity*, as the physician takes the patient's pulse, counting as he looks at his watch with his back turned to the patient. This model lends itself to certain attitudes and behaviors between the patient and clinician: the patient is to act as if he were an object to be studied or a "thing" to be treated. This not only distances the patient from his own lived experience, but equally depersonalizes the patient as a scientific experiment subjected to hypothesis testing.[44 [pp. 50–51]] While we extol the importance of science in medicine, this should not be the main model for the patient–clinician relationship because healing cannot be compressed to reductionist mechanisms of causation and intervention.[45] Healing includes science, but even more fundamentally it involves a critical connection between humans as sick person and healer in a caring relationship.

The economic is a second relational type that perceives the medical encounter in terms of a market exchange of goods. In this model, the patient is encouraged to act like a buyer of health and healing commodities. The clinician is a seller of expert knowledge and techniques and provides access to medicines to satisfy the patients' desires. This view suggests that the chief manner in which to interpret the patient–clinician interaction is in terms of a *buyer–seller* relationship. Though economic considerations have always been inevitable for the success of medicine, this model should not be a primary lens for the patient–clinician relationship because illness and healing are dimensions of human experience that should not be for sale.[46,47] Economic rationality based on market forces introduces hostile relational factors into a healing relationship of trust and need. Patients who are facing serious illness turn to clinicians not primarily in *desire*, but in fear, existential crisis, physical pain, and a basic disruption of living. Allowing money to serve as the leading lens of meaning takes advantage of persons who have entered a deeply vulnerable situation. In contrast, the patient–clinician relationship must remain a relational connection based in dependence and trust, with finances always remaining secondary.[48,49] While economic factors are critical for medicine, embracing the economic as the primary model for the relationship would introduce an economic rationality, undermining trust within the patient–clinician relationship. Patients would be objectified into dollar signs. Medical recommendations would be under suspicion for financial gain through under- or overtreatment, whichever would most benefit the clinician or hospital. For healing to flourish, the patient–clinician relationship needs to be shielded from economic rationality as a primary motivation. Economic considerations should not be allowed to become a primary factor within the patient–clinician relationship or its immediate context since this will directly undermine the act of healing. More than any other factor presently, this emphasis on financial gain jeopardizes American medicine.

Third, the bureaucratic and managerial model—which operates as a handmaid to economic forces—envisions clinicians as parts of a larger institutionalized healthcare delivery system. Medical tasks are divided into specific roles within a highly complex organizational structure, which has arisen because of economic factors and increasing specialization driven by developments in medical technology. When this model becomes primary, clinicians are envisioned as specialists with circumscribed roles, as parts of a larger healthcare team. For example, clinicians may spend more time staring at computer screens or filling out paperwork than in looking, talking, touching, or knowing the patient.[50,51] Patients are imagined in terms of itemized boxes to be checked and completed.[viii] The bureaucratization of medicine turns patients into *users*[38] and clinicians into health managers and administrators. While the organizational dimension of care is increasingly necessary considering the financial and scientific complexities of modern medicine, it also threatens the human connection in the healing encounter if it becomes the primary influence on the clinical encounter. When it does, it subverts the healing relationship, as suggested by Acar and others,[38] creating a difficult system for patients to navigate and an equally onerous one for clinicians to practice within.

From Hostility to Hospitality

Contrasting with these impersonal forces informing the patient–clinician relationship is a fourth model framed by the practice of hospitality (Table 16.1). In nuancing our broader definition as it pertains to the context of illness, *hospitality is an individual and collective practice in which the ill stranger in need is graciously received*.

Understanding medicine through the lens of hospitality is hardly a new proposal; rather, it is one based in ancient wisdom grounded especially in the experience of illness. Among a taxonomy of patient–clinician models,[43] hospitality uniquely stands out because it combines characteristics that are authoritarian, patient-centered, mutually interactive, and covenantal. It also provides a fitting corrective to certain contemporary forces threatening patient care and provides clarification on the engagement between clinicians and patients.[ix] From the rich perspective of hospitality, patients are imagined predominantly as subjects, not objects, and the clinical encounter prioritizes personal rather than impersonal relations. Hospitality has been a deemphasized model within Western medicine, yet one especially in need of recovery because of (1) its adeptness in describing the social dynamics at play in providing care for the sick, (2) its power to name persons, and (3) the clarity it offers concerning human motives in seeking the common good for the sick.

We briefly describe each of these three characteristics.

Hospitality and Medicine's Social Context

Although the term "hospitality" currently sounds quaint, tame, and has been coopted more recently by the "hospitality industry,"[x] the concept of hospitality remains a unique way to understand the social relations within the medical encounter. There are multiple congruencies where hospitality captures the human dynamics of medical care of the serious ill and thus offers patients and clinicians a normative manner guiding expectation, social obligation, and ways of action. We argue that hospitality is most adequately understood as a deep practice,[xi] which carries within it an internal logic of motivation and action necessary to receiving sick persons.[52 [p. 187]] It is a framework that fits contemporary medicine in four important ways.

1. *The stranger relationship*. Modern medicine is an encounter between strangers.[xii] Patients and clinicians seldom have a long-term relationship and yet often meet, converse, and engage within intense human crisis and suffering. American medicine will increasingly become an encounter among strangers: various factors (e.g., population growth, urbanization, specialization, etc.) have rendered single-practice medicine largely obsolete. Prior conceptual models that describe the medical encounter with an implicit reliance on ongoing neighbor-like familiarity between patient and clinician (e.g., paternal, priestly, friendship, or neighbor)[43 [pp. 277–300]] are inadequate models because the logic of those relationships assumes a familiarity that does not and will likely not exist again in medicine's future. While we mourn the loss of familiarity in the patient–clinician relationship, hospitality provides a framework for strangers that facilitates deep engagement on a personal level,

cultivating listening, respect, care, and compassion. A meeting between strangers does not necessitate, as some think,[42] an impersonal medicine if hospitality serves as the central model of care. While other patient–clinician models (Table 16.1) reinforce the relational distance of the medical encounter, hospitality simultaneously recognizes that metaphors of familiarity are unrealistic,[xiii] but that a different form of human intimacy and connection is achievable. Hospitality assumes and structures the foreignness of the relationship between patient and clinician.

2. *Power differences*. Intrinsically embedded within the patient–clinician relationship is a power difference. The patient is in a position of need. The clinician is in possession of knowledge, technical skill, and resources to engage the patient's need. Models that deny, attempt to mitigate, or eliminate this fundamental difference (e.g., legal and contractual)[43 [pp. 277–300]] ultimately may distort healing rather than correct misuse of power.[xiv] While checks and balances such as patient autonomy and informed consent are a positive development keeping at bay older, paternalistic practices, these checks are largely based on external forms of legal and contractual logic alien to the healing relationship. By contrast, hospitality recognizes a power differential between host and guest. In fact, the literal Latin meaning of hospitality likely means "master over a stranger" (*hosti* = stranger; *pit* = *power* or *master*).[53] As a framework, hospitality necessitates that hosts use their power to receive their vulnerable guests in such a manner that welcomes rather than suppresses the patient's personhood and agency. Like hospitality more generally, the clinician's power is to be exercised within a dynamic of humility, mutuality, and true consent of the guest.[54] The point is not to deny the power differential, but for clinicians, like hosts, to exert that power in humility and welcome those being received. Hospitality recognizes and structures the power difference between patient and clinician.

3. *Covenantal commitment*. The practice of medicine has historically involved covenantal expressions of binding commitment,[47] most visibly expressed in a physician's oath.[55 [pp. 89–112]] In Ancient Near Eastern and Biblical terms, a covenant comprised a triangulated relationship consisting of, not two parties as in a human contract, but three: a suzerain, a vassal, and the god who held both human parties responsible for their pledge.[56] Covenants often involved an uneven distribution of power and responsibility based, not in a reciprocal exchange of goods or rights, but a generous kindness and pledge of fidelity grounded in love.[57,58,xv] Traditionally, a physician's oath binds the clinician within a moral and spiritual practice that is motivated first by compassion and hospitality. A patient could confide and trust in the clinician because the clinician was bound before a transcendent god, and physicians called curses upon themselves if they abused their power by proving themselves inhospitable or uncaring to the patient. This was the point of the Hippocratic physicians swearing before Asclepius and other Greek gods. Similarly, Christian clinicians bound themselves before the Triune God in Jesus Christ.[59] The physician's oath sworn before the gods is covenantal by nature as the physician's failure to abide by the oath invites divine judgment. The covenant-shape of medical practice mirrors the implicit covenantal framework of a guest who enters into a stranger's home in need of protection. Hospitality entails an implicit covenantal

framework that pledges protection and fidelity of the powerful (a healthy clinician) to the weak patient.

4. *Limited resources.* The primary motivation for a host or a clinician is based on the same internal covenant logic: care and compassion. Derrida once extolled the untamed human virtue of unconditional hospitality in which hosts receive those in desperate need without condition or expectation.[21] Lesser forms of hospitality are mired in restrictive conditions pertaining to an ability to pay, worry over limited supplies, questions concerning the merit of the person in need, and other rule-focused boundaries and obligations that depersonalize and ultimately harm the relationship. Without authentic human care, the feelings that accompany hospitality erode and ultimately undermine welcome or healing. Even so, it is a perennial struggle for hosts to discern how much they can give or where boundaries must be drawn to protect limited resources.[60 [pp.127-149]] Similarly, clinicians face these dynamics when there is too much human need and too little personal energy or shared resources for the sick. Clinicians constantly face pressures to turn in on themselves and shut out the sick for the sake of their own well-being. Here, temptations arise where hospitality and care become replaced by external concerns such as money, comfort, honor, or sheer obligation. Limited resources create temptations so that hosts stop hosting and clinicians stop caring. These tensions and temptations risk destroying the beautiful and truly human expressions of compassion seen in both the traditional hospitality of welcoming a pilgrim into the home and the clinician receiving the patient in dignity and compassion. Nevertheless, even amid human finitude and resource limitations, it is in the keeping of human care and compassion as primary values that moves our actions from conditional to unconditional hospitality. Hospitality provides clinicians an ongoing historical narrative that explains the true limitations of their personhood and craft, but also the deep, almost inexplicable summoning to give oneself away in care and hospitality.

In summary, the concept of hospitality uniquely fits and describes the patient–clinician relationship since both parties in this interaction are strangers, meeting in circumstances with vastly distinct levels of power, and called upon to be guided by an implicit covenant of care and compassion despite human limits. The social expectations that guide hospitality in general are the same expectations that provide deep guidance to medicine. Unlike other descriptive models proposed for the patient–clinician relationship,[43 [pp. 279-297]] which tend to be theoretical or fail to adequately account for basic human concerns in the contemporary patient–clinician relationship, hospitality is universally understandable as a cross-culturally experienced human expression toward strangers in need. Although it is a practice under siege because of Western individualism and the tendency to isolate ourselves from those we do not know, hospitality remains a model that is understandable across time and culture. Hospitality remains the best model for today's medicine.

Terms of Hospitality

Recovering the framework of hospitality also includes attention to terminology pertaining to roles and context. The choice of terms reflects cultural beliefs about the patient–clinician relationship, and it socializes others into that particular system. The language produced by hospitality emphasizes the patient, the clinician, and the hospital.

Patient. The Latin meaning of patient refers to one who suffers with endurance and patience.[61 [p. 426]] This is principally moral language based in virtues that highlight fortitude, courage, and patience, all of which are necessary in pain and tribulation.[xvi] By recognizing someone primarily as a sufferer or patient, clinicians recognize personhood, the trial being experienced, and the necessity for physicians and nurses to come alongside as persons. In addition, this vocabulary appropriately recognizes that the sick person is active (holding moral agency in responding to illness) and passive (needing to rely on others for care and support). Some dismiss the term "patient" as paternalistic, but this may be because there has been a cultural loss of religious perspectives around serious illness and dying (see Chapter 6), perspectives which have emphasized the active dimensions of agency, decision-making, and moral growth within illness.[62,63] "Patient" also depicts how serious illness incapacitates the person to circumstances outside his or her thought and control, so that calling for absolute patient autonomy[42] poorly represents the experience or desire of those who are actually suffering. No English term better captures these active and passive dynamics than the traditional term of "patient." As it was traditionally conceived, a patient is a person called to actively grow and suffer within illness.

Clinician. While the terms "physician" and "nurse" describe the actions of providing medicine and nursing,[xvii] the term *clinician* is especially consistent with a framework of relational meaning. "Clinician," which we have used throughout this volume to refer to nurses and physicians, holds two interrelated senses that pertain to the sick. First, it has been widely used to refer to a medical person who is at the bedside, derived from the Greek word *klinē*, which translates as "bed." A clinician is one who attends at the *bedside*. Even more importantly, the verb form associated with "clinician" is the Greek term *klinō*, translated "to incline," "to bend," or "to bow down."[xviii] The verbal meaning of "to bend" or "to bow" is especially congruent with early religious insights, which framed the encounter with the sick as an encounter with the sacred. Rather than being one who attends at the bedside, which could suggest a towering over an inclined patient, the "clinician" is characterized by the disposition of reverence and awe, as the lesser (the clinician) bows (*klinō*) before the greater (the patient). If clinicians understood collectively their identity as those who bow down before their patients, healthcare itself would be transformed. A framework of hospitality invites terminology that accurately depicts the relationship of strangers, and, hence, it highlights "patient" and "clinician" as capturing the moral and spiritual aspects of these roles.

Hospital. Within the Western tradition, the term indicates a framework of meaning oriented around the concept of *hospitality*, which literally refers to the care and compassion shown to strangers.[xix] Whereas hospitality to strangers was widely valued in many cultures in the Ancient Near East and in Hellenistic cultures, the sick were stigmatized and shunned as strangers unworthy to be received.[64] Christianity played a principle role in reimagining the meaning of illness and in birthing the institution of the hospital as a new form of hospitality to the sick. Eminent medical historian Gary Ferngren notes that "The hospital was, in origin and conception, a distinctively Christian institution, rooted in Christian concepts of charity and philanthropy."[64] [p. 124] The ill were sacred before God and thus deserving of reverence and special kindness. Up until about the sixteenth century, hospitals were houses administering "mercy, refuge, and dying."[65] [p. 675] Emphasis was on spiritual comfort, in partnership with Hippocratic medicine, which upheld the centrality of compassion and hospitality. Many hospitals were associated with religious and monastic life that upheld receiving guests, especially the sick, within a sacred framework of receiving the divine presence.

In contrast to the language of hospitality, there is a growing movement in the United States to move away from calling our healing institutions "hospitals." Some have been renamed "medical centers" or some similar variant that removes *hospital* from the organization's name.[xx] This rebranding largely stems from market and industrial considerations whereby institutions seek to convey to the public that their organization offers a suite of innovative and comprehensive health services, creating distance from terminal illness or dying (as described in Chapter 6). Rebranding reflects these deeper institutional rationalities that have medicalized the hospital and demonstrate a dominance of the business model now increasingly governing these organizations.

How society sees the patient, clinician, and its institutional context holds enormous consequences for both patients and clinicians. Without clarity, the patient–clinician encounter is unmoored from personal relationship and the centrality of healing and becomes an instrumental means to some other non-healing, external goal. Our view is that hospitality, in its rich meaning and vocabulary, remains the most potent framework of meaning for medicine. If Western medicine loses this tradition of unconditional welcome to strangers in need, then the depersonalization of healing will near its completion and the icy world of disenchantment that Weber forewarned will be the only heritage remaining to the sick and dying.[8] This is not hyperbole, but a bitter and silent battle still waging within medicine. Traditional spiritualities that cherish hospitality still have a word to speak. There is a better future to be imagined.

The Host–Guest Model of Care

Embracing hospitality as a model for medicine and healthcare, in contrast to scientific, economic, and bureaucratic models, is not merely about terminology but is about upholding three basic activities that comprise the practice of medicine: *Receiving* strangers, *Seeing* the sacred, and, finally, *Repenting* from disordered motives.

Receiving. The practice of hospitality is centered on welcoming or receiving a stranger into one's own abode. The stranger normally has material needs because he is a pilgrim on a journey, far from personal resources. In response, hospitality includes a set of human actions, often performed collectively with others, whereby someone unknown and in unfamiliar territory is in temporary need of some combination of food, hearth, a bed, protection, kindness, and possibly wisdom and direction. As a metaphorical journey,[41,66] [p. 195] illness places the sick into unfamiliar territory, within physically vulnerable circumstances, and by necessity requires dependence on virtual strangers. The circumstances in which the ill turn to clinicians are not akin to a contractual relationship but are more like what Kleinman describes as an unfamiliar and dangerous journey.[41,66] [p. 195] Patients turn to clinicians because they are in bodily—and thus also, existential—desperation and need. Clinicians receive the sick into their "homes" of resource and protection in order to provide for immediate corporeal needs and the existential ones connected to it. The act of receiving the sick is to personally welcome them into one's medical power, meeting the patient's needs, but also going beyond the physical dimension in offering one's self in a gesture of kindness and love. The act of receiving can never be limited to body alone, since the perilous journey of illness involves the sick person's whole world experience (see Chapter 2). Likewise, the act of receiving cannot be limited to providing physical resources, but must equally provide a human connection that responds to all that has been imperiled. Thus, medicine at its most basic level is an individual and collective practice in which the ill stranger in need is graciously received. The medical arts are merely tools intended to be used within a larger context of hospitality aimed to support and care for the ill stranger in need. Medicine must always remember that it serves the care of patients.

Seeing. In most world religions, the practice of hospitality is linked with hosting the divine.[xxi] This is especially true within Christianity, based on the seminal teaching of Jesus, who connected the receiving of the sick stranger with the receiving of Jesus himself (Matthew 25:31–46). This was a unique way of seeing the sick that transformed cultural attitudes and responses to illness.[64] Such a framework suggests that clinicians see and receive the sick *as if they were seeing and receiving the divine presence.* Reflecting on this teaching, Sulmasy writes that clinicians need "to recover the sense that the encounter with the patient is an encounter with the holy mystery of God. . . . [Clinicians] may ask, 'Lord when did we see you sick and comfort you?' And the Lord answers, 'Whenever you did something for the least of my brothers and sisters, you did it for me."[67 [p. 50]]

To gaze at the suffering stranger is an interpretative act. Who is this stranger? Some see merely an object, others see a person like themselves, some see an object of terror that reminds them of the fact that they, too, will become sick and die, and still others see a mystery and wonder infinitely greater than themselves. How we individually and collectively respond to this question is rooted in our interpretation of what we see. The framework of hospitality suggests not only receiving but rightly seeing the patient as a special guest. In terms of the medical "gaze" that Picasso illustrated in *Science and Charity* and Foucault lamented, the patient is observed at a distance and fully described as an objectified medical concept.[68] But most agree that this depersonalized gaze is far too narrow, like the cyclops without peripheral vision. Some see the patient as a reminder of the death and suffering that affects every human being and attempt to hide away the terminally ill and dying in distant hospital wards. Others glimpse themselves as they see the patient, and this moves them to kindness. As right as this understanding may be, the interpretative lens of hospitality points beyond the ideal of humanizing the patient. Hospitality sees a mystery of the sacred revealed in the suffering of the patient. In this gaze, the only valid response from nurses and physicians is to bow in humility and gratitude for the privilege to serve.

A clinician's reverence before the patient is captured in Benedict of Nursia's *Rule*, which called for greeting guests, especially the poor and sick, "with all humility, with the head bowed down or the whole body prostrate on the ground, adoring Christ in them, as you are also receiving him."[69 [ch. 53] xxii] The posture of a clinician bowing (klinō) before the patient is also subtly intimated in Fildes' portrait of *The Doctor* (see Figure 1.1 and front cover). From this perspective, the only adequate response to the sacredness of the patient is humility and heartfelt compassion on the part of clinicians. Thus, it is with open eyes that the clinician bows in humility before the presence of the divine revealed in the sick person. In beholding the sacredness of the patient, an equally surprising irony unfolds within the hospitality model. The clinician no longer sees himself as holding the role of host, but realizes that he is the patient's guest.[xxiii] So what could appear to be a model that advances a power difference of clinicians over the patient in an unexpected manner reverses roles, interpreting power to be held by the patient over the clinician.

Repenting. Repentance simply means a turning away from the wrong direction and going the better way. The term comes from the Greek *metanoia*, which means to have a change of mind. Many clinicians and medical organizations are first drawn into medicine out of a heartfelt desire to care for the sick and to respond with loving deeds to those who are suffering. In time, however, these motivations are too often confused and blurred by an array of other external incentives. Health organizations and individual clinicians are susceptible to motivations such as ambition, greed, power, and more often now than ever, reduced to a survival mentality. While ulterior motives arise for many understandable and complex reasons, the important point is that these undermine the spirit of hospitality. Hospitality is based in a spirit of generous receiving and seeing correctly. The crucial focus is on gift-giving rather than what will be received. We know our claim sounds hollow within today's healthcare debates and utterly naïve in light of the economic preeminence of medicine in the United States.[70] Yet economics are driven by the combination of our culture's fear of death[71] and that fear's willingness to relocate exorbitant hope in the salvific power of science and technology (see Chapter 6). Immanence has perpetuated a false hope that blinds us to our mortality. It is these latter claims that hospitality challenges as naïve myths. No amount of the gross domestic product or technological hope can remove the sting of our mortality. Thus, our cultural attention must return to hospitality as medicine's foundational framework. Science, technology, and bureaucracy have an important and proper place in today's medicine. But they should not serve as the primary framework for medicine, as they have become, but as servants advancing compassion, relationship, and trust in the context of deep suffering and loss. Hospitality is a unifying framework for clinicians and health organizations to embrace the care of patients.

As argued in Part III, embracing hospitality and reordering impersonal social forces requires a new medical–religious partnership. This partnership must involve varied spiritual traditions in a way that includes their beliefs, practices, symbol systems, and communities. The wisdom embedded in these traditions, their thick network of relationships and institutional breadth are the only available counterforces able to resist and reorder the market, bureaucracy, or technology. For some, of course, reintroducing religion into medicine is a radical proposal that arouses profound fear of religious hegemony. Contrastingly, we argued in Chapter 15 that the United States has an intellectual and cultural heritage able to navigate issues of religious freedom and provide adequate protection against coercion while still also empowering religious communities and religious energies to partner in the care of the sick. Most religious communities in America are willing to participate within medicine's structures in a spirit of hospitality without vying for hegemony. But this demands the willingness of the most influential spiritual traditions in American medicine, especially Christian, Jewish, and Humanist, to resist the pathway of power struggle and culture wars and reimagine a shared medical space for the sake of patients and clinicians. Structural pluralism is a plausible solution if we move forward, as described in Chapter 15, in small, incremental steps and in partnership with science that emphasizes an open process of hypothesis-testing research.

What are the chances of such a cultural and professional turn away from problematic motivations caused by fear, money, ambition, or simply confusion that comes with lost vision? At the current moment, chances appear slim partly because there are so many hands in the money pot of medicine, the camouflaging of death remains a preeminent cultural power, and rival traditions too often trust in political means to adjudicate difference. Similarly, overwhelming social forces seem impenetrable and unstoppable. Even yet, *repentance* can include the most unexpected people and occur at the most surprising of times. For the sake of both patients and clinicians, we hold out hope that a change of mind and heart is still possible.

Considering our proposal of structural pluralism and the respiriting of medicine through hospitality, what concrete steps might be taken? Table 16.2 offers preliminary suggestions in practical next steps to be taken considering the direction of our argument.

New Portraits for Painting?

As Sir Luke Fildes's painting of *The Doctor* (Figure 1.1) illustrated the heart and gaze of a true healer in nineteenth-century England, even so contemporary medicine waits for new portrayals. Here, we close with one such portrait, which is based on a true account of a well-respected senior physician caring for cancer patients at a Harvard teaching hospital.

The inpatient was a young woman in her 30s. She was bedridden with excruciating cancer pain, so that she lay moaning on her side in a fetal position. The patient's family stood in the room perplexed and made anxious by her condition. After the attending physician entered the hospital room, trailed by two Harvard Medical students, she greeted the family and saw the cancer's devastation on her patient's face. In only a few months' time in being cared for by the oncologist, her face seemed old and exhausted. She no longer had strength to speak.

As the clinician made eye contact with the patient, she said, "We are going to make immediate changes to your medications to help you feel more comfortable. OK?"

Then the doctor's actions caught the family and medical students by surprise. The attending physician stooped down in her skirt and lay on her bare knees before the patient on the hard floor. The clinician was now face-to-face with this sufferer, placing her hand on her quivering body.

"I'm so sorry for what you are going through," she said. "I'll be back a little later this afternoon to check on you. Hopefully with these new medicines the pain will subside in the next hour or so."

The patient could only respond by locking eyes for a moment with her clinician.

Table 16.2 **Next steps implementing structural pluralism and the vision of hospitality**[xxiv]

If you are a . . .	*Then Possible Responses May Be To:*
Clinician	• Consider 1–2 small gestures that reintroduce or retain hospitality in your patient encounters. • Share those gestures with your coworkers and healthcare team to create a more hospitable environment. • Write a blog about these experiences and how they change you. • Find and meet with other healthcare workers and clinicians who share your spiritual tradition in your work context and work with a chaplain to provide tradition-specific patient- and family-centered care. • Identify the faith traditions of your colleagues and encourage them to provide tradition-specific patient- and family-centered care.
Medical Educator	• Develop competency-based objectives that promote structural pluralism and hospitality under the domains of patient care, communication, professionalism, and systems-based practice. • Design modules to address these competency-based objectives in various courses like physician diagnosis or doctor–patient courses. • Develop assessments for these objectives, especially for clinical students and residents. • Develop an Entrustable Professional Activity (EPA) around the theme of hospitality.
Patient	• Identify a primary care physician and communicate your expectation that the relationship is covenantal not transactional. • Give positive feedback to your clinician when you experience his or her hospitable care. • Ask if tradition-specific patient- and family-centered care is available in a hospital setting if that is important to you.
Health Systems Leader	• Create an advisory board with local religious leaders. Invite them to offer their expertise in promoting tradition-specific patient- and family-centered care. • Form ad hoc committee (clergy, administrators, clinicians) to study the issue and offer solutions to implementing these ideas. • Do a cost analysis of inviting a partnership with local congregations to improve the health of a patient population. • Put out a request for proposals for tradition-specific initiatives within your hospital that is evaluated by your advisory board. • Create awards and recognition for teams of clinicians that exercise hospitality in their clinic, unit, etc. • Do a study within your hospital of systems and specifics that mitigate hospitality.

Table 16.2 **Continued**

If you are a . . .	Then Possible Responses May Be To:
Researcher	• Develop a survey instrument that evaluates the hospitality of a clinician or clinical experience on a unit or within a clinic (conducted among patients, peers, and/or coworkers). • Work with a tradition-specific innovation to help define operational definitions of healthcare delivery for research purposes. • Conduct a study of outcomes (health, quality of life, cost, patient satisfaction, physician wellness) comparing a tradition-specific clinic and a clinic that practices medicine based on a model of Immanence.
Hospital Chaplain	• Identify and train tradition-specific teams of healthcare workers for patient- and family-centered care. • Identify clinicians who embody hospitality and encourage and support them. • Create a course for community clergy that trains them on how to hospitably navigate the biomedical context and provide local networks encouraging lay hospital visitation.
Community Clergy	• Train congregants to think about healing and the nature of medicine based on your spiritual tradition. • Teach your congregation about their role in exercising hospitality to the sick. • Create a plan to consult with families faced by the end of life. • Provide congregants opportunities to plan ahead by discussing legal wills, appointment of health proxies, and encouraging congregants to communicate their wishes with family members and their legal health proxies. • Develop teams in your congregation that provide hospitality for the sick in partnership with local physicians and hospitals.

Before rising, the doctor gave a slight squeeze with her hand, and slowly whispered, "I am with you."

This portrait is both gruesome and sacred. It captures some of the immense hostility faced by suffering patients. Serious illness is awful. Yet it also expresses how hospitality, though it cannot ultimately remove our finitude or completely shield us from pain, creates a holy space of human love that contains mystery and power. For a medical student to witness this encounter leaves a mark that is hard to forget. Perhaps therefore some (though certainly not all) are persuaded that human love, and ultimately divine love, transcend suffering and death. Medicine has a sacramental-like nature that at its best points beyond immanent ends toward something mysterious and ultimately healing. The argument of this book is that this spiritual relationship is more important than all the money or technology we might throw at illness. Nor is it something that can be "fixed" with money, better technology, or greater bureaucratic measures. This is an old portrait, writ large upon the professions, organizations, and structures of healing, that needs to be repainted for a medicine that is called to engage patients' physical and spiritual needs and resocialize its clinicians to receive and see the true nature of their patients.

Only hospitality will overcome the hostility.

Notes

i. From a positive perspective, these moral and religious identities could enable patients to more clearly understand, trust, and dialogue with their caregivers around serious illness, including more clearly navigating moral and spiritual questions. Clinicians could express their traditions within secular hospitals either subtly or overtly, depending on tradition emphasis, clinician preference, and local conditions. While in current practice these traditions remain present but hidden, structural pluralism will enable patients to more clearly understand the motives and worldview that inform an individual clinician since the clinician would be overtly connected with some tradition.

ii. If structural pluralism were adopted, it is foreseeable that physician-assisted suicide may likely be permitted as a legal option. The medical profession in general would take a stand of neutrality, but each moral or religious medical tradition would provide the larger public with clarity on how its clinicians approach issues concerning patient requests to die. Presumably, some patients would desire physicians who are willing to consider this option. Especially pertaining to issues of euthanasia, other patients might trust only those physicians unwilling to participate in physician-assisted suicide because they believe this is an immoral practice. However, the voluntary nature of patient consent that we described in Chapter 15 militates against nonvoluntary and involuntary euthanasia. At the beginning of life, the issue of abortion is distinct from either physician-assisted suicide or voluntary euthanasia as the unborn cannot give consent to their own abortion. Denying a fetus status of personhood circumvents issues of consent, but this goes against the sensibility that most religious traditions uphold in protecting the weak. Thus, structural pluralism may allow for physician-assisted suicide and voluntary euthanasia, but place the issue of abortion in a different category since the rules of consent are violated.

iii. In regards to health and illness, most spiritual traditions generally share similar presuppositions with the empirical sciences, and this enables substantial agreement between the findings of the medical sciences and most spiritual traditions. Broadly speaking, most traditions overlap in their acceptance of the medical sciences. With equal importance, however, postmodern accounts have clarified that the human knower is part of the process of knowledge production, undermining positivism and suggestive that science always moves forward based partly in personal or tacit knowledge.[18]

iv. Although MacIntyre understood large-scale traditions ("A living tradition then is a historically extended, socially embodied argument, and an argument precisely in part about the goods which constitute that tradition,"[52 [p. 222]] to be incommensurable, he also argued that traditions could renew themselves through constant reexamination and engage one another in a form of empathic critique (see A. MacInytre, Whose Justice? Which Rationality? University of Notre Dame Press, 1988). Here, we are merely suggesting that the scientific method holds an important role in both tradition-mediated rationality about the nature of health, illness, and healing and cross-tradition dialogue. Science cannot settle these disputes on its own but plays an important role of triangulation as "reality" can and does speak back to each tradition.

v. This plurality is often hidden by advocacy for a unified medical profession, which does sometimes flare into public hostility. With technological capacities expanding, there will be mounting conflict over definitions of health, the ethical uses of medical technology, and the ends of medicine.[11] Consensus over these issues is unlikely. This collectively leaves us with two choices. Either the more dominant group exerts power over the other, forcing it to accept limits or expansion of medical technologies (depending on which group is currently in power) and ultimately threatening removal from the profession. (This is exactly the view advocated here: J. Savulescu. Conscientious objection in medicine. *BMJ*. 2006;332(7536):294–297; and R. Y. Stahl, Emanuel E. J. Physicians, not conscripts—conscientious objection in healthcare. *N Engl J Med*. 2017;376(14):1380–1385). Or, contrastingly, we move toward a structural pluralistic approach that openly acknowledges distinct moral and spiritual traditions.[37]

vi. While creating a *spiritual monopoly* over medicine's institutions and professions may not be an intended aim, it does not appear possible to create a spiritually neutral medical system because the nature of medicine is an activity that interfaces with human weakness, suffering, and mortality. These touch on core human meanings that inherently require and produce religious-like values and responses, both from the ill and those who care for them. While a position of religious neutrality was an understandable goal for medicine, the evidence suggests that this is implausible when it comes to the context of serious illness.

Immanence monopolizes the structures of medicine to the degree that it holds sole authority over medicine's structures, whereas traditional spiritualties have been privatized to the individual level. Should this monopoly be tolerated? For the past century or so it has been increasingly accepted on the grounds that immanence is truly neutral toward religion, neither favoring one or disfavoring another. Our contention, however, is that a *spirituality of immanence* is in fact favored by medicine's structures and that all other traditional spiritualties have been increasingly marginalized. Conceptually flawed understandings around spirituality and religion have enabled immanence to overtake medicine's social structures, and the Abrahamic traditions accepted their lessened role under the understanding that immanence was a value-neutral system. Nevertheless, immanence has produced an entire system that intensely values bodily health, cure, and physical comfort as its chief love or telos. This system empowers a death-denying culture, tolerance for the expansion of impersonal medicine, and the medical system's avoidance of patients' religious experience of illness. The shift in the United States is not from a religiously informed medicine to a religiously neutral one, but from a spirituality congruent with Western monotheism to a monopoly of a religious-like system we call a *spirituality of immanence*.

vii. Each of the relational frameworks is an "ideal" type because they provide a pattern of often unconscious attitudes and behavior but are seldom the only model informing the patient–clinician relationship. In other words, all the frameworks may be operative under the surface, and the critical concern is identifying which one is most dominant, controlling the other types.

viii. This is a common way that medical interns and residents describe their own conscious experience of patient care. See, for example, recent articles by Nathaniel Morris, "A new doctor discovers the 'gritty' downside of modern medicine," *Washington Post*, June 18, 2017; and Levinson, Price, and Saini, "Death by a thousand clicks: leading Boston doctors decry electronic medical records" (March 12, 2017) in http://www.wbur.org/commonhealth/2017/05/12/boston-electronic-medical-records.

ix. Some argue that a discussion of models for the patient–clinician relationship is a fruitless exercise (see Marcum[43] for an extended discussion). Contrastingly, we believe that models reflect social consciousness and action, enabling moral comparison and evaluation. What is medicine exactly? Should medicine be like a business or more like a lab? Or is the dynamic of illness and the care of the sick akin to some other commonly shared human dynamic, one that provides clues on the norms that we should seek in patient care? Consideration of models of care forces important reflection on the systems that we have inherited from those who have gone before. Without considering models, it is impossible to evaluate the social structures that form medicine. By considering models of care, we can step back with some greater clarity, enabling us to ask if our social systems of care really reflect what we believe in the care of the seriously ill.

x. The concept of hospitality is not to be confused with the hospitality industry, which is a for-profit commodified service based in the desire and wants of a customer who is purchasing a fine meal, hotel, resort accommodations, or a cruise. As part of customer service, this form of hospitality refers to a warm and generous reception toward paying customers. We would suggest that if economic factors are the primary motivation for hospitality, then its meaning is coopted. The motivation behind what we mean by hospitality is not economic or financial gain. This is alien to the rationale of traditional hospitality.

xi. Here, we follow MacIntyre in his definition of practice: "By a practice I am going to mean any coherent and complex form of socially established cooperative human activity through which goods internal to that form of activity are realized in the course of trying to achieve those standards of excellence which are appropriate to, and partially definitive of, that form of activity, with the result that human powers to achieve excellence, and human conceptions of the ends and goods involved, are systematically extended."[52] Practices require certain internal virtues that are necessary in order to complete or meet the aims of a practice. Hospitality is a practice in that it holds within it a certain internal logic, requiring those who participate in it to be formed within that logic. One must also resist external rationalities that fail to bring about the ends of hospitality. Thus, in the context of illness, cure cannot be medicine's telos, since cure can at best temporarily put off dying, but most will still get sick and die from their diseases. Even within terminal illness, medicine has a responsibility to act. Nor is the basis of that action, *pace* Leon Kass ("Regarding the end of medicine and the pursuit of health," *Interest*. 1975;40:11–42), toward the ends of health, since on its face physical health does not appear congruent with the care of the terminally ill and dying. Rather, in the context of illness, health and cure are important secondary aims of medicine, but they do not supplant medicine's first aim, *the gracious reception of strangers in physical need because of illness*. Likewise, financial matters are important considerations within the care of the sick, but for hospitality to take place, motivations around money-making are alien to the internal logic of receiving strangers in need. When financial matters become central to medicine (as they threaten to in our time), the practice of hospitality toward the sick becomes impossible. It introduces a logic within medicine that objectifies patients as means to an end, rather than the end in themselves.

xii. The Greek for "strangers" is *xenos*. While xenophobia is the fear of strangers, hospitality refers to the receipt of strangers (*xenodocheō*) or the love of strangers (*philoxenia*).

xiii. Curlin and Hall's metaphor of "friend" may serve as a clarifying and instructive description of how physicians and patients might relate (F. A. Curlin and Hall, D. E. Strangers or friends? A proposal for a new spirituality-in-medicine ethic. *J Gen Intern Med*. 2005;20(4), 370–374). As a metaphor, its meaning does not imply a close affection or long-standing familiarity, as friendship might imply today. Rather, it focuses on the physician working with the patient in discerning and desiring the patient's true good. One strength of this metaphor is that it based in an Aristotelian view of friendship and also endorsed within the Judeo-Christian literature: "make friends with the physician for he is good for you" (Ben Sira 38:1). Another strength is that it recognizes and challenges the larger social framework that is commodifying and industrializing medicine. The friendship metaphor counteracts this cultural tendency. A third strength is that it emphasizes a nonauthoritarian relationship, stressing mutuality between physician and patient.

However, there are also some drawbacks to a friendship metaphor. Modern healthcare, especially that in urbanized, bureaucratized academic medical centers, leads to medical relationships more typically associated with strangers. The actual lack of time and bonding that most patients and physicians have with one another is very distant from what most true friendships enjoy or ideally pursue. In addition, the difference in knowledge and wisdom between physician and patient concerning the experience of illness and the complexity of medical knowledge is real. If the relationship were epitomized as friendship, it would not be a friendship based on equality—which is arguably an important dynamic among friends. For these reasons, we advocate for the concept of hospitality as better fitting the nature of the patient–clinician relationship.

xiv. We would conjecture that a diminishment of the hospitality model within medicine created an imbalance of authority toward either paternalism or autonomy. No matter the pleas among many contemporary bioethicists to swing authority away from clinicians and toward patient autonomy, most patients will find themselves journeying in an unfamiliar world, somewhat incapacitated by their condition, and wanting to be both heard, understood, and given clear direction. The neutering of a clinician's moral judgments[42] is not only impossible (since the act of caring itself is a moral judgment), but instead fastens clinicians into an instrumental framework of economic-bureaucratic moral values. This does not remove values from the larger medical system but instead ensconces immanence into every strand of twenty-first-century medicine.

xv. While William F. May's view of covenant is generally helpful,[47] his definition of covenant often does not reflect some ancient characteristics of most covenant-making, including those in Hittite culture, Near Eastern marriage covenants, or the major covenants in the Bible, where one party does not hold an obligation to the other party (see Gordon P. Hugenberger. *Marriage as a covenant.* New York: E. J. Brill; 1994; and W. A. Elwell, and Beitzel, B. J. (1988). Covenant. In: *Baker encyclopedia of the Bible* (vol. 1, p. 535). Grand Rapids, MI: Baker Book House). The suzerain is not obligated to enter covenant with the lesser, but does so out of compassion, love, and/or a hospitable spirt.[57]

xvi. Kleinman argues that "sick person" is a better term than "patient"[41 [pp. 3-4]] but also admits that it may be too artificial or inefficiently cumbersome to employ *sick person* consistently. In our view, Kleinman's dislike of the term does not fully consider the morally positive meaning implied by the Latin, the intrinsic personhood embedded in the term, or the moral activity required to long-suffer in sickness. Instead, the meaning of *patient* carries the core values that Kleinman rightly wants to highlight.

xvii. In Greek, Latin, and English, the term used for physicians has been primarily descriptive of those who practice the art of healing based in the Hippocratic tradition. Thus, they were called *iatros* in Greek, which is related to the verb *iaomai*, "to heal." The same pattern occurs in Latin (*medicus*), the person who practices *medici*; or, in early English, *physician*, a practitioner of *physic*. Similarly, the root for "nurse" is a reference to one who nurses a child at her bosom. Thus, these titles are derived from the roles and instruments related to their activity. As titles, they describe what a physician or nurse *does*, but they do not adequately describe the larger social *meaning*.

xviii. Κλίνω can mean to "lie down," as in the English word re-*cline*, but it also carries the sense of "to bow." The Septuagint, the Greek translation of the Hebrew Bible, used *klinō* in this sense of bowing in worship in Ezra 9:5 ("[I] fell upon my knees and spread out my hands to the Lord my God"). The New Testament employs a similar meaning in the Gospel of Luke (24:5) in which the disciples bowed (Κλίνω) their faces in reverence and awe before two angels announcing the resurrection of Jesus. For a discussion of the term, see W. Arndt, Danker, F. W., Bauer, W., and Gingrich, F. W. *A Greek-English lexicon of the New Testament and other early Christian literature*, 3rd ed. Chicago: University of Chicago Press; 2000: 549.

xix. "Hospital," "hospice," "hospitality," and "host" are all derivative from similar Latin meanings (*hosti·pit*), in which *hosti* refers to a stranger and *pit*, which refers to either a "feeder of" guests or a "master over" guests. For an extended discussion, see Margoliouth et al.[53 [pp. 808–809]]

xx. For example, consider the Boston Medical Center, one of the hospitals surveyed in the RSCC study. The former "Boston City Hospital" and "Boston University Medical Center Hospital" merged in 1996, and were renamed "Boston Medical Center," dropping the language of hospital completely. This is an ironic change since both joining institutions held only two words in common within their titles: "Boston" and "Hospital." "Boston" was retained in the new name but "hospital" dropped from the title.

xxi. In Buddhism, although not a theistic religion, there is pervasive emphasis on compassion and loving-kindness: the good monk should "Everywhere identify himself with all, he is pervading the whole world with a mind full of loving-kindness" (Buddha, as quoted in *The Buddhist Dictionary*). This includes strangers, beggars, and the sick. In the *Vinaya-Pitaka*, the Buddha finds a monk suffering from dysentery and admonishes the assembled monks who have neglected him: "Monks, you have not a mother, you have not a father who might tend you. If you, monks, do not tend one another, who is there who will tend to you? Whoever, monks, would tend me, he should tend the sick."

In Hinduism, the *Taittiriya Upanishad* (one of the older Vedic texts, from approximately the sixth century B.C.E.) offers this instruction on how to live a good life as a householder: "Treat your mother like a god. Treat your father like a god. Treat your guests like gods" (1.11.2). This belief is still prevalent throughout modern India; modern sources attest to the lavish welcome of guests into Hindu homes (Melwani, p. 34). This emphasis on hospitality has strong parallels in Indian and south Asian worship forms: "In Hindu forms of worship, God is the divine guest and rituals recreate, mostly symbolically, the kind of hospitality that is generally offered to an honored guest in India."[36 [p. 147]] The same things offered to a guest—food, water, clothing—are also offered to the gods and goddesses, creating a close parallel between welcoming God and welcoming the stranger.

In Judaism, receiving of strangers may include the surprise of receiving God's self. The earliest example of this experience is told in the story of Abraham, who expressed kindness to three visitors (Genesis 18), bowing before them (18:2), and offering them food, shelter, and conversation. These strangers turned out to be angelic visitors, including the Lord himself. Such hospitality is commanded within the Torah at least 24 times by calling Israelites to love the stranger just as God loves strangers (see, for example, Exodus 22:21, Leviticus 19:33–34, and Deuteronomy 10:18–19). Because God "loves" (*'āhēb*) the stranger, even so God's people are to love strangers since they, too, were strangers from their homes.

(We thank our research assistant, Alexandra Nichipor, for gathering the information presented in this footnote.)

xxii. In the Christian tradition, hosting a guest and caring for the sick—which can become simultaneous activities—take on even greater significance based on Christ's teaching. The guest is to be received and cared for as if he or she were Christ himself. The host–guest relationship was an important dynamic in Benedictine communities that followed *The Rule of St. Benedict*. It was within the monastic context of receiving strangers and caring for the sick that the very concept of *hospital* emerged—a place for showing Christian love to vulnerable strangers. "Many monks studied medical subjects as part of their general education," and many abbots became renowned healers. The Benedictines provide an especially adequate illustration for both the host–guest relationship and its implications for spiritual care. "Life in the monastery was fostered by a unique therapeutic environment." Historian Guenter Risse further illustrates Benedictine care of the dying in the following account: "Some brethren remained with the dying inmate throughout the day and night, praying and reading from the Scriptures by candlelight. The point of this vigil was to ensure 'proper passing'; nobody should be left to die alone. If death became imminent, the whole monastic community was summoned and the monks congregated around the sick on both sides of the bed alternately to pray and sing, using music to 'unbind' the pain and thus provide the departing with spiritual nourishment for the journey to the beyond."[65[p. 105]]

xxiii. Both in Greek and in Latin, the terms "host" and the "guest" (*xenos, hospes*) are the same term, which verbally demonstrates how, among the ancient Greeks and Romans, the two roles were immediately reversible because both parties were strangers to the other. With the same term referring to either role as host and guest, the theological reversal introduced by Jesus in Matthew 25:35 ("I was a stranger [*xenos*] and you welcomed [*synagō*] me") is semantically more intuitive to hearers of Matthew's Gospel in Greek. Christ could play both roles as the guest who is welcomed and the host who gathers those who follow him.

xxiv. This table was drafted with Dr. Bill Pearson, a medical educator at the Medical College of Georgia. It is used with his permission.

References

1. Tyler J. Vanderweele. Religion and health: a synthesis. In: Michael Balboni, Peteet John, eds. *Spirituality and religion within the culture of medicine*. New York: Oxford University Press; 2017:357–401.
2. T. A. Balboni, Balboni M., Enzinger A. C., Gallivan K., Paulk M. E., Wright A., Steinhauser K., VanderWeele T. J., Prigerson H. G. Provision of spiritual support to patients with advanced cancer by religious communities and associations with medical care at the end of life. *JAMA Intern Med*. 2013;173(12):1109–1117.

3. T. A. Balboni, Paulk M. E., Balboni M. J., Phelps A. C., Loggers E. T., Wright A. A., Block S. D., Lewis E. F., Peteet J. R., Prigerson H. G. Provision of spiritual care to patients with advanced cancer: associations with medical care and quality of life near death. *J Clin Oncol.* 2010;28(3):445–452.

4. T. Balboni, Balboni M., Paulk M. E., Phelps A., Wright A., Peteet J., Block S., Lathan C., Vanderweele T., Prigerson H. Support of cancer patients' spiritual needs and associations with medical care costs at the end of life. *Cancer.* 2011;117(23):5383–5391.

5. F. A. Curlin, Lantos J. D., Roach C. J., Sellergren S. A., Chin M. H. Religious characteristics of US physicians: a national survey. *J Gen Intern Med.* 2005;20(7):629–634.

6. M. J. Balboni, Sullivan A., Amobi A., Phelps A. C., Gorman D. P., Zollfrank A., Peteet J. R., Prigerson H. G., Vanderweele T. J., Balboni T. A. Why is spiritual care infrequent at the end of life? Spiritual care perceptions among patients, nurses, and physicians and the role of training. *J Clin Oncol.* 2013;31(4):461–467.

7. M. J. Balboni, Sullivan A., Enzinger A. C., Epstein-Peterson Z. D., Tseng Y. D., Mitchell C., Niska J., Zollfrank A., VanderWeele T. J., Balboni T. A. Nurse and physician barriers to spiritual care provision at the end of life. *J Pain Symptom Manage.* 2014;48(3):400–410.

8. H. H. Gerth, Mills C. Wright. *From Max Weber: essays in sociology.* New York: Oxford University Press; 1946.

9. Paul Starr. *The social transformation of American medicine.* New York: Basic Books; 1982.

10. Jonathan B. Imber. *Trusting doctors: the decline of moral authority in American medicine.* Princeton, NJ: Princeton University Press; 2008.

11. Farr Curlin, Hall Daniel. Red medicine, blue medicine: pluralism and the future of healthcare. *The Religion & Culture Web Forum* [http://divinity.uchicago.edu/martycenter/publications/webforum/052005/commentary.shtml]. 2005. Accessed October 1, 2017.

12. M. J. Balboni, Sullivan A., Smith P. T., Zaidi D., Mitchell C., Tulsky J. A., Sulmasy D., VanderWeele T. J., Balboni T. A. The views of clergy regarding ethical controversies in care at the end of life. *J Pain Symptom Manage.* 2018;55(1):65–74.

13. Gary B. Ferngren. *Medicine and religion: a historical introduction.* Baltimore: Johns Hopkins University Press; 2014.

14. Gary B. Ferngren. *Science and religion: a historical introduction.* 2nd ed. Baltimore: Johns Hopkins University Press; 2017.

15. Roy Wood Sellars. *Critical realism; a study of the nature and conditions of knowledge.* Chicago: New York, Rand; 1916.

16. Ian G. Barbour. *Issues in science and religion.* London: S. C. M. Press; 1966.

17. Roy Bhaskar. *The possibility of naturalism: a philosophical critique of the contemporary human sciences.* 4th ed. London; New York: Routledge, Taylor & Francis Group; 2015.

18. Michael Polanyi. *The tacit dimension.* Gloucester, MA: Peter Smith; 1983.

19. Francis. Clooney. Food, the guest, and the Taittiriya Upanisad: hospitality in the Hindu traditions. In: R. Kearney, ed. *Hosting the stranger: between religions.* New York: Continuum; 2011.

20. Elizabeth Burns Coleman, White K. *Medicine, religion, and the body.* Boston: Brill; 2010.

21. Jacques Derrida, Dufourmantelle Anne. *Of hospitality.* Stanford, CA: Stanford University Press; 2000.

22. Phil Halligan. Caring for patients of Islamic denomination: critical care nurses' experiences in Saudi Arabia. *J Clin Nurs.* 2006;15(12):1565–1573.

23. Isaline Horner. *The book of the discipline (Vinaya-Pitaka).* London, 1962.

24. Edward Kaplan. The open tent: angels and strangers. In: R. Kearney, ed. *Hosting the stranger: between religions.* New York: Continuum; 2011.

25. Joseph Mitsuo Kitagawa. Buddhist medical history. In: L. E. Sullivan, ed. *Healing and restoring: health and medicine in the world's religious traditions.* Basingstoke, UK: Macmillan; 1989.

26. Douglas Kohn. Judaism. In: S. Sorajjakool, Carr M. F., Bursey E. J., eds. *World religions for healthcare professionals.* United Kingdom: Francis; 2017; Chapter 10.

27. John Makransky. The awakening of hospitality. In: R. Kearney, ed. *Hosting the stranger: between religions.* New York: Continuum; 2011:109–114.

28. Lavinia Melwani. Hospitality: how guests are treated as god in the Hindu home. *Hinduism Today.* 2013;1 Oct. 2013:34–43.

29. Nyanatiloka. *Buddhist dictionary: manual of Buddhist terms and doctrines.* Chiang Mai, Thailand: Silkworm Books; 2007.

30. Norm Phelps. *The great compassion: Buddhism and animal rights.* Herndon, VA: Lantern Books; 2004.

31. Stephen R. Prothero. *God is not one: the eight rival religions that run the world--and why their differences matter.* San Francisco: HarperOne; 2011.

32. Fazlur Rahman. Islam and health/medicine. In: L. E. Sullivan, ed. *Healing and restoring: health and medicine in the world's religious traditions.* Basingstoke, UK: Macmillan; 1989.

33. Andy Rotman. Buddhism and hospitality: expecting the unexpected and acting virtu-ously. In: R. Kearney, ed. *Hosting the stranger: between religions.* New York: Continuum; 2011:115–122.

34. Śaṅkarācārya, Satchidanandendra Saraswati. *The Taittiriya upanishad.* Karnataka, India: Adhyatma Prakasha Karyalaya; 1st ed 1961.

35. Houston Smith. *The world's religions.* New York: HarperCollins Publishers; 2009.

36. Swami Tyagananda. God as guest: hospitality in Hindu culture. In: R. Kearney, ed. *Hosting the stranger: between religions.* New York: Continuum; 2011:147–150.

37. Diana L. Eck. Prospects for pluralism: voice and vision in the study of religion. *J Am Acad Relig.* 2007;75(4):743–776.

38. M. Acar. Do we need a new word for patients? What's in a name, after all? *BMJ.* 1999;319(7222):1437.

39. What's in a name? *Lancet.* 2000;356(9248):2111.

40. A. Mariotto, De Leo D., Realdon P., Callegaro G. What's in a name. *Lancet.* 2001;357(9262):1133.

41. Arthur Kleinman. *The illness narratives: suffering, healing, and the human condition.* New York: Basic Books; 1988.

42. Robert M. Veatch. *Patient, heal thyself: how the new medicine puts the patient in charge.* Oxford/New York: Oxford University Press; 2009.

43. James A. Marcum. *An introductory philosophy of medicine: humanizing modern medicine.* Dordrecht: Springer; 2008.

44. Jeffrey Paul Bishop. *The anticipatory corpse: medicine, power, and the care of the dying.* Notre Dame, IN: University of Notre Dame Press; 2011.

45. Eric J. Cassell. *The nature of suffering and the goals of medicine.* 2nd ed. New York: Oxford University Press; 2004.

46. Michael J. Sandel. *What money can't buy: the moral limits of markets.* London: Penguin; 2013.

47. William F. May. *The physician's covenant: images of the healer in medical ethics.* 2nd ed. Lexington, KY: Westminster John Knox Press; 2000.

48. E. D. Pellegrino. Toward a reconstruction of medical morality. *Am J Bioeth.* 2006;6(2):65–71.

49. Edmund D. Pellegrino, Thomasma David C. *Helping and healing: religious commitment in health care.* Washington, DC: Georgetown University Press; 1997.

50. L. Chen, Guo U., Illipparambil L. C., Netherton M. D., Sheshadri B., Karu E., Peterson S. J., Mehta P. H. Racing against the clock: internal medicine residents' time spent on electronic health records. *Grad Med Educ.* 2016;8(1):39–44.

51. L. Block, Habicht R., Wu A. W., Desai S. V., Wang K., Silva K. N., Niessen T., Oliver N., Feldman L. In the wake of the 2003 and 2011 duty hours regulations, how do internal medicine interns spend their time? *J Gen Intern Med.* 2013;28(8):1042–1047.

52. Alasdair C. MacIntyre. *After virtue: a study in moral theory.* 2nd ed. Notre Dame, IN: University of Notre Dame Press; 1984.

53. D. S Margoliouth. Hospitality. In: J. Hastings, Selbie J. A., & Gray L. H., eds. *Encyclopædia of religion and ethics.* Vol 6. Edinburgh: T. & T. Clark; New York: Charles Scribner's Sons; 1926.

54. Jay Katz. *The silent world of doctor and patient.* New York: Free Press; Collier Macmillan; 1984.

55. Daniel P. Sulmasy. *The rebirth of the clinic: an introduction to spirituality in health care.* Washington, DC: Georgetown University Press; 2006.

56. J. T. Hamme, and Laney, J. C. Covenant, critical issues. In: J. D. Barry, ed. *The Lexham Bible dictionary*. Bellingham, WA: Lexham Press; 2016.

57. M. Weinfeld. The covenant of grant in the Old Testament and in the ancient near East. *J Am Orient Soc*. 1970;90(2):184–203.

58. Gordon Paul Hugenberger. *Marriage as a covenant: a study of biblical law and ethics governing marriage, developed from the perspective of Malachi*. Leiden/New York: E. J. Brill; 1994.

59. Allen Verhey. The doctor's oath—and a Christian swearing it. In: S. E. Lammers, Verhey A., eds. *On moral medicine*. Grand Rapids, MI: W. B. Eerdmans; 1998:108–119.

60. Christine D. Pohl. *Making room: recovering hospitality as a Christian tradition*. Grand Rapids, MI: W. B. Eerdmans; 1999.

61. Walter William Skeat. *An etymological dictionary of the English language*. Oxford: Clarendon Press; 1898.

62. Allen Verhey. *The Christian art of dying: learning from Jesus*. Grand Rapids, MI: W. B. Eerdmans; 2011.

63. Lydia S. Dugdale. *Dying in the twenty-first century: toward a new ethical framework for the art of dying well*. Cambridge, MA: MIT Press; 2015.

64. Gary B. Ferngren. *Medicine & health care in early Christianity*. Baltimore: Johns Hopkins University Press; 2009.

65. Guenter B. Risse. *Mending bodies, saving souls: a history of hospitals*. New York: Oxford University Press; 1999.

66. Arthur Kleinman. What really matters: living a moral life amidst uncertainty and danger. New York: Oxford University Press; 2006.

67. Daniel P. Sulmasy. *A balm for Gilead: meditations on spirituality and the healing arts*. Washington, DC: Georgetown University Press; 2006.

68. Michel Foucault. *The birth of the clinic*. London: Routledge; 1989.

69. Timothy Fry, ed. *The rule of St. Benedict in English*. Collegeville, MN: The Liturgical Press; 1982.

70. Elizabeth H. Bradley, Taylor Lauren A. *The American health care paradox: why spending more is getting us less*. 1st ed. New York: PublicAffairs; 2013.

71. Ernest Becker. *The denial of death*. New York: Free Press; 1973.

INDEX

Note: Page numbers followed by f indicate figures; page numbers followed by t indicate tables; page numbers followed by b indicate boxes